Surgical Oncology Nursing

Edited by
Gail Wych Davidson, MS, NP-C, OCN®
Joanne L. Lester, PhD, CNP, AOCN®
Meghan Routt, RN, MSN, GNP/ANP-BC, AOCNP®

Oncology Nursing Society
Pittsburgh, Pennsylvania

ONS Publications Department
Executive Director, Professional Practice and Programs: Elizabeth Wertz Evans, PhD, RN, MPM, CPHQ, CPHIMS, FHIMSS, FACMPE
Publisher and Director of Publications: William A. Tony, BA, CQIA
Managing Editor: Lisa M. George, BA
Technical Content Editor: Angela D. Klimaszewski, RN, MSN
Staff Editor II: Amy Nicoletti, BA
Copy Editor: Laura Pinchot, BA
Graphic Designer: Dany Sjoen
Editorial Assistant: Judy Holmes

Library of Congress Cataloging-in-Publication Data
Surgical oncology nursing / edited by Gail Wych Davidson, Joanne L. Lester, Meghan Routt.
    p. ; cm.
    Includes bibliographical references.
    ISBN 978-1-935864-29-5 (alk. paper)
    I. Davidson, Gail Wych, editor of compilation. II. Lester, Joanne, editor of compilation. III. Routt, Meghan, editor of compilation. IV. Oncology Nursing Society, issuing body.
    [DNLM: 1. Neoplasms–nursing. 2. Perioperative Nursing–methods. WY 156]
    RC266
    616.99'40231–dc23
2013046672

Publisher's Note
This book is published by the Oncology Nursing Society (ONS). ONS neither represents nor guarantees that the practices described herein will, if followed, ensure safe and effective patient care. The recommendations contained in this book reflect ONS's judgment regarding the state of general knowledge and practice in the field as of the date of publication. The recommendations may not be appropriate for use in all circumstances. Those who use this book should make their own determinations regarding specific safe and appropriate patient-care practices, taking into account the personnel, equipment, and practices available at the hospital or other facility at which they are located. The editors and publisher cannot be held responsible for any liability incurred as a consequence from the use or application of any of the contents of this book. Figures and tables are used as examples only. They are not meant to be all-inclusive, nor do they represent endorsement of any particular institution by ONS. Mention of specific products and opinions related to those products do not indicate or imply endorsement by ONS. Websites mentioned are provided for information only; the hosts are responsible for their own content and availability. Unless otherwise indicated, dollar amounts reflect U.S. dollars.

ONS publications are originally published in English. Publishers wishing to translate ONS publications must contact ONS about licensing arrangements. ONS publications cannot be translated without obtaining written permission from ONS. (Individual tables and figures that are reprinted or adapted require additional permission from the original source.) Because translations from English may not always be accurate or precise, ONS disclaims any responsibility for inaccuracies in words or meaning that may occur as a result of the translation. Readers relying on precise information should check the original English version.

Printed in the United States of America

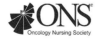

Integrity • Innovation • Stewardship • Advocacy • Excellence • Inclusiveness

Contributors

Editors

Gail Wych Davidson, MS, NP-C, OCN®
Nurse Practitioner, Surgical Oncology
Arthur G. James Cancer Hospital and Richard J.
  Solove Research Institute
The Ohio State University Comprehensive
  Cancer Center
Columbus, Ohio
Chapter 1. Overview

Joanne L. Lester, PhD, CNP, AOCN®
Senior Researcher, Department of Psychology,
  College of Arts and Sciences
The Ohio State University
Columbus, Ohio
Chapter 8. Surgical Care of Breast Cancer; Chapter 13. Surgical Care of Cancers of the Male Pelvis and Urologic Cancers; Chapter 24. Survivorship Issues in Surgical Oncology Nursing

Meghan Routt, RN, MSN, GNP/ANP-BC, AOCNP®
Inpatient Nurse Practitioner, Surgical Oncology
Arthur G. James Cancer Hospital and Richard J.
  Solove Research Institute
The Ohio State University Comprehensive
  Cancer Center
Columbus, Ohio
Chapter 6. Geriatric Implications in Surgical Oncology

Authors

Susan D. Bell, MS, CNRN, CNP
Nurse Practitioner, Neurosurgery
The Ohio State University Wexner Medical Center
Columbus, Ohio
Chapter 15. Surgical Care of Brain Tumors

Kelli Bergstrom, RN, BSN, ET, CWOCN
Nursing Administration
Arthur G. James Cancer Hospital and Richard J.
  Solove Research Institute
The Ohio State University Comprehensive
  Cancer Center
Columbus, Ohio
Chapter 23. Surgical Wounds and Ostomy Care

Lynne Brophy, RN-BC, MSN, AOCN®
Oncology Clinical Nurse Specialist
Bethesda North Hospital–TriHealth
Cincinnati, Ohio
Chapter 11. Surgical Care of Lower Gastrointestinal Cancers

Sue A. Burke, BSN, RN, CNOR
Nursing Staff Development Coordinator
Arthur G. James Cancer Hospital and Richard J.
  Solove Research Institute
The Ohio State University Comprehensive
  Cancer Center
Columbus, Ohio
*Chapter 4. Perioperative Care of the Patient
With Cancer; Chapter 20. Intraoperative Radiation Therapy*

Frances Cartwright-Alcarese, PhD, RN-BC, AOCN®
Senior Director of Nursing Oncology Services
New York University Langone Medical Center
New York, New York
*Chapter 12. Surgical Care of Cancers of the
Female Pelvis*

JoAnn Coleman, DNP, ACNP, AOCN®, GCN
Acute Care Nurse Practitioner
Clinical Program Coordinator
Sinai Center for Geriatric Surgery
Sinai Hospital
Baltimore, Maryland
*Chapter 17. Surgical Care of Neuroendocrine
and Other Endocrine Cancers*

Gail M. Egan, MS, ANP
Nurse Practitioner
Interventional Radiology
Community Care Physicians
Albany, New York
*Chapter 19. Interventional Radiology: Diagnosis
and Treatment*

Sarah E. Ferrari, MSN, RN, CNS, CPHON®
Clinical Nurse Specialist
Bass Center for Childhood Cancer and Blood
  Diseases
Lucile Packard Children's Hospital at Stanford
Palo Alto, California
*Chapter 5. Pediatric Implications in Surgical
Oncology*

Catherine L. Levy, MS, RN
Clinical Trials Specialist
Division of Blood Diseases and Resources
National Heart, Lung, and Blood Institute
National Institutes of Health
Bethesda, Maryland
Chapter 14. Surgical Care of Skin Cancer

Deborah Anne Miller, RN, MSN
Nurse Educator/Consultant
Upper Arlington, Ohio
Chapter 21. Reconstructive Surgery

Michael J. Miller, MD
Professor of Plastic Surgery, Chair of Department of Plastic Surgery
The Ohio State University Wexner Medical Center
Columbus, Ohio
Chapter 21. Reconstructive Surgery

Kristin Moore, RN, BSN
Outpatient Patient Care Resource Manager
Musculoskeletal Oncology
Arthur G. James Cancer Hospital and Richard J.
  Solove Research Institute
The Ohio State University Comprehensive
  Cancer Center
Columbus, Ohio
Chapter 16. Surgical Care of Bone Cancers

**Sally W. Morgan, MS, RN, ANP-BC, ACNS-BC,
GNP-BC**
Perioperative Nurse Practitioner
The Ohio State University Wexner Medical Center
Columbus, Ohio
*Chapter 3. Preoperative Care of the Patient With
Cancer*

Kathleen E. Morton, MSN, RN
Senior Clinical Research Nurse Specialist
Surgery Branch, Immunotherapy Section
Center for Cancer Research
National Cancer Institute
National Institutes of Health
Bethesda, Maryland
Chapter 14. Surgical Care of Skin Cancer

Terezie Tolar Mosby, EdD, MS, RD, IBCLC, LDN
Clinical Dietitian III
St. Jude Children's Research Hospital
Memphis, Tennessee
*Chapter 22. Nutritional Care of the Surgical
Patient*

Donna Owen, RN, MS, CFNP, CPNP
(at the time of writing)
Nurse Practitioner
The Ohio State University Center for Advanced
  Robotic Surgery
Columbus, Ohio
(at the time of publication)
Nurse Practitioner, Pediatrics
Mary Rutan Hospital
Bellefontaine, Ohio
Chapter 18. Robotic Minimally Invasive Surgery

Lisa Parks, MS, RN, CNP
Gastrointestinal/Hepatobiliary Nurse Practitioner
Division of Surgical Oncology
Arthur G. James Cancer Hospital and Richard J.
  Solove Research Institute
The Ohio State University Comprehensive
  Cancer Center
Columbus, Ohio
Chapter 10. Surgical Care of Upper Gastrointes-
tinal Cancers

Kara L. Penne, RN, MSN, ANP, AOCNP®
Nurse Practitioner
Surgical Oncology
Duke Cancer Institute
Durham, North Carolina
Chapter 2. Diagnosis of Cancer

Molly Pierce, RN, BSN, ET, CWOCN
Coordinator, Enterostomal Therapy
Arthur G. James Cancer Hospital and Richard J.
  Solove Research Institute
The Ohio State University Comprehensive
  Cancer Center
Columbus, Ohio
Chapter 23. Surgical Wounds and Ostomy Care

Raymond J. Scarpa, DNP, AOCN®
Supervising Advanced Practice Nurse
Department of Otolaryngology Head and Neck
  Surgery
University Hospital, University of Medicine and
  Dentistry of New Jersey
Newark, New Jersey
Chapter 7. Surgical Care of Head and Neck Cancers

Christine E. Smith, MSN, RN, CNS, CNOR
Perioperative Clinical Nurse Specialist/Educator
Lucile Packard Children's Hospital at Stanford
Palo Alto, California
Chapter 5. Pediatric Inplications in Surgical
Oncology

Catherine Wickersham, BSN, RN, OCN®
Clinical Nurse IV
Memorial Sloan-Kettering Cancer Center
New York, New York
Chapter 9. Surgical Care of Lung Cancer

Louise Williams, BSN, RN, CNOR
Staff Nurse
Arthur G. James Cancer Hospital and Richard J.
  Solove Research Institute
The Ohio State University Comprehensive
  Cancer Center
Columbus, Ohio
Chapter 4. Perioperative Care of the Patient
With Cancer; Chapter 20. Intraoperative Radia-
tion Therapy

Disclosure

Editors and authors of books and guidelines provided by the Oncology Nursing Society are expected to disclose to the readers any significant financial interest or other relationships with the manufacturer(s) of any commercial products.

A vested interest may be considered to exist if a contributor is affiliated with or has a financial interest in commercial organizations that may have a direct or indirect interest in the subject matter. A "financial interest" may include, but is not limited to, being a shareholder in the organization; being an employee of the commercial organization; serving on an organization's speakers bureau; or receiving research from the organization. An "affiliation" may be holding a position on an advisory board or some other role of benefit to the commercial organization. Vested interest statements appear in the front matter for each publication.

Contributors are expected to disclose any unlabeled or investigational use of products discussed in their content. This information is acknowledged solely for the information of the readers. The contributors provided the following disclosure and vested interest information:

Joanne L. Lester, PhD, CNP, AOCN®: National Comprehensive Cancer Network, research funding

Gail M. Egan, MS, ANP: AngioDynamics, Interrad Medical, Genentech, Medcomp, Teleflex, and Semprus BioSciences, consultant or advisory role; Interrad Medical, stock options; Interrad Medical and Elcam Medical, research funding

Contents

Preface

Nurses' experiences involving surgical patients with cancer can vary significantly based on geographic setting, institution size, large (or small) pool of oncology nursing peers, and relationships with members of the collaborative oncology multidisciplinary team. In large cancer-focused institutions, it is common to have separate, specialized care centers for surgical oncology patients, both inpatient and outpatient. In most facilities, however, these specialized units staffed with specially trained and certified oncology nurses are obsolete because of the changing financial climate. Therefore, surgical oncology patients are often on mixed units with similar surgical patient populations and often are cared for by staff with little knowledge of oncology nursing care. The differing treatment trajectory, expectations, and needs of the surgical oncology patient clearly point to the need for the provision of specialized care. Similar to our physician colleagues and the Society of Surgical Oncology, the additional education, training, and passion to care for this unique patient population must be committed with a similar nursing workforce.

Surgery remains the mainstay of treatment for the patient diagnosed with a solid tumor. Care of the patient with cancer before and after surgery continues to evolve with the integration of expanding multidisciplinary teams and new diagnostic, interventional, and surgical procedures. Healthcare providers and members of the oncology-related healthcare teams can no longer work within silos but must actively interact, collaborate, and communicate with all members of the team. Patients who receive neoadjuvant and intraoperative chemotherapy or radiation therapy require a surgical oncology RN or advanced practice nurse (APN) who has a specialized skill set and body of knowledge to safely, competently, and compassionately provide care. The multimodal treatment plan for the patient with cancer must be implemented by an empathetic team with a clear understanding of the complete cancer trajectory and unique needs of the surgical oncology patient, family, and caregiver.

The editors of this text represent a few of the diverse roles within surgical oncology. Each career path has been unique, each perspective a bit different, yet each passionate about the guiding principles of oncology nursing and the special role of the surgical oncology nurse. Each role offers a glimpse into comprehensive care delivery.

Oncology case managers or navigators offer a unique role to ensure patients and families timely access to services across the care continuum. As nurses combine a collaborative relationship with the multimodality oncology team, local area resources, and third-party payer contracts, the oncology case manager can play a key role to facilitate quality care at the right time and in the right place. Navigation of the complex healthcare environment should not be diverted to the patient/family/caregiver; rather, nurses must develop caring, trusting relationships with their patients and navigate their paths to networking opportunities within the institution and in the community. Coordinated care across the cancer continuum is critical to optimal outcomes.

The APN role within the surgical oncology team is constantly evolving. The oncology nurse practitioner (NP) provides expert care across all practice settings. The NP works collaboratively with surgical oncologists to deliver care to patients across the perioperative continuum. Additionally, NPs conduct survivorship clinics and closely monitor patients wherever they are on the cancer trajectory. Oncology clinical nurse specialists (CNSs) are charged to develop, implement, and evaluate programs and ensure standards for quality care. CNSs facilitate staff education and patient education programs and help RNs to provide nursing care to complex patient populations. APNs work within the multidisciplinary team to facilitate and afford excellent, personalized patient care.

Care of the surgical oncology patient must be based on the evidence, best practice, and the desires, dreams, and hope of our survivors. Clinical problems that cannot be solved with existing evidence should be transformed into burning questions with a hunger to find the answer. Nurse researchers have the skill set to develop studies to find answers to uncharted survivorship issues and unsolved symptom management issues. In addition, nurse researchers can mentor APNs and RNs to think every day about the evidence and how to improve patient care. Existing evidence and new research findings should rapidly travel to the bedside and transform care for our survivors.

The challenge of nursing professionals to update their knowledge and to keep pace with new developments is both a personal responsibility and the responsibility of the leadership team. Leaders must ensure access to current materials and education, and staff must seek opportunities to learn, to educate colleagues, and to translate the impact of the treatment plan to patients, families, and caregivers. Whether care is provided in an oncology-only setting or within a diverse patient care environment, the nurse must be knowledgeable and adapt care to the unique needs of the patient. *Surgical Oncology Nursing* bridges concepts and information unique to surgical oncology nursing and the important patient populations in our care. It is an honor to work with surgical oncology patients and their families. Every day, they impress us with their strength, intensity, and hope—a hope to cure cancer and a hope to prevent it. We are fortunate as nurses to have the privilege to share our worlds with these inspiring survivors.

Gail Wych Davidson, MS, NP-C, OCN®
Joanne L. Lester, PhD, CNP, AOCN®
Meghan Routt, RN, MSN, GNP/ANP-BC, AOCNP®

CHAPTER 1

Overview

Gail Wych Davidson, MS, NP-C, OCN®

History of Surgical Oncology

Surgery is the oldest form of cancer treatment for solid tumors, and today, for many cancers it offers the greatest chance for cure. Until recently, surgery was the only treatment that could offer a cure (Rosenberg, 2011). The description of the surgical treatment of cancer can be traced to circa 1600 B.C. in Egypt with documentation of events back to 3000 B.C. (see Figure 1-1). These teachings described tumors that could be cured by surgery, but cautioned to not treat lesions that could be fatal. Hippocrates (460–375 B.C.) used the same caution with his descriptions of the clinical symptoms related to cancer and favored quality of life to surgical intervention. For the next 1,500 years, surgery was reserved for traumatic injuries, as few would elect to undergo painful surgeries in the absence of anesthetics, and most patients died from sepsis (Niederhuber, 2008). A new interest in cancer treatment developed in the 18th century when pathologists described cancer as a local occurrence that spreads to other anatomic sites. A deeper understanding of human physiology occurred with ongoing pathologic discoveries at autopsy (Pollock, Choti, & Morton, 2010).

Early Leaders

Several breakthroughs in the 19th century allowed for the advancement of cancer surgery. In 1809, Ephraim McDowell removed a 22-pound ovarian tumor from a patient who survived for 30 years. This inspired interest in the exploration of elective cancer surgery (Pollock et al., 2010). In the mid-1800s, Louis Pasteur described a germ theory of disease, which became the premise for Joseph Lister's development of antisepsis using carbolic acid and heat to clean surgical instruments. Robert Wood Johnson invented an

1

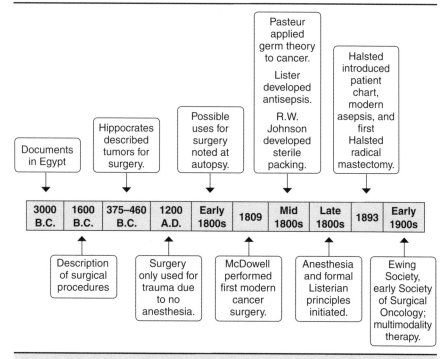

Figure 1-1. Timeline of the History of Surgical Oncology

individualized sterile wound packing, which further controlled wound infection (Pollock et al., 2010). These developments in addition to the use of ether and chloroform as anesthetics would advance the field of surgery (Rutkow, 2012). In the late 1800s, with the utilization of the Listerian principles (disinfection of hands, instruments, and field of operation, as well as scrupulous surgical technique and gentle handling of tissues), infection rates decreased (Rutkow, 2012).

William Halsted, MD

William Stewart Halsted used meticulous tissue handling and aseptic technique and developed the principle of en bloc resection as seen in the radical mastectomy (Rosenberg, 2011). Beyond his talent as a surgeon, Halsted showed great interest in the education for future surgeons. He is credited with the development of the residency system for training surgeons. Surgeons learned both scientific and practical aspects of surgery with the intent to raise the standard of surgical science (Rutkow, 2012). Halsted's collaboration with fellow cancer colleague Sir William Osler marked one of the earliest examples of providing multidisciplinary care.

James Ewing, MD

Dr. James Ewing is credited as the father of the multidisciplinary approach for the treatment of cancer (Society of Surgical Oncology [SSO], n.d.). Ewing was a pioneer in the field of oncology, from his expertise as a pathologist, interest in new treatment modalities, and role in the advancement of radiation therapy. Beyond his clinical skills, Ewing's administrative talents allowed him to recruit and organize medical doctors and surgeons to provide multidisciplinary care for patients with cancer. In 1940, the James Ewing Society began as an alumni association of graduates to showcase his cancer-focused, multimodality medical program at Memorial Hospital in New York (which later became Memorial Sloan-Kettering Cancer Center). Over the years, physicians and scientists from other institutions were eligible to join the group, which became SSO and gained national recognition from the American Medical Association. With a focus on medical education, training, research, and patient care, SSO (n.d.) is committed to the advancement of the science and practice of surgical oncology worldwide.

Surgical Oncology Today

A physician who provides care for surgical oncology patients requires extensive specialized training and education related to the principles of cancer surgery. The surgeon must have a complete understanding of the biology of cancer, the role of systemic chemotherapy, radiation therapy, immunotherapy, clinical trials, cancer prevention, and the care available through the multidisciplinary team. Likewise, the nurse who cares for surgical oncology patients must also be educated to provide appropriate care.

The Oncology Nursing Society (ONS, n.d.) was founded in 1975 to support the specialty profession of oncology nursing. ONS is dedicated to excellence in patient care, education, research, and administration in oncology nursing and aims to set the standard of nursing care for patients with cancer. The Society's mission is to promote excellence in oncology nursing and quality cancer care. Nurses have access to best practice clinical care standards and supporting evidence and research to develop knowledge and practice patterns related to this specialty. The ONS Surgical Oncology Special Interest Group (chartered in 1991) provides nurses working in any aspect of the surgical care continuum with networking and collaborative opportunities.

Principles of Oncology Surgery

Principles of cancer surgery are based on the goal of surgery (e.g., prevention, cure, palliation), the functional importance of the organ or structure, the ability to reconstruct the area, and the patient's condition to undergo the procedure. Other key components include the technical ability of the surgeons and surgical team, the availability of adjuvant therapies, and the biology of the disease (Wagman, 2009).

The terms *operable* and *resectable* are used to describe surgical cases. *Operable* describes the patient's physiologic condition to undergo surgery, and *resectable* is the possibility of the tumor to be surgically removed (Wagman, 2009). Cancer surgery can be performed for several reasons, including prevention, diagnosis, cure, rehabilitation, and palliation (Lester, 2007).

Goals of Surgical Procedures

Prevention

The surgical oncology team must also be proficient in the prevention of certain cancers as designated by risk factors such as personal and family history and possible or true genetic mutations. Some genetic mutations indicate a high risk of cancer development. Similarly, when these risk factors are known, patients are monitored very closely to detect any changes in condition. Some patients may choose to have the organs removed, for example, prophylactic bilateral mastectomies in a woman with risk factors such as a genetic mutation of *BRCA1* or *BRCA2* (Rosenberg, 2011). When the gene mutation for multiple polyposis is identified, the patient may desire to undergo a total colectomy to prevent the development of colon cancer (Rosenberg, 2011). Knowledge of genetic research and a relationship with a genetic counselor is essential for the surgical oncologist, nurse, and patient and family.

Diagnosis

The diagnostic role of surgery is the removal of tissue for histologic examination (Rosenberg, 2011). When a lesion or mass is found, it must be biopsied to determine pathology—benign (nonmalignant) or cancerous (malignant). Additional cellular and genetic features are incorporated to form the final diagnosis. Biopsies can be performed with a fine needle (e.g., fine needle aspiration) or with a retractable core needle device that punctures the tumor and removes small amounts of tissue (Mills, White, Diggs, Fortino, & Vetto, 2013). If a larger amount of tissue is required for diagnosis, an incisional biopsy (i.e., an open procedure to remove part of a lesion) or excisional biopsy (i.e., an open procedure to remove the entire lesion, mass, or lymph node) may be done. Another surgical tool is the diagnostic laparoscopy. When the extent of disease is unclear or symptoms do not match pathologic or radiographic evidence, a diagnostic laparotomy may be performed. Through small incisions in the anatomic area of concern, a laparoscope is placed so the surgeon can visualize internal structures and identify any irregularities. An ultrasound probe may also be used to explore area densities. Tissue and fluids can be gathered for pathology, histology, and cytology. These techniques can aid in the diagnosis and staging of disease. Laparoscopic surgery also has the benefit of sparing the patient the large incision and extended healing time associated with open-and-close surgery.

Cure

Surgery for the removal of a primary cancer includes resection of the entire tumor as well as a margin of normal tissues around the mass. This resection may also include adjacent blood vessels and lymphatic tissue or other organs the tumor may abut. Surgery for metastatic disease may be performed if the outcome has a potential for cure. General principles in surgical technique involve an adequate incision to visualize and remove the tumor, with the least potential for scarring and trauma to surrounding tissue.

The malignancy is removed with adjacent vessels and lymphatics and at least 1 cm of uninvolved tissue (known as a *clear margin*) with limited handling. Adequate clear margins are a critical aspect of cancer surgery and are defined as "a complete resection of normal tissue around a primary lesion, complete removal of involved regional lymph nodes, resection of adjacent affected organs, and en bloc resection of biopsy tracts and tumor sinuses" (Niederhuber, 2008, p. 414). Frozen sections during surgery are used to evaluate tissue margins when complete resection is a concern (Niederhuber, 2008). A positive margin with cancer cells at the edges of the pathologic specimen equates to an incomplete or noncurative resection.

Reconstruction and Rehabilitation

Quality of life is an important aspect in surgical oncology care. As specialists perform complex and radical surgeries to eradicate disease, the potential exists for a loss of function or disfigurement. Oncoplastic surgeons have become important members of the multidisciplinary team for their expertise of microsurgery, reconstruction, restoration of function, and repair of defects from radical cancer surgery (Li et al., 2014). A major source of psychological distress in patients with cancer is coping with a diagnosis that has a potential impact on body image (Reed, 2009). The utilization of muscle flaps, free flaps with bone grafts, skin grafts, and tissue transfers at the time of the initial surgical intervention can alleviate some distress related to cosmetic defects. In addition, the functional impact of surgery is an important consideration in the need for prosthetics and ultimate rehabilitation to improve patients' quality of life.

Palliation

Nearly all cancers can cause distress and symptoms because of tumor progression or lack of response to treatment (Reed, 2009). Palliative surgery is performed with the goal of comfort, not cure. Palliative surgery can involve debulking, decompression, or diversion from the tumor. *Debulking* refers to removal of a bulky tumor or cytoreductive surgery. This surgery may be executed to decrease tumor burden in anticipation of chemotherapy or radiation therapy that would be more effective on the smaller amount of residual disease (Niederhuber, 2008). *Decompression* is performed to decrease pressure on a structure, such as placement of a gastrostomy tube to allow gastric juices to drain when a gastric outlet obstruction exists. A *diversion* may be done if an area is obstructed, such as creating a colostomy for bowel obstruction or placing an esophageal stent for esophageal blockage. Procedures also can assist with decreasing pain or helping with symptom management. The goal of palliative surgery is to decrease suffering and facilitate comfort. Palliative surgery is an important tool to promote quality and dignity. It is vital that the patient, family, and caregivers understand the intent and impact of the surgery.

Types of Surgical Interventions and Procedural Care

Patients with cancer undergo many interventions that require technical skill and care. In the past, these interventions or procedures were performed exclusively by surgeons; however, today, the interventional radiologist and team may complete the procedure and related care. Procedures such as biopsies, vascular access device placement, drain and stent placement, and tumor embolization and ablation are often accomplished within a procedural suite by these specially trained physicians. With radiographic imaging as a guide and appropriate levels of conscious sedation of patients, these professionals can safely, efficiently, and effectively render care.

Minimally Invasive Surgery

Minimally invasive surgery was once unthinkable in surgical oncology because the belief was that a wide incision was necessary to fully visualize and explore a cancerous growth and adjacent tissue. However, inventive technology now allows a skilled surgeon to fully explore the human anatomy through the use of laparoscopic and robotic devices. Operative tools to enhance laparoscopes and robotic arms are continually evolving to allow smaller access ports and greater dexterity than a surgeon's hand may achieve in direct contact with the patient (Halabi et al., 2013). The potential for smaller incisions and minimal manipulation within the operative field may result in easier recovery, improved outcomes, and rapid return to daily life and meaningful activities.

Open Surgery

Traditionally, surgical oncologists used an open approach to surgical resection. Large, wide incisions were made in the anatomic area of the tumor to visualize the tumor, adjacent tissue, vessels, and lymphatics and minimize manipulation of the cancer upon removal. This approach remains relatively common today, but as technology advances and surgical skills are developed, the need for an open approach will likely diminish. Complications from extensive wound healing can lead to a delay in beginning adjuvant therapy, as well as the patient's return to a meaningful quality of life and activities.

The Surgical Team in the Perioperative Arena

Safe surgical interventions require the dedication of multiple staff across the patient care continuum. When a surgical intervention is indicated, the physician and clinical team must ensure the patient will tolerate the procedure. Once this is established and informed consent obtained, the patient will enter the perioperative arena.

The preoperative area is responsible for final preparations prior to entrance into the operating room (OR). The surgeon and anesthesiologist will often see the patient in the preoperative area, and nursing staff will complete final preparations. The OR team consists of (a) a surgeon, who is in charge of the planned operation and any deviations from the plan, (b) a surgical first assistant or assisting surgeons, who assist with the procedure and perform commands as directed by the surgeon, (c) a scrub nurse or surgical technician, who maintains the sterile field and instruments directly around the patient, (d) a circulating nurse, who readies sterile packages and deploys necessary equipment to the sterile surgical field (via the scrub nurse) and is responsible for documentation and all sponge and instrument counts, and (e) an anesthesiologist or nurse anesthetist, who provides analgesia, sedation, anesthesia, intubation, ventilation, hemodynamic monitoring, and vital sign and medication management.

After completion of the surgery, the patient is moved to the postanesthesia (recovery) room and is intensively monitored by a nurse for effects of extubation and anesthesia. The nurse and anesthesiologist collaborate to ensure the patient has stabilized (i.e., vital signs have returned to baseline and the patient is hemodynamically stable) before the patient moves to the next level of care. The patient will be discharged or moved to the appropriate nursing unit for ongoing care.

The patient may receive care on a unit prepared to take care of surgical patients, a unit prepared to take care of patients with cancer, or a unit prepared to care for patients having specific cancer surgeries. The nurse must be prepared to care for the patient based on the diagnosis and surgical intervention. General postsurgical principles will apply and include monitoring vital signs; providing hydration and nutrition; assessing incisions, tubes, and drains; and assisting with activity and pulmonary toilet. The nurse should also understand the patient's cancer trajectory, which includes the anticipated stage of cancer, other treatments the patient has had or will receive, and the goals of the surgical procedure and planned outcomes, as well as functional and physiologic challenges that the patient may face postoperatively. The nursing plan of care must address and educate the patient, family, and caregivers on important needs related to short- and long-term care.

Morbidity and Mortality

Surgical morbidity and mortality can be quite high following extensive cancer surgery if physiologic and biochemical deficiencies are not corrected (Pollock et al., 2010). Because of the age at diagnosis, debility, and wasting characteristics of the disease, patients with cancer may not be in optimal condition prior to surgery. Care must be taken to improve protein stores and nutrition, fluid volume, and blood and electrolyte levels prior to the surgical procedure. *Operative mortality* is defined as mortality that occurs within 30 days of a surgical procedure (Pollock et al., 2010). A complete physiologic, biochemical, and metastatic evaluation should occur prior to surgery, as well as maximum treatment of any comorbid diagnoses. In patients with cancer, the underlying disease is a major determinant of operative mortality (Rosenberg, 2011). Mortality related to complications from anesthesia is attributed to the presurgical physical status of the patient (Niederhuber, 2008). This risk has decreased substantially with the advent of anesthesia patient classification, standardized practices, and improved supervision in the OR. The risk-benefit ratio, the goals of surgery, and alternative options and outcomes must be well-defined, discussed, and understood by the surgeon and the patient, family, and caregivers to ascertain the choice of intervention.

Outcomes and Quality of Life

Outcome studies generally review data to discern the effectiveness of treatment with the ultimate indicators of death, time to recurrence or disease-free interval, and morbidity measures. More recently, functional status, quality-of-life indicators (e.g., patient-reported outcome assessments), and cost and cost-effectiveness have become increasingly important (Earle & Schrag, 2011). Oncology nursing-sensitive outcome classifications are symptom experience, functional status, safety (e.g., preventable adverse events), psychological distress, and cost/economics (Given et al., 2004). Quality care and outcomes are measured with the oncology patient across the full continuum of care. Examples within the perioperative setting include time-out and surgical infection control procedures used with each patient to ensure quality care. Inpatient nursing staff must be vigilant about prevention of falls and pressure ulcers, and accuracy of medication administration. Outpatient staff must measure appropriateness of testing, timeliness of care provision, time for education, and survivorship care. Nurses who care for patients with cancer must consider both provider and patient/caregiver outcomes and the impact of quality nursing care. As more patients become long-term cancer survivors, the impact of cancer treatment across the life span must take into account the lasting consequences.

Nursing Care of the Surgical Oncology Patient

Care of the patient with cancer in the midst of a surgical intervention requires a blend of oncology and surgical nursing skills. Immediate physical needs may mostly include surgically focused care, yet the patient's psychosocial care needs cannot be forgotten. Although the surgical intervention may physically take place outside of the oncology department, it still requires specific oncology care. Today's patient with cancer may receive neoadjuvant or adjuvant chemotherapy, biotherapy, or radiation therapy, and the impact of these treatments must be understood by all caregivers. Cancer site–specific guidelines are provided by the National Comprehensive Cancer Network and include the medical and supportive plans of care. Other resources for cancer care are provided by the National Cancer Institute, the American Cancer Society, and ONS. From prevention and early detection, through the medical and surgical care trajectory, to rehabilitation, palliation, or survivorship, nurses play a key role in the education, support, and care of the patient with cancer. It is essential that nurses interact with the surgical oncology team as well as the patient, family, and caregiver and are knowledgeable of the impact of current and future care needs.

Conclusions

The nurse with comprehensive relationship skills will be crucial to the ongoing development of nursing practice and the care of the patient with cancer. Collaboration with the expanding multidisciplinary teams is critical to the optimization of oncology care. The past decade has demonstrated advances in surgical technology, from microvascular oncoplastic surgery to minimally invasive and robotic surgical techniques. With these advances comes the increased need to nurture the relationships with the oncology team to ensure best patient outcomes. The oncology nurse must advocate for nursing research to develop evidence-based approaches to patient care inclusive of the surgical arena, optimizing outcomes for the cancer survivor. The oncology nurse must remain current and forward-looking to assist the patient to navigate the complex, multifaceted world of cancer care.

References

Earle, C.C., & Schrag, D. (2011). Health services research and economics of cancer care. In V.T. DeVita Jr., T.S. Lawrence, & S.A. Rosenberg (Eds.), *Cancer: Principles and practice of oncology* (9th ed., pp. 345–358). Philadelphia, PA: Lippincott Williams & Wilkins.

Given, B., Beck, S., Etland, C., Gobel, B.H., Lamkin, L., & Marsee, V. (2004, July). Nursing-sensitive patient outcomes—Description and framework. Retrieved from http://www2.ons .org/Research/NursingSensitive/Description

Halabi, W.J., Kang, C.Y., Jafari, M.D., Nguyen, V.Q., Carmichael, M.C., Mills, S., ... Pigazzi, A. (2013). Robotic-assisted colorectal surgery in the United States: A nationwide analysis of trends and outcomes. *World Journal of Surgery, 37*, 2782–2790. doi:10.1007/s00268-013-2024-7

Lester, J. (2007). Surgery. In M.E. Langhorne, J.S. Fulton, & S.E. Otto (Eds.), *Oncology nursing* (5th ed., pp. 337–345). St. Louis, MO: Elsevier Mosby.

Li, P., Shen, L., Li, J., Liang, R., Tian, W., & Tang, W. (2014). Optimal design of an individual endoprosthesis for the reconstruction of extensive mandibular defects with finite element analysis. *Journal of Cranio-Maxillofacial Surgery, 42*, 73–78. doi:10.1016/j.jcms .2013.02.005

Mills, J.K., White, I., Diggs, B., Fortino, J., & Vetto, J.T. (2013). Effect of biopsy type on outcomes in the treatment of primary cutaneous melanoma. *American Journal of Surgery, 205*, 585–590. doi:10.1016/j.amjsurg.2013.01.023

Niederhuber, J.E. (2008). Surgical interventions in cancer. In M.D. Abeloff, J.O. Armitage, J.E. Niederhuber, M.B. Kastan, & W.G. McKenna (Eds.), *Abeloff's clinical oncology* (4th ed., pp. 407–416). Philadelphia, PA: Elsevier Churchill Livingstone.

Oncology Nursing Society. (n.d.). About ONS. Retrieved from http://www.ons.org/about-ons

Pollock, R.E., Choti, M.A., & Morton, D.L. (2010). Principles of surgical oncology. In R.C. Bast Jr., W.N. Hait, D.W. Kufe, R.E. Pollock, & R.R. Weichsel (Eds.), *Holland-Frei cancer medicine* (8th ed., pp. 499–509). Shelton, CT: Peoples Medical House Publishing-USA.

Reed, M. (2009). Principles of cancer treatment by surgery. *Surgery, 27*, 178–181. doi:10.1016/ j.mpsur.2009.01.003

Rosenberg, S. (2011). Surgical oncology: General issues. In V.T. DeVita Jr., T.S. Lawrence, & S.A. Rosenberg (Eds.), *Cancer: Principles and practice of oncology* (9th ed., pp. 268–275). Philadelphia, PA: Lippincott Williams & Wilkins.

Rutkow, I. (2012). History of surgery. In C.M. Townsend Jr., R.D. Beauchamp, B.M. Evers, & K.L. Mattox (Eds.), *Sabiston textbook of surgery* (19th ed., pp. 2–18). Philadelphia, PA: Elsevier Saunders.

Society of Surgical Oncology. (n.d.). About the Society of Surgical Oncology. Retrieved from http://www.surgonc.org/about-sso

Wagman, L. (2009). Principles of surgical oncology. In D.G. Haller, L.D. Wagman, K.A. Camphausen, & W.J. Hoskins (Eds.), *Cancer management: A multidisciplinary approach*. Retrieved from http://www.cancernetwork.com/cancer-management-11

CHAPTER 2

Diagnosis of Cancer

Kara L. Penne, RN, MSN, ANP, AOCNP®

Introduction

An accurate and complete diagnosis of malignancy is the cornerstone of cancer treatment. Diagnosis includes history and physical examination, radiographic evaluation based on the affected body system, laboratory evaluation, and biopsy. Suspicious tissue or cells must undergo histologic evaluation to determine presence of malignancy, degree of differentiation, and tumor genetics before therapy can be initiated (Lin et al., 2013). These characteristics play a key role in both diagnosis and classification of malignancy. The surgical team is often the first group to assess the patient, specifically in solid tumors. Once a cancer diagnosis has been made, the treatment plan is discussed with the multidisciplinary team. Often surgery is the next intervention in order to remove or debulk the tumor and determine the pathologic stage.

Staging is crucial in treatment decision making and prognosis determination. Ideally, the stage of the malignancy should be established prior to treatment, although the surgical intervention may be necessary to determine the stage of solid tumors (Park et al., 2013). Staging procedures include history and physical examination, radiologic evaluation based on disease site, pathology specimens, and serum studies. This chapter will briefly discuss the components of diagnosis and staging.

History and Physical Examination

The clinical evaluation begins with a thorough history and physical examination. A comprehensive patient history includes evaluation of symptoms related to the chief presenting complaint with details about development and associated events. Medical, surgical, and family history are obtained. If malignancy is of concern, a focused social and family history is recorded (Baer et al., 2013). Active or passive exposure to environmental carcinogens (e.g., asbestos, cadmium, benzenes, other chemicals), work history, tobacco and alcohol use, and prior and current illnesses are explored. A systems-focused review is conducted to assess cancer-related symptoms, such as frequent infections, rectal or vaginal bleeding, hemoptysis, cough, shortness of breath, gastrointestinal (GI) changes, unexpected weight loss or gain, palpable masses, or skin changes (National Cancer Institute [NCI], n.d.). Vital signs are evaluated for evidence of fever and respiratory or cardiac abnormalities. A skin examination is performed to assess for skin lesions, masses, or ulcerations. Lymphatic examination (e.g., bilateral cervical, axillary, supra- and infraclavicular, groin, popliteal areas) includes palpation of lymph nodes to identify nodular, shotty, or diffuse changes (Sharma, Shinde, & Luyun, 2013). Chest examination includes auscultation of breath sounds in anterior and posterior quadrants for presence of wheezing, coarse rhonchi, or absence of breath sounds, which may indicate malignant effusion. Abdominal examination includes auscultation of bowel sounds and palpation for areas of tenderness, hepatomegaly, splenomegaly, or masses. The musculoskeletal examination includes assessment of extremities for peripheral edema, evaluation of range of motion, and palpation of the spine for tenderness (NCI, n.d.).

In men, bilateral testicular examination is performed to assess for abnormalities of the scrotum or testicles; however, its effectiveness is controversial. It is not routinely recommended because outcomes are typically favorable in the absence of screening and testicular cancer has a low incidence (Agency for Healthcare Research and Quality, 2012). Digital rectal examination should be performed to assess for enlarged prostate or prostatic nodules, rectal masses, or presence of blood (Goldberg, 2008). The female examination should include inspection of the vulva for masses, vaginal and adnexal examination with cervical specimens, and digital rectal examination. Breast examination should include inspection of the skin for induration or erythema, palpation of breast tissue for masses, and inspection of nipples for inversion or bleeding (Bryan & Snyder, 2013; Goldberg, 2008). Performance status is a critical assessment factor that influences treatment recommendations, clinical trial inclusion criteria, and prognosis. Common performance status scales include the Karnofsky Performance Status (KPS), an 11-point scale (0%–100% function), and the Eastern Cooperative Oncology Group (ECOG) scale, which uses a 5-point scale (0 = fully functional, 5 = dead) (Mallick, 2007).

Laboratory Studies

During the initial evaluation of a patient with suspected malignancy, baseline laboratory studies are helpful to assess organ function and other possible abnormalities associated with cancer-related diagnoses. Laboratory evaluation includes complete blood count, liver function panel, renal panel, and coagulation studies. Tumor markers can be measured in blood, urine, stool, body fluids (e.g., ascites, pleural effusion, spinal fluid), and tumor tissue. Patterns of gene expression and DNA changes can also be detected in tumor tissue (Moldovan, Mitroi, Petrescu, & Aschie, 2013). Tumor markers are used to evaluate baseline disease status, develop treatment plans, determine patterns of recurrence, and measure response to treatment (NCI, 2011).

Imaging Studies

Imaging studies (see Table 2-1) are ordered to identify the location and extent of disease and to monitor response or recurrence after therapeutic interventions. The types of studies used are based on the cancer location, possible metastatic sites, and the sensitivity and specificity of the study. *Sensitivity* refers to the potential of the test to identify an abnormality; *specificity* is the ability to accurately identify the disease.

Prior to administrating contrast in any scan, assessing the patient's renal status (e.g., creatinine) and allergy profile is critical. Allergies to iodine or

Table 2-1. Common Imaging Studies Used in Cancer Diagnosis and Staging

Study	Brief Explanation
Plain radiograph/x-ray	Screening films to determine what scans are needed
Computed tomography	Used frequently; provides two-dimensional images
Nuclear scan	Scan that requires radioactive tracers
Positron-emission tomography (PET) scan	Uses radioactive tracer to tag cancer cells; very sensitive, but not always specific, depending on cancer
Single photon emission computed tomography scan	Similar to PET scan; uses radioactive tracer for three-dimensional images; used in prostate cancer
Magnetic resonance imaging	Uses magnetic and radiofrequency fields to provide three-dimensional images
Mammogram	Provides two-dimensional imaging of breasts; low radiation
Barium x-ray	X-ray of digestive tract using barium to trace structures

shellfish may require premedication with corticosteroids and antihistamines to prevent or reduce allergic reaction or may indicate the need to avoid contrast altogether. Patients on diabetic medications such as metformin may require dose adjustment or stopping the medication to prevent acute renal failure (Clinical Pharmacology, 2011).

Plain Radiographs

Plain films are used as a first look to determine abnormalities. Plain films are also useful to evaluate bone malignancies or metastatic disease. Plain radiographs are not as sensitive as nuclear bone scans in detecting bony metastasis but may be used to identify pathologic fractures (Costelloe et al., 2009). These studies are relatively inexpensive and require no patient preparation except removal of metal items (e.g., belts, bras, jewelry) that may obscure the film.

Computed Tomography

Computed tomography (CT) scans are used frequently in diagnostic evaluation of suspected and known malignancies. CT imaging uses two-dimensional images to produce three-dimensional x-ray images of the body and its internal organs. CT scans can also be performed with contrast for better visualization of anatomy and abnormalities. Contrast media can be administered orally, intravenously, or rectally based on the type of CT scan and the focus of evaluation. CT can be used to detect a tumor or abnormality, evaluate the tumor size and characteristics, guide biopsy of abnormal tissue, help plan therapeutic intervention, and evaluate disease response to therapies (Ross, Galban, & Rehemtulla, 2011). Specialized CT scans such as spiral, or helical, CT have higher resolution and can be used to examine difficult areas such as the spine or in emergency situations when a brisk scan is necessary to detect abnormalities, for example, pulmonary embolism (Ross et al., 2011).

Nuclear Scans

Nuclear scans include imaging that is completed with the use of radioactive tracers; the images are from the inside out. Before the test, the patient is injected with a tagged radioactive tracer. The nuclear scanner uses a special camera that detects energy from the tracers and creates images on film. Uptake on the scans may indicate an abnormal process such as cancer, infection, or bony disease. Nuclear scans can be combined with other specialized scans to provide distinct images (e.g., single photon emission computed tomography [SPECT]). Common nuclear medicine scans include bone scan, myocardial perfusion scan, parathyroid and thyroid scans, and hepatobiliary iminodiacetic acid (expressed as HIDA) scan (Xie, Padhy, & Wong, 2012).

Positron-Emission Tomography

Positron-emission tomography (PET) scans involve the injection of a radioactive tracer, usually glucose (F-fluorodeoxyglucose [F-FDG]), to tag tumor cells (Ross et al., 2011). Tumors that are metabolically active absorb the glucose and are visualized on gamma camera images. Certain tissues (e.g., brain, kidney) can uptake glucose, which may limit accuracy for the scan. Furthermore, some tumors do not attract glucose, such as thyroid cancer, and therefore PET cannot be used for definitive evaluation. PET scans can be helpful to determine malignancies of unknown primary. Roh et al. (2008) demonstrated that F-FDG PET scan sensitivity was significantly higher (87.5%) than CT scan alone (43.7%) in detecting primary tumors in patients (N = 44) who presented with cervical metastases from unknown origin. PET scans are often combined with CT or magnetic resonance imaging (MRI) to provide both anatomic and metabolic information (Ross et al., 2011).

Single Photon Emission Computed Tomography Scan

SPECT scans are similar to PET scans. They also use radioactive tracers to provide three-dimensional images and are used primarily to identify metastases from prostate cancer (Beheshti, Langsteger, & Fogelman, 2009).

Magnetic Resonance Imaging

MRI uses magnetic and radiofrequency fields to provide three-dimensional images and is especially useful in imaging of brain and spinal cord tumors. Innovative contrast modalities now allow for visualization of antiangiogenic effects as in the dynamic contrast-enhanced functional MRI (DCE-MRI). This imaging provides rapid image sequences that allow visualization of the microvascular and pathophysiologic characteristics of tumors (O'Connor, Jackson, Parker, & Jayson, 2007).

Mammogram

A screening mammogram involves two low-radiation x-rays of the breasts to screen for breast cancers. Mammograms are 80% effective in detecting palpable and nonpalpable tumors as well as microcalcifications (American Cancer Society, 2012). If a lump or abnormality is found, a diagnostic mammogram can be performed, with or without the addition of ultrasound or MRI (Drukteinis, Mooney, Flowers, & Gatenby, 2013; Taneja et al., 2009). Screening mammography has been shown to reduce the number of deaths from breast cancer among women ages 40–74 (American Cancer Society, 2012; Tabár et al., 2011).

Barium X-Rays

A barium test (e.g., esophagram, upper GI study) is a radiographic examination used to evaluate the esophagus, stomach, and small bowel. The images provide information about the function and anatomy of the digestive tract such as the presence of peptic ulcer disease, reflux disease, or cancer. Patients must fast prior to the test, and upon arrival are given oral barium contrast to ingest. Barium can cause constipation; therefore, the patient should be given instructions to prevent or improve constipation. Barium can also be given rectally in a balloon to examine the colon and rectum. Barium enema is used only when a virtual or surgical colonoscopy cannot be performed (Halligan et al., 2013).

Diagnostic and Staging Procedures

Diagnostic and staging procedures (see Table 2-2) are used to obtain tissue for cytologic examination and, in some cases, to visualize the tumor and surrounding area (e.g., lymph nodes). The following procedures are considered minimally invasive because existing orifices are used for entry, or tiny

Table 2-2. Common Diagnostic and Staging Procedures

Procedure	Brief Explanation
Upper esophagogastro-duodenoscopy	Scope of upper gastrointestinal tract to duodenum
Endoscopic ultrasound	Scope to obtain biopsy of tissue in gastrointestinal tract
Endoscopic retrograde cholangiopancreatography	Scope to examine biliary structures and part of small intestine
Sigmoidoscopy	Limited scope of distal colon/rectum
Colonoscopy	Scope to examine large intestine and distal small intestine
Laparoscopy	Surgical procedure to visualize internal anatomy or obtain tissue through tiny port holes in abdomen
Bronchoscopy	Scope of trachea and bronchi
Mediastinoscopy	Surgical scope through upper sternal incision to examine mediastinal structures and lymph nodes
Thoracoscopy	Surgical scope to examine pleural and thoracic cavities

incisions are used as portholes for instrumentation. Nursing management is required for pre-, peri-, and postexamination education and to monitor for side effects such as bleeding, infection, or pain. If conscious sedation or general anesthesia is used, the patient must be accompanied by someone who can ensure the patient's safe return to home.

Prior to contrast administration in any scan, it is critical to assess the patient's renal status (e.g., creatinine) and allergy profile. Allergies to iodine or shellfish may require premedication with corticosteroids and antihistamines to prevent or reduce allergic reaction or may preclude contrast altogether. Patients on diabetic medications such as metformin may require dose adjustment or stopping the medication to prevent acute renal failure (Clinical Pharmacology, 2011).

Upper Esophagogastroduodenoscopy

Upper esophagogastroduodenoscopy (EGD) is used to examine the upper GI tract to the level of the duodenum and to biopsy areas of suspicion. With the patient under sedation, a thin endoscope is inserted through the mouth and maneuvered through the upper GI tract to explore for areas of abnormality and potential tissue biopsy (Waxman, 2011).

Endoscopic Ultrasound

Endoscopic ultrasound (EUS) is used to biopsy a suspicious area for a definitive diagnosis of cancer. EUS may identify small masses undetected by CT scan but suspected in clinical findings. During EUS, a thin lighted tube with a small ultrasound probe is passed through the patient's mouth into the stomach and the duodenum; IV contrast may be used. Ultrasound images show the size and location of abnormal masses or lesions in the esophagus, stomach, or pancreas, as well as the presence of vascular involvement (Waxman, 2011).

Transrectal ultrasound (TRUS)-guided biopsy can be useful in evaluation and diagnosis of pelvic cancers. TRUS is a standard diagnostic test for patients with suspected prostate cancer (Symons et al., 2013). Fine needle aspiration of abnormal masses or lesions can be obtained with conscious sedation or general anesthesia based on coexisting patient comorbidities.

Endoscopic Retrograde Cholangiopancreatography

Endoscopic retrograde cholangiopancreatography (ERCP) uses a thin endoscope that is guided through the upper GI tract. A catheter is threaded through the endoscope into the bile and pancreatic ducts, and dye is injected. Subsequent images assess any duct narrowing or blockage from tumor or other condition (Waxman, 2011).

If bile duct blockage or narrowing is a clinical concern as indicated by jaundice, a biliary or pancreatic duct stent may be placed to improve bile flow; if indicated, biopsies can be obtained. IV contrast may be used during the ERCP; therefore, patients should be assessed for contrast or iodine allergies and renal status. Patients are often given a course of antibiotics following the procedure to prevent infection when a stent is placed (Waxman, 2011).

Sigmoidoscopy

Flexible and rigid sigmoidoscopy procedures are endoscopic examinations of the distal portion of the colon. Biopsies of abnormal lesions and any suspicious polyps can be removed at the same time as this procedure. Preparation includes an enema 30–60 minutes before the examination.

Colonoscopy

A colonoscopy is the endoscopic examination of the large intestine and distal small intestine for detection of polyps and precancerous or cancerous lesions. Lesions can be removed or biopsied at the time of colonoscopy for pathologic review (Walker et al., 2013). Preparation for colonoscopy includes a low-fiber, clear liquid diet the day before the procedure and a thorough bowel cleansing.

Laparoscopy

Diagnostic laparoscopy is a surgical evaluation of the abdomen or pelvis via small port incisions and a small camera that is entered into the cavity. Abnormal tissue may be biopsied for diagnostic purposes. Laparoscopy may be performed to rule out occult metastatic disease prior to surgical resection (Leake et al., 2012). General anesthesia is used.

Bronchoscopy

Bronchoscopy is the use of a scope to visualize the trachea and bronchi for abnormalities including tumors, infection, and inflammation. The procedure is performed with conscious sedation. Specimens can be obtained using a needle, forceps, or brushings for culture, cytologic, and pathologic review. Bronchoscopy is a standard component combined with PET/CT for clinical staging of non-small cell lung cancer (Muehling et al., 2011).

Mediastinoscopy

Mediastinoscopy is a diagnostic procedure performed under general anesthesia to diagnose and stage lung cancer or lymphoma. A mediastinoscope is inserted through a small incision above the sternum that enables examination of tissue and lymph nodes within the mediastinum; if abnormal, biopsies can be obtained. The combination of mediastinoscopic biopsy and PET/CT demonstrated a greater chance of detecting lung cancer compared to PET/CT alone, which demonstrated a 25% false-positive rate (Darling, Dickie, Malthaner, Kennedy, & Tey, 2011).

Thoracoscopy

Thoracoscopy is a surgical procedure that includes visualization, biopsy, and resection of masses within the pleural and thoracic cavities. Video-assisted thorascopic surgery (VATS) uses a small video camera that is inserted into the thoracic cavity through a small incision. A retrospective review of patients (N = 145) who underwent lobectomy the using the VATS procedure had significantly fewer side effects with reduced blood loss, shorter hospitalization, and shorter recovery period than patients undergoing the standard open thoracotomy (Shigemura & Yim, 2007).

Cancer Staging

Cancer staging is a description of the location of cancer, tumor size, lymph node status, and presence or absence of metastatic spread. The most common staging system is the TNM Classification of Malignant Tumors, which was developed by the International Union Against Cancer (see Figure 2-1) (Edge et

T = Tumor
TX—Primary tumor cannot be evaluated.
T0—No evidence of tumor
Tis—In situ or noninvasive tumor
T1, 2, 3, 4—Size of tumor based on specific cancer

N = Nodal status
NX—Lymph node status cannot be evaluated in regional lymph nodes.
N0—No evidence of tumor in regional lymph nodes
N1, 2, 3—Amount of disease in regional nodes; list by number groups

M = Spread of disease beyond tumor site (metastasis)
MX—Metastatic potential or condition cannot be evaluated.
M0—No evidence of metastasis
M1—Cancer has spread to a distant part of body.

Figure 2-1. TNM Staging Guidelines for Solid Tumors

Note. Based on information from National Cancer Institute, 2013.

al., 2010). Today, all solid tumors use the tumor, node, metastasis (TNM) staging system, whereas tumors such as non-Hodgkin lymphoma use the Ann Arbor staging system, and Hodgkin lymphoma uses the Cotswolds staging system. Leukemias are classified as acute and chronic, and subclassified as in remission, recurrent, or untreated (Edge et al., 2010).

Different categories of staging exist to assist descriptions of the tumor status. *Clinical staging* is based on the clinical presentation of the tumor as found on physical examination, radiographic studies, and positive biopsy results. *Pathologic staging* is the most accurate type of staging and is performed after surgery with removal of the tumor, surrounding structures, and lymph nodes, if applicable. *Restaging* is done if the tumor recurs and additional surgery is performed (Edge et al., 2010). The pathologic stage of a tumor never changes; however, the clinical presentation or recurrence of disease may change based on interventions or presentation.

Conclusions

As research advances cancer treatment and technology, it is likely that diagnostic procedures will continue to become less invasive. Progress is ongoing to lower patient risk, improve patient care, and reduce healthcare costs, which are parallel to the development of minimally invasive procedures. It is crucial that surgical oncology nurses pursue continuing education and maintain a level of knowledge that will enhance patient care and support ongoing research.

References

Agency for Healthcare Research and Quality. (2012). *Guide to clinical preventive services, 2012* (AHRQ Pub. No. 12-05154). Retrieved from http://www.ahrq.gov/professionals/clinicians -providers/guidelines-recommendations/guide/guide-clinical-preventive-services.pdf

American Cancer Society. (2012). *Breast cancer facts and figures 2011–2012.* Retrieved from http:// www.cancer.org/acs/groups/content/@epidemiologysurveilance/documents/document/ acspc-030975.pdf

Baer, H.J., Schneider, L.I., Colditz, G.A., Dart, H., Andry, A., Williams, D.H., ... Bates, D.W. (2013). Use of a Web-based risk appraisal tool for assessing family history and lifestyle factors in primary care. *Journal of General Internal Medicine, 28,* 817–824. doi:10.1007/s11606-013-2338-z

Beheshti, M., Langsteger, W., & Fogelman, I. (2009). Prostate cancer: Role of SPECT and PET in imaging bone metastases. *Seminars in Nuclear Medicine, 39,* 396–407. doi:10.1053/ j.semnuclmed.2009.05.003

Bryan, T., & Snyder, E. (2013). The clinical breast exam: A skill that should not be abandoned. *Journal of General Internal Medicine, 28,* 719–722. doi:10.1007/s11606-013-2373-9

Clinical Pharmacology. (2011). Metformin. Retrieved from http://clinicalpharmacology-ip .com/Forms/Monograph/monograph.aspx?cpnum=379&sec=moncontr

Costelloe, C.M., Rohren, E.M., Madewell, J.E., Hamaoka, T., Theriault, R.L., Yu, T., ... Ueno, N.T. (2009). Imaging bone metastases in breast cancer: Techniques and recommendations for diagnosis. *Lancet Oncology, 10,* 606–614. doi:10.1016/S1470-2045(09)70088-9

Darling, G.E., Dickie, A.J., Malthaner, R.A., Kennedy, E.B., & Tey, R. (2011). Invasive mediastinal staging of non-small cell lung cancer: A clinical practice guideline. *Current Oncology, 18,* e304–e310. Retrieved from http://www.current-oncology.com/index.php/oncology/article/view/820/777

Drukteinis, J.S., Mooney, B.P., Flowers, C.I., & Gatenby, R.A. (2013). Beyond mammography: New frontiers in breast cancer screening. *American Journal of Medicine, 126,* 472–479. doi:10.1016/j.amjmed.2012.11.025

Edge, S.B., Byrd, D.R., Compton, C.C., Fritz, A.G., Greene, F.L., & Trotti, A., III. (Eds.). (2010). *AJCC cancer staging manual* (7th ed.). New York, NY: Springer.

Goldberg, C. (2008). A practical guide to clinical medicine: Male genital and rectal exam. Retrieved from http://meded.ucsd.edu/clinicalmed/genital.htm

Halligan, S., Wooldrage, K., Dadswell, E., Kralj-Hans, I., von Wagner, C., Edwards, R., ... Atkin, W. (2013). Computed tomographic colonography versus barium enema for diagnosis of colorectal cancer or large polyps in symptomatic patients (SIGGAR): A multicentre randomised trial. *Lancet, 381,* 1185–1193. doi:10.1016/S0140-6736(12)62124-2

Leake, P.A., Cardoso, R., Seevaratnam, R., Lourenco, L., Helyer, L., Mahar, A., ... Coburn, N.G. (2012). A systematic review of the accuracy and indications for diagnostic laparoscopy prior to curative-intent resection of gastric cancer. *Gastric Cancer, 15*(Suppl. 1), S38–S47. doi:10.1007/s10120-011-0047-z

Lin, H.Y., Amankwah, E.K., Tseng, T.S., Qu, X., Chen, D.T., & Park, J.Y. (2013). SNP-SNP interaction network in angiogenesis genes associated with prostate cancer aggressiveness. *PLOS One, 8,* e59688. doi:10.1371/journal.pone.0059688

Mallick, I. (2007, July 18). What is the performance status? Retrieved from http://lymphoma.about.com/od/stageandprognosis/f/performance.htm

Moldovan, L., Mitroi, A., Petrescu, C., & Aschie, M. (2013). Classification of breast carcinomas according to gene expression profiles. *Journal of Medicine and Life, 6,* 14–17. Retrieved from http://www.ncbi.nlm.nih.gov/pmc/articles/PMC3624639

Muehling, B., Wehrmann, C., Oberhuber, A., Schelzig, H., Barth, T., & Orend, K.H. (2011). Comparison of clinical and surgical-pathological staging in III-A non-small cell lung cancer patients. *Thoracic Oncology, 19,* 89–93. doi:10.1245/s10434-011-1895-9

National Cancer Institute. (n.d.). SEER training modules: History and physical exam. Retrieved from http://training.seer.cancer.gov/diagnostic/history.html

National Cancer Institute. (2011, December 7). Tumor markers. Retrieved from http://www.cancer.gov/cancertopics/factsheet/detection/tumor-markers

National Cancer Institute. (2013, May 3). Cancer staging. Retrieved from http://www.cancer.gov/cancertopics/factsheet/Detection/staging

O'Connor, J.P.B., Jackson, A., Parker, G.J.M., & Jayson, G.C. (2007). DCE-MRI biomarkers in the clinical evaluation of antiangiogenic and vascular disrupting agents. *British Journal of Cancer, 96,* 189–195. doi:10.1038/sj.bjc.6603515

Park, H.J., Kim, D.W., Yim, G.W., Nam, E.J., Kim, S., & Kim, Y.T. (2013). Staging laparoscopy for the management of early-stage ovarian cancer: A meta-analysis. *American Journal of Obstetrics and Gynecology, 209,* 58.e1–58.e8. doi:10.1016/j.ajog.2013.04.013

Roh, J.-L., Kim, J.S., Lee, J.H., Cho, K.-J., Choi, S.-H., Nam, S.Y., & Kim, S.Y. (2008). Utility of combined ^{18}F-fluorodeoxyglucose-positron emission tomography and computed tomography in patients with cervical metastases from unknown primary tumors. *Oral Oncology, 45,* 218–224. doi:10.1016/j.oraloncology.2008.05.010

Ross, B.D., Galban, C.J., & Rehemtulla, A. (2011). Functional imaging. In V.T. DeVita Jr., T.S. Lawrence, & S.A. Rosenberg (Eds.), *Cancer: Principles and practice of oncology* (9th ed., pp. 666–675). Philadelphia, PA: Lippincott Williams & Wilkins.

Sharma, P., Shinde, S.S., & Luyun, R.F. (2013). Waxing and waning lymphadenopathy. *American Journal of Medicine, 126*, e3–e4. doi:10.1016/j.amjmed.2013.01.009

Shigemura, N., & Yim, A.P. (2007). Variation in the approach to VATS lobectomy: Effect on the evaluation of surgical morbidity following VATS lobectomy for the treatment of stage I non-small cell lung cancer. *Thoracic Surgical Clinics, 17*, 233–239. doi:10.1016/j.thorsurg.2007.03.009

Symons, J.L., Huo, A., Yuen, C.L., Haynes, A.M., Matthews, J., Sutherland, R.L., … Stricker, P.D. (2013). Outcomes of transperineal template-guided prostate biopsy in 409 patients. *BJU International, 112*, 585–593. doi:10.1111/j.1464-410X.2012.11657.x

Tabár, L., Vitak, B., Chen, T.H., Yen, A.M., Cohen, A., Tot, T., … Duffy, S.W. (2011). Swedish two county trial: Impact of mammographic screening on breast cancer mortality during three decades. *Radiology, 260*, 658–663. doi:10.1148/radiol.11110469

Taneja, C., Edelsberg, D., Weycker, D., Guo, A., Oster, G., & Weinreb, J. (2009). Cost-effectiveness of breast cancer screening with contrast-enhanced MRI in high-risk women. *Journal of the American College of Radiology, 6*, 171–179. doi:10.1016/j.jacr.2008.10.003

Walker, A.S., Nelson, D.W., Fowler, J.J., Causey, M.W., Quade, S., Johnson, E.K., … Steele, S.R. (2013). An evaluation of colonoscopy surveillance guidelines: Are we actually adhering to the guidelines? *American Journal of Surgery, 205*, 618–622. doi:10.1016/j.amjsurg2012.12.006

Waxman, I. (2011). Cancer diagnosis: Endoscopy. In V.T. DeVita Jr., T.S. Lawrence, & S.A. Rosenberg (Eds.), *Cancer: Principles and practice of oncology* (9th ed., pp. 596–602). Philadelphia, PA: Lippincott Williams & Wilkins.

Xie, W., Padhy, A.K., & Wong, W.Y. (2012). Unusual presentation of extraosseous metastases on bone scintigraphy. *Clinical Nuclear Medicine, 37*, 793–797. doi:10.1097/RLU.0b013e31824c5ec0

CHAPTER 3

Preoperative Care of the Patient With Cancer

Sally W. Morgan, MS, RN, ANP-BC, ACNS-BC, GNP-BC

Introduction

The preoperative evaluation of the patient with cancer can be challenging because of the additional burden that cancer and cancer treatments impose. Nurses may prepare patients in the preoperative area for diagnostic procedures to obtain tissue for diagnosis and treatment planning; curative procedures to remove the cancer; palliative procedures to relieve discomfort and improve quality of life; or brachytherapy to implant radioactive devices into or near the tumor to provide cure or palliation. A preoperative evaluation includes a detailed history of the nature of the cancer, previous and current treatments with side effects, and comorbid conditions.

Preparation for Surgery

Cardiopulmonary System

The five cardiac risk factors identified in noncardiac surgeries are history of stroke, angina or myocardial infarction, heart failure, renal insufficiency, and diabetes (Guyatt, Akl, Crowther, Gutterman, & Schünemann, 2012). Patients who have undergone chemotherapy may require additional cardiovascular evaluation because of potential side effects from chemotherapy that may affect the cardiovascular system. Chemotherapy-induced myocardial ischemia is more likely to develop in patients with existing coronary artery disease (CAD) because of their decreased coronary flow reserve. Some chemotherapeutic agents can induce myocardial ischemia, with typical signs and symptoms resembling those of an acute coronary syndrome: chest pain, dyspnea, arm/jaw pain, ischemic electrocardiogram (ECG) changes, and elevated cardiac enzymes (Broder, Goettlib, & Lepor, 2008).

Pulmonary disease can adversely affect patients with cancer because of the increased risk for pneumonia, pleural effusions, and chemotherapeutic toxicity. Patients with any type of malignancy are at increased risk for pneumonia because of impaired host defenses, especially patients with hematologic malignancies, such as lymphoma, multiple myeloma, and leukemia. Cancers of the aerodigestive tract are associated with aspiration pneumonia, and intrathoracic malignancies are associated with bronchial occlusion and postobstructive pneumonia. Patients with mesothelioma or other cancers who develop malignant pleural effusions may undergo preoperative thoracentesis to optimize lung function prior to surgery. Chemotherapeutic agents such as bleomycin can be associated with pulmonary toxicity, placing patients at risk for interstitial pneumonitis that may lead to pulmonary fibrosis. These patients should undergo careful anesthetic and postoperative oxygen management and avoid high concentrations of inspired oxygen, which can exacerbate bleomycin pulmonary toxicity.

Hematologic Disease

Patients with cancer are at an increased risk for perioperative bleeding as a consequence of chemotherapy, malnutrition, anticoagulation medications, or malignant infiltration of the liver or bone marrow. Given the significant risk of these problems, patients with cancer may need to be screened for coagulation factor deficiency with prothrombin time and partial thromboplastin time. Patients with malnutrition or liver disease may need to be treated with vitamin K and fresh frozen plasma before surgery (Pereira & Phan, 2004).

Reversible causes of anemia should be treated prior to surgery. Blood transfusions are indicated for patients with symptoms of anemia or anemia with an anticipated large surgical blood loss. Elective surgery should be postponed until chemotherapy has been completed and absolute neutrophil count (ANC) is more than 1,000 cells/mm³. A platelet count of at least 50,000/mm³ is usually adequate for most surgical procedures.

Patients with cancer account for about 20% of all reported cases of venous thromboembolism (VTE), and 15% are patients undergoing chemotherapy. VTE is one of the leading causes of cancer death after the cancer itself (Khorana, Francis, Culakova, Kuderer, & Lyman, 2007). Risk factors for VTE include the time period of three to six months after diagnosis, chemotherapy, hormone therapy, metastatic disease, cancer procoagulants, thrombophilia, length and complications of cancer surgery, presence of central venous catheters, age greater than 40 years, and debilitation and slow recovery (Spyropoulos et al., 2008).

Gastrointestinal System

Patients with any cancer have the potential to develop gastrointestinal (GI) complications. Eating and drinking can be impaired by pain, nausea, stomatitis, or tumors involving the oropharynx or GI tract; patients with cancer may become significantly malnourished. Anemia due to bleeding and malabsorption with vitamin D deficiencies and coagulopathy can occur. Improvement or correction of these nutritional deficiencies prior to surgery may positively affect outcomes related to healing, infection, and ultimate progression of disease. Most often when tumors obstruct the alimentary tract, IV fluids with corrective nutrients or hyperalimentation may be required to correct severe deficiencies. Otherwise, surgery may need to be delayed until deficiencies can be corrected by medications or oral supplementation.

Surgery should generally not be delayed for intensive nutritional support with the exception of severely malnourished patients as characterized by a body weight loss greater than 15%, cachectic in appearance with a low body mass index, and serum albumin level below 2.5 mg/dl. Because of the higher complication rate associated with total parenteral nutrition, enteral nutrition (oral or via feeding tube) is the most feasible route for providing nutrition (Malone & Weed, 2008).

Hepatic Disease

Substantial liver disease can be detected by history and on examination with palpable ascites, icterus, encephalopathy, and spider angiomata. The preoperative patient with liver disease may present with myriad complications, including obstructive jaundice, acute and chronic hepatitis, and cirrhosis. Although patients present with well-compensated liver disease preoperatively, decreased intraoperative and perioperative oxygen delivery to the liver can occur as a result of hemorrhage, hypoxemia, hypotension, use of hepatotoxic medications, and the patient's position during the procedure, thus increasing morbidity and mortality.

Renal Disease

Kidney disease is defined by five stages (see Figure 3-1) (Bellomo, Ronco, Kellum, Mehta, & Palevsky, 2004). Hemodialysis should be scheduled the day before surgery to correct hyperkalemia and fluid overload and to reduce the risk of excessive bleeding (Trainor, Borthwick, & Ferguson, 2011). Heparin used during hemodialysis has a residual anticoagulant effect that can last two to three hours after the procedure (Favero & McMahon, 2010). Uremia can cause platelet dysfunction resulting in increased perioperative bleeding.

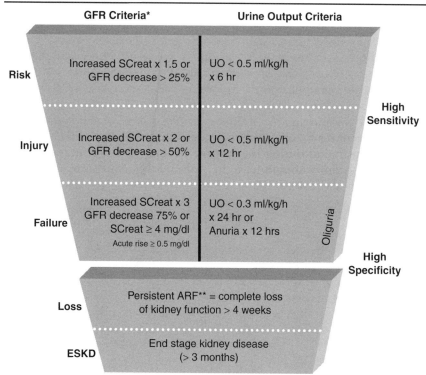

GFR Criteria*	Urine Output Criteria	
Risk	Increased SCreat x 1.5 or GFR decrease > 25%	UO < 0.5 ml/kg/h x 6 hr
Injury	Increased SCreat x 2 or GFR decrease > 50%	UO < 0.5 ml/kg/h x 12 hr
Failure	Increased SCreat x 3 GFR decrease 75% or SCreat ≥ 4 mg/dl Acute rise ≥ 0.5 mg/dl	UO < 0.3 ml/kg/h x 24 hr or Anuria x 12 hrs
Loss	Persistent ARF** = complete loss of kidney function > 4 weeks	
ESKD	End stage kidney disease (> 3 months)	

High Sensitivity

High Specificity

Oliguria

Proposed classification scheme for acute renal failure (ARF). The classification system includes separate criteria for creatinine and urine output (UO). A patient can fulfill the criteria through changes in serum creatinine (SCreat) or changes in UO, or both. The criteria that lead to the worst possible classification should be used. Note that the F component of RIFLE (Risk of renal dysfunction, Injury to the kidney, Failure of kidney function, Loss of kidney function and End-stage kidney disease) is present even if the increase in SCreat is under three-fold as long as the new SCreat is greater than 4.0 mg/dl (350 μmol/l) in the setting of an acute increase of at least 0.5 mg/dl (44 μmol/l). The designation RIFLE-F$_C$ should be used in this case to denote "acute-on-chronic" disease. Similarly, when the RIFLE-F classification is achieved by UO criteria, a designation of RIFLE-F$_O$ should be used to denote oliguria. The shape of the figure denotes the fact that more patients (high sensitivity) will be included in the mild category, including some without actually having renal failure (less specificity). In contrast, at the bottom of the figure the criteria are strict and therefore specific, but some patients will be missed. *GFR = Glomerular Filtration Rate; **ARF = Acute Renal Failure

Figure 3-1. Five Stages of Renal Failure Based on Glomerular Filtration Rate or Urine Output Criteria

Note. From "Acute Renal Failure—Definition, Outcome Measures, Animal Models, Fluid Therapy and Information Technology Needs: The Second International Consensus Conference of the Acute Dialysis Quality Initiative (ADQI) Group," by R. Bellomo, C. Ronco, J.A. Kellum, R.L. Mehta, P. Palevsky, and the ADQI Workgroup, 2004, *Critical Care, 8,* p. R206. doi:10.1186/cc2872. Copyright 2004 Bellomo et al.; licensee BioMed Central Ltd. This is an Open Access article: verbatim copying and redistribution of this article are permitted in all media for any purpose, provided this notice is preserved along with the article's original URL.

Patients with end-stage kidney disease generally have minimal or no urine output. IV fluids should be restricted to optimize cardiac output. Antibiotics and other medications should be mixed in a minimal volume of fluid for piggybacks or given as an IV push whenever possible (Favero & McMahon, 2010).

Patients receiving peritoneal dialysis should exchange the dialysate before the start of the surgery. For short procedures, dialysate usually can remain in the peritoneum. An intraoperative exchange may be required for longer procedures to adjust the dialysate concentrations to manage excess fluid administration during the surgery. Patients who are undergoing abdominal procedures should have the dialysate drained completely just before the surgical procedure (Kohli, 2006).

Endocrine System

The preoperative goal for the patient with diabetes is to achieve glycemic control prior to the start of the surgery. Perioperative uncontrolled diabetes can lead to complications, such as volume depletion and electrolyte imbalance from osmotic diuresis, diabetic ketoacidosis, nonketotic hyperosmolar state, and increased surgical site infections. A serum glucose concentration of less than 40 mg/dl (2.2 mmol/L) may induce transient cognitive deficits or cardiac events such as arrhythmias. A strict glycemic control range, to maintain the serum glucose readings above 100 mg/dl and below 180–200 mg/dl, has recently been recommended for patients undergoing cardiac surgery (Lazar, 2012). Outcomes related to this strict control continue to be monitored. Insufficient evidence exists to use these strict guidelines with all surgical procedures (Kao, Meeks, Moyer, & Lally, 2009).

Pregnancy

Ideally, nonurgent surgery should be performed in the second trimester when preterm contractions and spontaneous abortion are least likely. In surgery, the fetal heart rate should be monitored and documented pre- and postoperatively. The decision to use intermittent or continuous intraoperative fetal monitoring should be based on factors such as gestational age and type of surgery. Fetuses that are greater than 23–24 weeks of gestation should be continuously monitored throughout surgery. The surgery should be performed at an institution with available neonatal and pediatric services and an obstetric care provider with Cesarean delivery privileges. Informed consent should be obtained from the mother to undergo an emergency Cesarean delivery prior to the cancer-related surgery in the event that an emergency would occur while the woman is under anesthesia (American College of Obstetricians and Gynecologists, 2011).

Preoperative Medication Guidelines

Over-the-Counter and Prescription Drugs

Surgeons and anesthesiologists advise patients to continue medications (see Table 3-1) that have a significant effect when withheld. Medications that could potentially interact with anesthetics and increase surgical risks should be discontinued during the perioperative period unless they are related to significant quality of life (Whinney, 2009).

Cardiovascular medications that are recommended to be continued include cardiac rhythmic drugs, beta-blockers, statins, calcium channel blockers, digoxin, and clonidine (Fleisher et al., 2009). Preoperative management of warfarin is usually based on the individual patient's condition, the risks of hemorrhage versus the risk of thromboembolism, the surgical procedure, and the type of surgery (e.g., elective, urgent, emergent). For low-risk procedures, warfarin is generally withheld for four to five days before the surgery (Guyatt et al., 2012). Patients considered to be at high risk for perioperative venous thrombosis may receive low-molecular-weight heparin once the warfarin has been stopped until 24 hours before the surgery (Jaffer, 2009). Thienopyridines are often used in patients who have experienced strokes, recent acute coronary syndromes, or recent percutaneous coronary interventions with stents. Patients with coronary stents who require surgery should remain on aspirin and clopidogrel through surgery if possible. If this is not possible because of bleeding risk, clopidogrel should be stopped five to seven days before surgery while aspirin therapy is continued perioperatively (Fleisher et al., 2009; Kover, 2012). Possible exceptions to continuing low-dose aspirin include intracranial surgery, spinal canal surgery, and posterior chamber of the eye surgery because of the potential dire consequences of bleeding and the difficulty of compressing these surgical sites. Nonsteroidal anti-inflammatory drugs should generally be held at least three to seven days because of antiplatelet effects. Ibuprofen may be given up to 24 hours preoperatively (Kover, 2012). Oral contraceptives, hormone replacement therapy, and selective estrogen receptor modulators can increase the risk of VTE (Levin, 2009).

Central nervous system drugs are usually safe to continue and include selective serotonin reuptake inhibitors, selective norepinephrine reuptake inhibitors, benzodiazepines, lithium, valproic acid, antiepileptic drugs, bupropion, and long-term opioid use. Antiparkinsonian drugs should be monitored closely, and antipsychotic drugs should be avoided (Levin, 2009).

Pulmonary drugs such as inhaled beta agonists, anticholinergics, leukotriene inhibitors, and glucocorticoids are generally given the day of surgery. Theophylline should be discontinued the evening before surgery (Levin, 2009). GI drug classifications of H_2 blockers and proton pump inhibitors should be taken preoperatively to reduce stress-related mucosal damage (Muluk & Macpherson, 2012).

Table 3-1. Guide for Preoperative Management of Patient's Self-Reported Over-the-Counter and Prescriptive Drugs

Drug or Preparation	Recommendation	Possible Negative Side Effects
Cardiac medications		
• Rhythmic drugs, beta-blockers, statins, calcium channel blockers, digoxin, and clonidine	Continue these medications as usual; take with sip of water the morning of surgery.	Diuretic-based cardiac drugs have risk of hypovolemia and electrolyte imbalance and should be avoided if possible.
• Angiotensin-converting enzyme inhibitors and angiotensin receptor blockers	Take day of surgery with small sip water if used to manage hypertension. If used for heart failure, hold until postoperative period.	Determine reason for drug and adjust accordingly. Want to control hypertension and avoid hypovolemia in people taking it for heart failure.
• Warfarin-containing drugs or other systemic blood thinners	Stop 4–5 days prior to surgery and check prothrombin time/international normalized ratio (for warfarin or low-molecular-weight drugs).	If not an emergent surgery, systemic blood thinners are stopped to prevent hemorrhage or clotting issues. Risk of stroke or thromboembolism. Heparin may be initiated at time of surgery pending risk of stroke or thrombus, or cardiac arrhythmias if taking for atrial fibrillation.
• Thienopyridines (e.g., clopidogrel, prasugrel, ticlopidine) for patients with history of stroke, recent acute coronary syndromes, or recent percutaneous coronary interventions with stents	Patients with drug-embedded coronary stents who are awaiting cardiac surgery should remain on aspirin and thienopyridines, if possible. If patient cannot stay on drugs because of bleeding risk, drug should be stopped 5–7 days before surgery with maintenance of aspirin therapy. Ticlopidine should be stopped 10–14 days preoperatively. Prasugrel should be stopped 7 days preoperatively and resumed postoperatively as soon as possible. Cilostazol should be held 48 hours preoperatively and can usually be resumed 48 hours postoperatively.	Risk of bleeding, hematoma formation, diffuse ecchymosis, or hemorrhage if drugs are maintained; risk of clot (e.g., localized or systemic) if drugs are stopped. Need to weigh the risk of bleeding versus the risk of thromboembolic events.

(Continued on next page)

Table 3-1. Guide for Preoperative Management of Patient's Self-Reported Over-the-Counter and Prescriptive Drugs *(Continued)*

Drug or Preparation	Recommendation	Possible Negative Side Effects
Nonsteroidal anti-inflammatory drugs	Hold 3–7 days before surgery. Ibuprofen may be given up to 24 hours before surgery.	Risk of hemorrhage or hematoma due to antiplatelet effects Risk of increased ecchymosis or hematoma
Oral contraceptives, hormone replacement therapy, and selective estrogen receptor modulators (e.g., tamoxifen, raloxifene)	Discontinue 4–6 weeks before surgery in patients who are at high risk for venous emboli formation. If taking for systemic treatment for breast cancer prevention, high-risk conditions, invasive breast cancer, or osteopenia or osteoporosis, stop 4 weeks before surgery. Consult oncologist prior to discontinuing drug.	Can increase risk of clot formation, specifically deep vein thrombosis or pulmonary embolus
Central nervous system drugs (e.g., selective serotonin reuptake inhibitors, selective norepinephrine reuptake inhibitors, benzodiazepines, lithium, valproic acid, antiepileptic drugs, bupropion, and long-term opioids)	Typically safe to continue through the pre-, peri-, and postoperative periods. Take the morning of surgery with sip of water.	Neuroleptic malignant syndrome, a serious condition characterized by altered consciousness, extrapyramidal signs, autonomic instability, fever, elevated creatinine, and leukocytosis
• Antiparkinsonian drugs		If blood level drops, neuroleptic malignant syndrome may occur.
Pulmonary agents (e.g., inhaled beta agonists, anticholinergics, leukotriene inhibitors, glucocorticoids)	Generally administered the day of surgery and as needed just prior to inhalation anesthesia.	Bronchospasms can occur if drugs are not used on routine basis. Increased stress can increase need of drug.
• Theophylline	Discontinue the evening before surgery.	

(Continued on next page)

Table 3-1. Guide for Preoperative Management of Patient's Self-Reported Over-the-Counter and Prescriptive Drugs *(Continued)*

Drug or Preparation	Recommendation	Possible Negative Side Effects
Gastrointestinal drugs (e.g., H$_2$ blockers, proton pump inhibitors)	Take preoperatively with sip of water.	Lack of routine medication may increase risk of stress-related mucosal damage. Decreased gastric volume and increased gastric fluid pH, which can reduce the risk of chemical pneumonitis from aspiration.
Antithyroid medications	Take the day of surgery.	Avoids drop in thyroid levels, although minimal concern for most patients
Corticosteroids	If taking for less than three weeks or on alternating-day schedule, should maintain dosing throughout surgical phases. Regular dosing of 5 mg daily or higher should continue, including day of surgery. May require an IV bolus or extra oral dose.	Avoid drop in blood levels, as this can cause physiologic stress. Patients who take corticosteroids on a routine basis can easily experience physiologic stress with multiple issues. All steroid use can negatively affect risk of systemic infection, surgical site infection, and rate and quality of wound healing.
Diabetic medications (oral agents for type 2 diabetes or to manage other conditions)	Discontinue oral hypoglycemic drugs or noninsulin injectables the morning of surgery. Ideally, diabetics, especially insulin-dependent diabetics should be the first cases of morning to avoid low glucose levels.	Long-acting drugs may drop serum glucose level due to nothing-by-mouth status.
• Metformin	Hold 24–48 hours prior to surgery if there is risk of renal failure or anticipated high blood loss.	
• Insulin-dependent type I diabetic drugs	Take one-third to one-half dose of long-acting insulin; omit short-acting insulin.	Decrease in dosage will decrease risk of ketoacidosis during surgery with precipitous and dangerous drops in serum glucose.

(Continued on next page)

Table 3-1. Guide for Preoperative Management of Patient's Self-Reported Over-the-Counter and Prescriptive Drugs *(Continued)*

Drug or Preparation	Recommendation	Possible Negative Side Effects
Over-the-counter herbal supplements	Assess patient and family for any over-the-counter herbal supplements, vitamins, and minerals. General recommendations are to stop herbal supplements 10–14 days prior to surgery; can resume with provider's approval once healed.	Often patients do not view these substances as reportable drugs and may not know the deleterious effects on surgical outcomes. May negatively impact anesthesia or operative procedure, most likely due to unknown pharmacokinetics and interactions and polypharmacy. Can cause cardiac instability, electrolyte imbalances, myocardial infarction, stroke, bleeding, and negative heart and blood pressure effects.

Note. Based on information from Fleisher et al., 2009; Guyatt et al., 2012; Heyneman, 2003; Killen et al., 2010; Kover, 2012; Lazar, 2012; Muluk & Macpherson, 2012; Whinney, 2009.

Antithyroid medications should be taken the day of surgery. Patients who have been taking glucocorticoids for less than three weeks or use alternate-day therapy should continue prescribed doses preoperatively. Patients who have taken prednisone 5 mg/day or greater for more than five days in the 30 days preceding surgery should continue scheduled medication through the day of surgery. A stress dose may also be required and is dependent on the severity of the operative stress (Muluk & Macpherson, 2012). Patients who manage type 2 diabetes with medications should discontinue oral hypoglycemic drugs or noninsulin injectables the morning of surgery. Metformin may be held 24–48 hours preoperatively if renal failure is a risk or high blood loss is anticipated (Kover, 2012). Patients with type 1 diabetes need to continue with some basal insulin even without eating to prevent ketoacidosis (Killen, Tonks, Greenfield, & Story, 2010; Lazar, 2012).

Herbal Medications

The ingestion of herbal medicines up to the day of surgery may negatively affect anesthesia and the operative procedure. Mortality and morbidity can occur in the perioperative period because of unknown polypharmacy. The potential for untoward drug-herb complications can include cardiac instability, electrolyte imbalances, myocardial infarction, stroke, bleeding, heart and blood pressure effects, prolonged or inadequate anesthesia, and changes in the body's interaction with other medicines (Heyneman, 2003). Because many patients do not consider herbal substances to be medications or are reluctant to admit to taking herbal medications, preoperative assessment needs to specifically include questions about these supplements (Flanagan, 2001).

Infection Precautions

If a patient complains of or presents with signs, symptoms, or any evidence of active infection during the preoperative evaluation, the surgeon should be notified immediately. Complete treatment of the infection may be required prior to elective surgical procedures to prevent complications of anesthesia administration or surgical outcomes. Precautions are particularly necessary if an artificial prosthesis will be placed, pneumonia exists, infection is present at the proposed site of surgery, or absolute neutrophil count is compromised (Williams, 2008). *Staphylococcus aureus* nasal carriers are three to six times more likely to develop healthcare-associated infections (Bode et al., 2010). Patients should undergo a standardized *Staphylococcus* nasal screening preoperatively to identify carriers of either methicillin-resistant *Staphylococcus aureus* (MRSA) or methicillin-sensitive *Staphylococcus aureus* (MSSA). Patients who test positive for *Staphylococcus aureus* are instructed to apply a 2% mupirocin ointment intranasally twice daily for five days. Nasal swabs should be obtained the day of admission for patients who did not have preoperative screening.

If the patient tests positive, mupirocin is administered immediately prior to surgery and continued postoperatively until the results are negative for either MSSA or MRSA. A 10-dose decolonization regimen is continued postoperatively among patients who subsequently were positive for either MSSA or MRSA. Patients who test positive for MRSA are treated preoperatively with vancomycin (Mehta et al., 2013).

Skin Preparation

Preoperative showering with 2% chlorhexidine the night before and the day of surgery is done to reduce bacterial colonization of the skin (Adamina, Gie, Demartines, & Ris, 2013). Patients should avoid hair removal with straight or electric razors or a depilatory on the operative site before surgery. Razors abrade the skin surface, and depilatories may cause skin reactions that can lead to skin infections. Body hair is no longer automatically removed unless the presence of hair will interfere with the procedure. If body hair needs to be removed before surgical incision, electronic clippers are recommended instead of straight razor shaving (Dizer et al., 2009).

Antibiotic Use

The appropriate use of antibiotics is important to minimize surgical site infections. National guidelines have been established for the appropriate selection of preoperative antibiotics that should be administered within one hour before the surgical incision is made and should be discontinued within 24 hours after surgery (Surgical Care Improvement Project [SCIP], 2012). SCIP is composed of national organizations that include the Centers for Medicare and Medicaid Services (CMS) and the Joint Commission, who are committed to an improvement of surgical care by a significant reduction in surgical complications. Indicators have been developed to measure improvement and to standardize the reporting and comparison of data (SCIP, 2012).

Common measures to reduce the incidence of surgical site infections include administration of an antibiotic within one hour of incision (two hours if vancomycin or quinolone are used), verification with documentation that antibiotic was received, and discontinuation of antibiotics within 24 hours of surgery end time or 48 hours for cardiac surgery (SCIP, 2012).

Effective October 2012, Medicare rewards hospitals that provide quality care through its Hospital Value-Based Purchasing Program. Hospitals will be paid based on the quality of acute care services provided and how they perform on seven of the SCIP measures and 18 other measures. The Joint Commission plans to tie scores to core measures of hospital accreditation.

Conclusions

Effective patient, family, and caregiver education is essential to improve health outcomes for patients undergoing surgery. Ideally patient education begins in the surgeon's office, continues in preadmission testing, and is completed in the preoperative area on the day of surgery. The preoperative evaluation of the patient with cancer is essential to the reduction of surgical morbidity. Evaluation is individualized to assess each patient's risk for surgery based on functional status and comorbidities. Patients need to be instructed about which medications that should be taken and which ones should be held. The surgical oncology nurse in the perioperative period ensures adherence to national standards to provide for optimal patient outcomes.

References

Adamina, M., Gie, O., Demartines, N., & Ris, F. (2013). Contemporary perioperative care strategies. *British Journal of Surgery, 100,* 38–54. doi:10.1002/bjs.8990

American College of Obstetricians and Gynecologists. (2011). Nonobstetric surgery during pregnancy. Committee opinion No. 474. *Obstetrics and Gynecology, 117,* 420–421. doi:10.1097/AOG.0b013e31820eede9

Bellomo, R., Ronco, C., Kellum, J., Mehta, R., & Palevsky, P. (2004). Acute renal failure—Definition, outcome measures, animal models, fluid therapy and information technology needs: The Second International Consensus Conference of the Acute Dialysis Quality Initiative Group. *Critical Care, 8,* 204–212. doi:10.1186/cc2872

Bode, L., Kluytmans, J., Wertheim, H., Bogaers, D., Vandenbroucke-Grauls, C., Roosendaal, R., … Vos, M. (2010). Preventing surgical-site infections in nasal carriers of *Staphylococcus aureus.* *New England Journal of Medicine, 362,* 9–17. doi:10.1056/NEJMoa0808939

Broder, H., Goettlib, R.A., & Lepor, N.E. (2008). Chemotherapy and cardiotoxicity. *Reviews in Cardiovascular Medicine, 9,* 75–83. Retrieved from http://www.ncbi.nlm.nih.gov/pmc/articles/PMC3723407/

Dizer, B., Hatipoglu, S., Kaymakcioglu, N., Tufan, T., Yava, A., Iyigun, E., & Senses, Z. (2009). The effect of nurse-performed preoperative skin preparation on postoperative surgical site infections in abdominal surgery. *Journal of Clinical Nursing, 18,* 3325–3332. doi:10.1111/j.1365-2702.2009.02885.x

Favero, H., & McMahon, M. (2010). Care of the adult chronic kidney disease patient in the perianesthesia setting. *Journal of PeriAnesthesia Nursing, 25,* 162–167. doi:10.1016/j.jopan.2010.03.009

Flanagan, K. (2001). Preoperative assessment: Safety considerations for patients taking herbal products. *Journal of PeriAnesthesia Nursing, 16,* 19–26. doi:10.1053/jpan.2001.20639

Fleisher, L.A., Beckman, J.A., Brown, K.A., Calkins, H., Chaikof, E.L., Fleischmann, K.E., … Robb, J.F. (2009). ACC/AHA 2009 guidelines on perioperative cardiovascular evaluation and care for noncardiac surgery. *Journal of the American College of Cardiology, 54,* e13–e118. doi:10.1016/j.jacc.2009.07.010

Guyatt, G.H., Akl, E.A., Crowther, M., Gutterman, D.D., & Schuünemann, H.I. (2012). Executive summary: Antithrombotic therapy and prevention of thrombosis (9th ed.). American College of Chest Physicians evidence-based clinical practice guidelines. *Chest, 141*(Suppl. 2), S7–S47. doi:10.1378/chest.1412S3

Heyneman, C.A. (2003). Preoperative considerations: Which herbal products should be discontinued before surgery? *Critical Care Nursing, 23,* 116–124. Retrieved from http://ccn.aacnjournals.org/content/23/2/116.long

Jaffer, A.K. (2009). Perioperative management of warfarin and antiplatelet therapy. *Cleveland Clinic Journal of Medicine, 76*(Suppl. 4), s37–s44. doi:103949/ccjm.76.s4.07

Kao, L.S., Meeks, D., Moyer, V.A., & Lally, K.P. (2009). Peri-operative glycemic control regimens for preventing surgical site infections in adults. *Cochrane Database of Systematic Reviews, 2009*(3). doi:10.1002/14651858.CD006806.pub2

Khorana, A.A., Francis, C.W., Culakova, E., Kuderer, N.M., & Lyman G.H. (2007). Thromboembolism is a leading cause of death in cancer patients receiving outpatient chemotherapy. *Journal of Thrombosis and Haemostasis, 5,* 632–634. doi:10.1111/j.1538-7836.2007.02374.x

Killen, J., Tonks, K., Greenfield, J.R., & Story, D.A. (2010). New insulin analogues and perioperative care of patients with type I diabetes. *Anaesthesia and Intensive Care, 38,* 244–249. doi:10.1111/j.1538-7836.2007.02374.x

Kohli, M. (2006). Chronic kidney disease. In S.L. Cohn, G.W. Smetana, & H.G. Weed (Eds.), *Perioperative medicine: Just the facts* (pp. 191–197). New York, NY: McGraw-Hill.

Kover, A. (2012). *Perioperative medication management.* Presentation at the 2012 Central Ohio PeriAnesthesia Nurses Seminar, Columbus, OH.

Lazar, H.L. (2012). Glycemic control during coronary artery bypass graft surgery. *International Scholarly Research Network: Cardiology, 2012,* 1–14. doi:10.5402/2012/292490

Levin, D. (2009). What is the appropriate use of chronic medications in the perioperative setting? *The Hospitalist.* Retrieved from http://www.the-hospitalist.org/details/article/423691/What_is_the_appropriate_use_of_chronic_medications_in_the_perioperative_setting.html

Malone, S., & Weed, H.G. (2008). Perioperative nutritional issues. In J. Yeung, C. Escalante, & R. Gagel (Eds.), *Medical care of cancer patients* (pp. 682–683). Shelton, CT: BC Decker.

Mehta, S., Hadley, S., Hutzler, L., Slover, J., Phillips, M., & Bosco, J.A., III. (2013). Impact of preopeative MRSA screening and decolonization on hospital-acquired MRSA burden. *Clinical Orthopaedics and Related Research, 471,* 2367–2371. doi:10.1007/s11999-013-2848-3

Muluk, V., & Macpherson, D.S. (2012). Perioperative medication management. [Literature review current through May 2013]. Retrieved from http://www.uptodate.com/home/index.html

Pereira, J., & Phan, T. (2004). Management of bleeding in patients with advanced cancer. *Oncologist, 9,* 561–570. doi:10.1634/theoncologist.9-5-561

Spyropoulos, A., Brotman, D., Amin, A., Deitelzweig, S., Jaffer, A.K., & McKean, S.C. (2008). Prevention of venous thromboembolism in the cancer surgery patient. *Cleveland Clinic Journal of Medicine, 75*(Suppl.), S17–S26. Retrieved from http://www.ccjm.org/content/75/Suppl_3/S17.long

Surgical Care Improvement Project. (2012). *Tips for safer surgery.* Retrieved from https://www.premierinc.com/safety/topics/scip/downloads/consumer-tips.pdf

Trainor, D., Borthwick, E., & Ferguson, A. (2011). Perioperative management of the hemodialysis patient. *Seminars in Dialysis, 24,* 314–326. doi:10.1111/j.1525-139X.2011.00856.x

Whinney, C. (2009). Perioperative medication management: General principles and practical applications. *Cleveland Clinic Journal of Medicine, 76,* S126–S132. doi:10.3949/ccjm.76.s4.20

Williams, M. (2008). Infection control and prevention in perioperative practice. *Journal of Perioperative Practice, 18,* 274–278.

CHAPTER 4

Perioperative Care of the Patient With Cancer

Sue A. Burke, BSN, RN, CNOR, and Louise Williams, BSN, RN, CNOR

Introduction

The three phases of care for all patients undergoing surgery are the preoperative, intraoperative, and postoperative phases. Each phase requires the nurse to be knowledgeable about the patient and family as well as the surgical procedure and the potential effects of anesthesia. A cancer diagnosis adds additional considerations, as patients enter the surgical arena at all stages of the cancer trajectory. Patient safety is imperative throughout all phases of care.

Perioperative Care

Safety

Improvements in operating room (OR) safety have evolved over time with the help of multiple agencies. Many initiatives have occurred and include the National Patient Safety Goals (NPSGs) developed by the Joint Commission, which later expanded to include the Universal Protocol for the Prevention of Wrong Site, Wrong Procedure, and Wrong Person Surgery (Joint Commission, 2012). In 2002, the Centers for Medicare and Medicaid Services and the Centers for Disease Control and Prevention introduced the Surgical Infection Prevention Project, which was developed to reduce surgical site infections and antibiotic usage. The Institute for Healthcare Improvement (2013) followed with a campaign to reduce surgical complications. The World Health Organization developed the Surgical Safety Checklist (World Alliance for Patient Safety, 2008). Many institutions have adapted this checklist to meet their organizational needs (see example in Figure 4-1).

Most recently the Surgical Care Improvement Project (SCIP) evolved, which is a national quality partnership of organizations focused on improved surgical care to significantly reduce surgical complications. It is a unique partnership that has proven to be a transformational change in health care (see Table 4-1). SCIP's goal was to reduce the incidence of surgical complications nationally by 25% by 2010. Implementation of the SCIP checklists and measures had a positive effect, as postoperative complication rates fell by 36% (Watson, 2011).

Perioperative Team

The perioperative patient care team is a multidisciplinary group of professionals working closely to provide optimal patient care (Phillips, 2013). The nursing team involves RNs in the preoperative and postoperative areas as well as in the OR. The RN in the OR functions in the circulator role, and another RN or surgical technologist performs the duties of the scrub role. Additional nurses also may monitor the patient undergoing surgery with the use of a local anesthetic agent only or assist the primary circulating nurse in operating technologic devices such as lasers or cell savers. Additional scrub personnel may be needed when two or more surgical teams operate at the

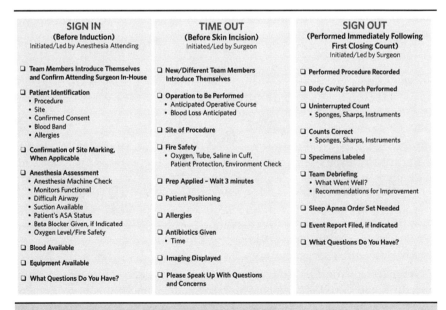

Figure 4-1. The Ohio State University Wexner Medical Center Surgical Safety Checklist

Note. Figure courtesy of The Ohio State University Wexner Medical Center. Used with permission.

Table 4-1. Surgical Care Improvement Project National Hospital Inpatient Quality Measures

Set Measure	Measure Name—Applicable for Q1–Q3 2014
Infection Quality Indicators	Prophylactic Antibiotic Received Within One Hour Prior to Surgical Incision
	Recommended Prophylactic Antibiotic Selection for Surgical Patients
	Prophylactic Antibiotics Discontinued Within 24 Hours After Surgery End Time—48 Hours for CABG and Other Cardiac Surgery
	Cardiac Surgery Patients With Controlled Postoperative Blood Glucose
	Surgery Patients With Appropriate Hair Removal
	Urinary Catheter Removed on Postoperative Day 1 (POD 1) or Postoperative Day 2 (POD 2) With Day of Surgery Being Day Zero
	Surgery Patients With Perioperative Temperature Management
Venous Thrombo-embolism Quality Indicator	Surgery Patients Who Received Appropriate Venous Thromboembolism Prophylaxis Within 24 Hours Prior to Surgery to 24 Hours After Surgery
Cardiac Quality Indicator	Surgery Patients on Beta-Blocker Therapy Prior to Arrival Who Received a Beta-Blocker During the Perioperative Period

CABG—coronary artery bypass graft

Note. Based on information from Joint Commission, 2014b.

same time. The surgical team can consist of an attending surgeon, fellow, resident, intern, physician assistant, RN first assistant, and medical students. Several surgical teams may be present, depending on the surgical procedure. For example, surgical oncology may perform a mastectomy, and the second surgical team (e.g., plastic surgery) may perform the immediate reconstruction. The anesthesia care team may involve an attending along with a fellow, a resident, a certified registered nurse anesthetist, or an anesthesia assistant.

Plan of Care

The plan of care starts in the physician's office when the surgical procedure is discussed and scheduled. Reservation forms may be sent to alert the OR staff to the specific needs for the planned surgical procedure such as equipment or supplies. Often patients may be enrolled in a research study or clinical trial. The study or trial may involve one, two, or all three perioperative phases and may include additional laboratory testing, imaging, tissue sampling, or medication administration. This information is included in the report to the next care provider.

Preoperative Phase and Anesthesia

The anesthesiologist will assign the patient an American Society of Anesthesiologists (ASA) status that describes the patient's preoperative health status. This ASA Physical Status Classification System (see Figure 4-2) is used worldwide (ASA, 2012). Types of anesthesia relevant to the surgery are discussed with the patient and can include general, regional, conscious sedation, and monitored anesthesia care. General anesthesia is an unconscious state with depressed or obtunded reflexes, analgesia, amnesia, and muscular relaxation. Regional anesthesia involves a nerve block to a specific area. Common types of regional anesthesia are spinal and epidural blocks. The patient may be awake but is free of pain and may be given additional medications to relieve stress and anxiety. Conscious sedation is defined as a drug-induced depression of consciousness, although patients respond appropriately to verbal commands (ASA, 2009). Monitored anesthesia care involves a local anesthetic agent at the surgical site and IV sedation, as provided by an anesthesia care provider (Spry, 2013). Local anesthesia involves the surgeon administering a local anesthetic into the operative site. An RN usually monitors the patient throughout the surgery or procedure.

Before the surgery, an IV site is identified. The site needs to accommodate the appropriate-size catheter in conjunction with the type of surgery and anesthesia. The site should be accessible and in an area that does not interfere with the surgery or patient's dominant side, if possible. The preoperative assessment is documented in the patient's medical record (see Figure 4-3).

The patient often experiences stress and anxiety during the perioperative process. Once questions and concerns are addressed, the patient may be premedicated with sedatives, anxiolytics, or narcotics. The preoperative nurse can also provide a calming environment for the patient.

ASA 1—Normal healthy patient
ASA 2—Patient with mild systemic disease
ASA 3—Patient with severe systemic disease
ASA 4—Patient with severe systemic disease that is a constant threat to life
ASA 5—Moribund patient who is not expected to survive without the operation
ASA 6—Declared brain-dead patient whose organs are being removed for donor purposes

Figure 4-2. American Society of Anesthesiologists Physical Status Classification System

Note. From "ASA Physical Status Classification System," by the American Society of Anesthesiologists, 2012. Retrieved from http://www.asahq.org/For-Members/Clinical-Information/ASA-Physical-Status-Classification -System.aspx. Copyright 2012 by the American Society of Anesthesiologists. Reprinted with permission.

- Time of assessment
- Patient verification
  - Banded (name and medical record number)
- Procedure verified (site and laterality)
- Blood ID band
  - Blood products available
- H & P completed
- Surgical consent (signed/dated/timed)
- Site marked
- DNR suspend form signed
- Sterilization consent signed
- Limb disposition consent obtained
- Pre-op lab/test drawn today
- Patient taking beta-blocker
- Voided prior to procedure
- Alerts:
  - Anesthesia alert (difficult airway, OSA)
  - Medical power of attorney
  - Cardiac device (pacemaker, AICD)
  - Pathology alert
  - Research protocol
  - Interpreter services needed
  - Transportation alert (ASU patient has ride home)
  - Bed alert
- Family
- Patient prep verification (bowel, CHG)
- Advance directives (POA, DNR-CC)

- Personal belongings
  - Dentures
  - Glasses
  - Clothing
- Prosthetics/implants
- NPO
- Allergies
- Medications
  - Medication review
  - Pre-op meds given
- Precautions:
  - Isolation precautions
  - Chemotherapy
  - Light precautions for photodynamic therapy
- Patient history
  - Pt status
  - Limitations
  - Vital signs (HR, BP, Resp, Temp)
  - Airway
  - Pain scale
- Skin assessment
  - Variations
  - Braden score
  - Preventive dressing placed
- Fall risk assessment
- Psychosocial needs
- Patient education
  - Education needs assessment
  - Preferred learning method
  - Orders reviewed and verified

Figure 4-3. An Example of a Preoperative Assessment

AICD—automatic implantable cardioverter defibrillator; ASU—ambulatory surgery unit; BP—blood pressure; CHG—chlorhexidine gluconate; DNR—do-not-resuscitate; DNR-CC—do-not-resuscitate comfort care; H & P—history and physical; HR—heart rate; NPO—nothing by mouth; OSA—obstructive sleep apnea; POA—power of attorney; Pt—patient; Resp—respiration rate; Temp—temperature

Intraoperative Phase

The intraoperative phase begins when the patient enters the OR and is completed upon transfer to a phase I recovery area such as a postanesthesia care unit (PACU) or phase II area such as an ambulatory surgery unit (Spry, 2013). The OR nurse will interview the patient prior to surgery, review the preoperative checklist, and receive a report from the preoperative nurse. Standardized methods of communication are preferred and may involve face-to-face or written methods (Association of periOperative Registered Nurses, 2013).

Preparation of the Operating Room

The room is prepared for the surgical procedure prior to the patient's arrival in the OR. The physician preference card is used to assist the OR staff with room organization. This is a written or electronic tool that lists the supplies, equipment, medications, and instruments necessary for a specific surgical procedure. It may also include correct positioning of the patient. It is important to use a suitable room that can accommodate the procedure. Some surgeries require the use of video systems, microscopes, robots, radiologic technologies, pneumatic tourniquets, and numerous surgical instruments. It is important to use the appropriate OR bed that can hold and position the patient properly and allow the surgeon to perform the procedure. Specific OR beds are available for neurologic, orthopedic, urologic, and outpatient surgeries, each with unique attachments such as head frames, arm boards, leg boards or stirrups, and padding. Each varies depending on the patient's weight. The OR beds may also need to rotate, flex, and tilt during the surgery (see Figure 4-4).

Nursing staff in the patient's OR will arrange the equipment and open required sterile supplies. The scrub person performs a surgical hand scrub and dons a sterile gown and gloves. The team prepares the sterile fields by organizing the surgical instruments, sutures, sponges, and solutions. Before the patient enters the OR, the nursing team confirms the sterility of the surgical instruments and supplies. They perform the sharp, sponge, and instrument counts as required. Initial counts are completed to establish a baseline for subsequent counts to promote safe patient outcomes and reduce the risk of a retained foreign body (Association of periOperative Registered Nurses,

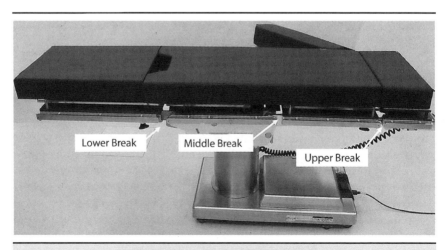

Figure 4-4. Operating Room Table

Note. Photo courtesy of Sue A. Burke, BSN, RN, CNOR. Used with permission.

2013). All medications and solutions delivered to the sterile field are verified and appropriately labeled.

The anesthesia care provider prepares for the patient. The anesthesia machine, monitors, and equipment are checked. The anesthesia care provider confirms the availability of the anesthetic agents that will be used. Additional supplies for induction and intubation may be assembled after completion of the preoperative interview. For airway management, a video laryngoscope or flexible fiber-optic scope may be requested. If an awake intubation is performed, the patient receives a topical anesthetic spray and gel to numb the area prior to insertion of the tube. If needed, an epidural catheter or hemodynamic monitoring lines may also be inserted.

Preparation for Surgery

Institutions that use a surgical safety checklist begin with the sign-in as the patient enters the OR. Prior to induction, deep vein thrombosis (DVT) preventive measures are ensured. Safety straps are placed across the patient's thighs and arms to secure them to the OR bed. When planned, the patient will go through induction and intubation. Once the airway is established and maintained, if ordered, a urinary drainage device is inserted. The patient's core body temperature may be monitored through an esophageal probe or urine temperature catheter.

Patient Positioning

Several positions are common for the patient during surgery: supine, lateral (e.g., for lung, hip, vascular, or kidney surgeries), prone (e.g., for spine, back, or posterior extremity), high lithotomy (gynecologic), low lithotomy (urologic or perineal), sitting (cranial, shoulder, or breast reconstruction), and jackknife (rectal) (see Table 4-2). Patients undergoing general anesthesia begin in the supine position for induction. Once the airway is secured, they are placed in the required position needed to perform the surgery. All patient positions require an assessment of correct body alignment, padding of bony prominences, and protection against nerve damage. Padding may consist of foam or gel products. Positioning devices include OR bed mattress, headrests, arm boards, wrist restraints, pillows, stirrups, Vac-Pac®, bean bag, laminectomy frame, chest rolls, axillary roll, shoulder braces, and footboards. A safety strap is needed in each position to assist in securing the patient to the OR bed. Correct patient positioning is the responsibility of the entire perioperative patient care team.

Each position has the potential to cause complications. Complications can range from pressure ulcers, shearing injury (caused by adjacent surfaces sliding along each other, such as skin remaining fixed on bed while internal structures slide downward [Treatment of Pressure Ulcers Guideline Panel, 1994]), nerve damage, DVT, diminished lung capacity, joint dislocation, and altera-

Table 4-2. Common Surgical Positions

Position	Description
Supine	Patient is flat on his or her back. Arms may be extended at various degrees (no greater than 90° at the axilla) on padded arm boards or secured at their sides. • Trendelenburg: Patient is tilted with the head lower than the feet. • Reverse Trendelenburg: Patient is tilted with the head higher than the feet.
Prone	Patient is on his or her abdomen. Arms are secured at the side or extended 90° at the elbow on padded arm boards.
Lateral	Patient is on his or her side; bottom leg is flexed at the knee. The top leg is straight or slightly flexed at the knee. A pillow is placed between the legs. The lower arm is secured to a padded arm board; the upper arm is secured on an elevated arm board, sling or pillow.
Lithotomy	Patient begins in the supine position. The hips/buttocks are located at the lower break in the surgical table. Legs are placed in stirrups (sling, boot, or knee crutch). The lower portion of the surgical table is removed. • High lithotomy: The legs are placed in sling stirrups. • Low lithotomy: The legs are placed in boot or knee crutch stirrups.
Sitting or Fowler's	Patient begins in supine position. The hips are at the middle break in the bed. The back of the bed is elevated to 45°. Knees are at the lower break in the bed. The knees are flexed by lowering the lower break of the surgical table.
Jackknife	Patient begins in a prone position. The hips are centered over the middle break in the surgical table. The table is flexed to 90° at the hips.

Note. Based on information from Association of periOperative Registered Nurses, 2013; Heizenroth, 2011; Phillips, 2013.

tions in blood pressure (Heizenroth, 2011). A preoperative baseline assessment is imperative to determine any possible complications. The circulating nurse assesses for skin integrity and potential contributing factors such as poor nutrition, impaired circulation, age, chemotherapy protocols, radiation treatments (external beam), and other disease processes (Walton-Geer, 2009). Pressure ulcers can develop on bony prominences that are in prolonged contact with the OR bed or positioning devices such as stirrups or arm boards. Shearing and joint dislocation can occur during positioning and patient transfer. Nerve damage, DVT, and alterations in vital signs can develop as a result of position, anesthetic agents, and prolonged surgery (see Table 4-3).

Skin and Device Preparations

The incision site is prepped after positioning is completed. This may include hair removal if it will interfere with incision. An antimicrobial solution should be applied to the intended surgical site and surrounding tissue

Table 4-3. Complications Related to Patient Positioning

Position	Pressure Areas	Nerve Damage	Vascular Compromise
Supine	Head/occiput Shoulders/scapula Elbow Spine: vertebra, coccyx, and sacrum Heels	Brachial plexus when arms > 90° at axilla Ulnar nerve	Deep vein thrombosis (DVT) Hypertension in Trendelenburg Diminished lung capacity in Trendelenburg Hypotension in reverse Trendelenburg
Prone	Face/cheek/eyes/ears Breast (females) Elbows Iliac crest Genitalia (males) Knees Toes	Shoulder Arm/upper extremity nerves	DVT Diminished lung capacity
Lateral	Ear Shoulder Ribs Ilium Hip/femoral head Knee Ankle	Brachial plexus Peroneal nerve	DVT Diminished lung capacity in the dependent lung
Lithotomy	Head/occiput Shoulders/scapula Elbow Hips Coccyx/sacrum Lateral legs Heels	Hip dislocation Sciatic nerve Peroneal nerve Saphenous nerve	DVT Diminished lung capacity
Sitting or Fowler's	Scapula Elbows Ischial tuberosity Coccyx/sacrum Back of knees Heels	–	DVT
Jackknife	Face/cheek/eyes/ears Breast (females) Elbows Iliac crest Genitalia (males) Knees Toes	Shoulder Arm/upper extremity nerves	DVT Diminished lung capacity

Note. Based on information from Association of periOperative Registered Nurses, 2013; Heizenroth, 2011; Phillips, 2013.

(Association of periOperative Registered Nurses, 2013). The selection of the solution is dependent on the location of the surgical site, patient allergies and skin condition, environmental risks such as fire, and other considerations (Zinn, Jenkins, Swofford, Harrelson, & McCarter, 2010). Sterile drapes are placed around the incision site by the surgical team members.

Prior to the start of the procedure, a time out from the surgical safety checklist (see Figure 4-1) is performed. It involves the entire perioperative patient care team. According to the Joint Commission (2014a), the time out allows a final assessment that the correct patient, site, and procedure are identified. All issues or discrepancies must be resolved prior to the start of surgery.

During Surgery

The perioperative team continually monitors aseptic technique throughout the surgery and is responsible for the correction of any violations. When thermal energy technology is used, such as electrosurgery, laser, or microwave ablation, the circulating nurse confirms that all safety precautions are followed. The circulating nurse anticipates the needs of the surgeon and provides any additional supplies. The nurse coordinates care with other surgeons or support teams such as radiology or pathology. When the tissue specimen is removed, the nurse labels the specimen and sends it to pathology. The type of testing is ordered by the surgeon and could include frozen section, lymphoma workup, permanent pathology, or culture. Frozen sections can assess for tissue diagnosis or margins (e.g., cancerous or noncancerous). This information will assist the surgeon with any further resection.

If chemotherapy is used intraoperatively, the patient is placed on chemotherapy safety precautions. Hyperthermic intraperitoneal chemotherapy, limb perfusion, and bladder instillation are examples of intraoperative chemotherapy.

When drains and dressings are ordered, the nurse delivers them to the sterile field. All care provided in the OR is documented on the patient's medical record. Before the patient leaves the OR, all surgical counts must be completed.

At the completion of the procedure, a sign out from the surgical safety checklist is completed. The circulating nurse provides an initial handoff report to the next care provider prior to the patient leaving the OR. A brief report may include respiratory, cardiac, and neurologic status; drains; and precautions. This gives the receiving unit time to prepare for any special equipment or supplies. The OR nurse may accompany the patient to the PACU and provide a detailed report.

Postoperative Phase and Postoperative Assessment

The postoperative phase begins when the patient is transferred to the PACU or designated post-procedure area and ends when this care is completed. The patient may be discharged to home, observed for less than 24 hours, or admitted to the hospital (Spry, 2013). Two postanesthesia phases of care exist, phase I and phase II. In phase I care, the focus is on providing postanesthesia nursing in the immediate postanesthesia period, whereas phase II care focuses on preparation for the home or an extended care environment (American Society of PeriAnesthesia Nurses, 2012–2014). When the patient arrives in the PACU, an immediate assessment is performed that includes ABC (evaluation of the airway, breathing, and circulation), vital signs, and a comprehensive report from the anesthesia care provider (Odom-Forren, 2011).

Once the report is completed, a thorough assessment is initiated. This includes a head-to-toe assessment of all body systems (see Figure 4-5). Vital signs and a pain assessment are typically taken every 5 minutes for the first 15 minutes, then every 15 minutes until discharge. Pain assessment and management is performed using an appropriate assessment tool. The anesthesia care provider primarily manages the care of the patient during the postanesthesia phase. The nurse must continually assess for possible complications related to the type of surgery the patient had, as well as the type of anesthesia. The SCIP measures continue in the postanesthesia phase. The PACU nurse will follow safe-handling precautions if the patient received chemotherapy in the OR.

Once the established discharge criteria are met, the anesthesiologist usually discharges the patient from the PACU. A common scoring system is the Aldrete score. Activity, respiration, circulation, consciousness, and oxygen saturation level are scored from 0 to 2. A total score of 8–10 is generally acceptable for PACU discharge (Aldrete, 1998). A report is given to the next care provider by telephone before the patient leaves the PACU or face-to-face after the patient reaches the unit. For certain procedures the receiving unit nurse may come to the PACU for a face-to-face report and direct observation of the patient. The report should include a preoperative history, pertinent information regarding the patient's surgery and recovery, medications the patient received, physician's orders, and any other appropriate information (Odom-Forren, 2011).

Conclusions

Perioperative nursing is a specialty practice area and requires continuing education and training to be knowledgeable about new technologies, procedures, and treatments. Certification should be encouraged for staff in all areas of care. It is important for the nurse to understand the type of care provided to the patient during surgery. Patient education is included throughout each phase of care but is done primarily in the preoperative and postoperative phases. Handoff communication is vital throughout the continuum of care to achieve the goal of providing quality and safe patient care.

Initial and ongoing assessment and documentation components include, but are not limited to:
1. Integration of data received at transfer of care
   a. Relevant preoperative status
   b. Anesthesia/sedation technique and agents
   c. Length of time anesthesia/sedation administered, time reversal agents given
   d. Pain and comfort management interventions and plan
   e. Medications administered
   f. Type of procedure
   g. Estimated fluid/blood loss and replacement
   h. Complications occurring during anesthesia course, treatment initiated, response
   i. Emotional status on arrival to the operating or procedure room
2. Vital signs[d]
   a. Airway patency, respiratory status, breath sounds, type of artificial airway, mechanical ventilator settings and oxygen saturation; end-tidal CO_2 (capnography) monitoring if available and indicated
   b. Blood pressure: non-invasive or arterial line
   c. Pulse: apical, peripheral
   d. Cardiac monitor rhythm documented per institutional protocol
   e. Temperature/route
   f. Hemodynamic pressure readings: central venous, pulmonary artery and wedge and intracranial pressure if indicated
   g. Pregnancy-related assessments
3. Pain level
4. Sedation level
5. Comfort level
6. Neurological function to include level of consciousness
7. Sensory and motor function as appropriate
8. Position of patient
9. Condition and color of skin
10. Patient safety needs[a]
11. Neurovascular: peripheral pulses and sensation of extremity(ies) as applicable
12. Condition of dressings and visible incisions
13. Type, patency, and securement of drainage tubes, catheters, and receptacles
14. Intake and output
    a. Amount and type of drainage (urine, drains, etc.)
    b. Fluid intake (IV, PO)
15. Pupillary response as indicated
16. Intravenous assessment: location of lines, condition of IV site, type of solution infusing
17. Medication management
18. Surgery/procedure specific assessments
19. Individualized plan of care
20. Nursing actions and/or interventions with outcome
21. Anticipation of any needed equipment for receiving unit (as appropriate)
22. Inclusion of family in care of patient as indicated

Figure 4-5. American Society of PeriAnesthesia Nurses Initial Assessment: Phase I Recovery

(Continued on next page)

(Continued)

23. Notification of patient care unit when patient is ready for discharge from PACU; provision of handoff report of significant events in the operating room and PACU
24. Postanesthesia scoring system if used[5,6,7]

Figure 4-5. American Society of PeriAnesthesia Nurses Initial Assessment: Phase I Recovery

[a] Patient safety needs could include, but not be limited to: institutional requirements for medication reconciliation, fall risk assessments, site verification, risk for suicide and medication management.

[d] Frequency of adult vital sign assessment during Phase I is institution specific. Practice varies across the country with frequency ranging from every five to every fifteen minutes. Expert opinion recommends that the frequency of vital sign assessment occurs a minimum of every fifteen minutes during Phase I as clinical condition requires.

In terms of postoperative pediatric assessment, close to 74% of survey respondents admitted that an initial blood pressure is always obtained from the pediatric patient on arrival to Phase I.

References

5. Joshi GP. New concepts in recovery after ambulatory surgery. Ambulatory Surg.2003;10:167-70.

6. Marshall SI, Chung F. Discharge criteria and complications after ambulatory surgery. Anesth Analg. 1999;88:508-17.

7. Saar LM. Use of a modified Postanesthesia Recovery Score in phase II perianesthesia period of ambulatory surgery patients. J PeriAnesth Nurs. 2001;16:82-9.

Note. From "Practice Recommendation 2, Initial and Ongoing Assessment: Phase I" (pp. 38–39), in *2012–2014 Perianesthesia Nursing Standards, Practice Recommendations and Interpretive Statements,* by the American Society of PeriAnesthesia Nurses (ASPAN), Cherry Hill, NJ: Author. Copyright © 2012–2014 by ASPAN. Reprinted with permission. All rights reserved.

References

Aldrete, J. (1998). Modifications to the postanesthesia score for use in ambulatory surgery. *Journal of PeriAnesthesia Nursing, 13,* 148–155.

American Society of Anesthesiologists. (2009). Continuum of depth of sedation: Definition of general anesthesia and levels of sedation/analgesia. Retrieved from http://www.asahq.org/ For-Members/Standards-Guidelines-and-Statements.aspx

American Society of Anesthesiologists. (2012). ASA physical status classification system. Retrieved from http://www.asahq.org/For-Members/Clinical-Information/ASA-Physical-Status -Classification-System.aspx

American Society of PeriAnesthesia Nurses. (2012–2014). *2012–2014 perianesthesia nursing standards, practice recommendations and interpretive statements.* Cherry Hill, NJ: Author.

Association of periOperative Registered Nurses. (2013). *Perioperative standards and recommended practices.* Retrieved from http://www.aorn.org/Books_and_Publications/Perioperative _Standards_and_Recommended_Practices/Perioperative_Standards_and_Recommended _Practices.aspx#axzz2DaUOE2LF

Heizenroth, P.A. (2011). Positioning the patient for surgery. In J.C. Rothrock (Ed.), *Alexander's care of the patient in surgery* (14th ed., pp. 144–173). St. Louis, MO: Elsevier Mosby.

Institute for Healthcare Improvement. (2013, April 2). Surgical Care Improvement Project. Retrieved from http://www.ihi.org/knowledge/Pages/OtherWebsites/SurgicalCare ImprovementProject.aspx

Joint Commission. (2012). Facts about the National Patient Safety Goals. Retrieved from http://www.jointcommission.org/standards_information/npsgs.aspx

Joint Commission. (2014a). National Patient Safety Goals effective January 1, 2014. Retrieved from http://www.jointcommission.org/assets/1/6/HAP_NPSG_Chapter_2014.pdf

Joint Commission. (2014b). Specifications manual for national hospital inpatient quality measures. Retrieved from http://www.jointcommission.org/specifications_manual_for_national _hospital_inpatient_quality_measures.aspx

Odom-Forren, J. (2011). Postoperative patient care and pain management. In J.C. Rothrock (Ed.), *Alexander's care of the patient in surgery* (14th ed., pp. 267–293). St. Louis, MO: Elsevier Mosby.

Phillips, N. (2013). *Operating room technique* (12th ed.). St. Louis, MO: Elsevier Mosby.

Spry, C. (2013). *Essentials of perioperative nursing* (4th ed.). Burlington, MA: Jones and Bartlett.

Treatment of Pressure Ulcers Guideline Panel. (1994, December). *Treatment of pressure ulcers* (AHCPR Clinical Practice Guidelines, No. 15). Rockville, MD: Agency for Health Care Policy and Research. Retrieved from http://www.ncbi.nlm.nih.gov/books/NBK63903/

Walton-Geer, P.S. (2009). Prevention of pressure ulcers in the surgical patient. *AORN Journal, 89*, 538–548. doi:10.1016/j.aorn.2008.12.022

Watson, D.S. (2011). *Perioperative safety*. St. Louis, MO: Elsevier Mosby.

World Alliance for Patient Safety. (2008). *WHO surgical safety checklist and implementation manual*. Retrieved from http://www.who.int/patientsafety/safesurgery/ss_checklist/en/

Zinn, J., Jenkins, J.B., Swofford, V., Harrelson, B., & McCarter, S. (2010). Intraoperative patient skin prep agents: Is there a difference? *AORN Journal, 92*, 662–671. doi:10.1016/j. aorn.2010.07.016

CHAPTER 5

Pediatric Implications in Surgical Oncology

Christine E. Smith, MSN, RN, CNS, CNOR, and Sarah E. Ferrari, MSN, RN, CNS, CPHON®

Introduction

Caring for children with cancer is a unique and dynamic pediatric specialty. Childhood cancers account for less than 1% of all cancers diagnosed in the United States (American Cancer Society, 2014), yet cancer remains one of the leading causes of death for children (Centers for Disease Control and Prevention, 2013). More than 15,000 individuals younger than 20 years old are expected to be diagnosed with cancer in 2014 in the United States, in contrast to 1.6 million adults (American Cancer Society, 2014). Cancer prevalence, risk factors, types, treatment facilities, and prognoses in children are all distinctly different from those in adults, as are the personalized treatment plans.

Treatment

Historically, pediatric cancer treatment was provided by surgeons and pathologists (Foley & Fergusson, 2011); surgery was the primary treatment modality. Today, multimodal therapies are used in most treatment protocols and include combinations of surgery, chemotherapy, biotherapy, radiation therapy, and stem cell transplantation (Rossetto, 2008). The number of surgical resections among the pediatric population has decreased (Foley & Fergusson, 2011).

Although the fundamental treatment modalities for adults and children are analogous, pediatric protocols are specific to the age of the child and the specific type of cancer. In addition, the majority of pediatric patients with cancer are enrolled in clinical trials; 60% enter studies at diagnosis. Additional research opportunities exist after the initial diagnosis related to growth and development, survivorship care, recurrent disease, or palliative care (CureSearch for Children's Cancer, 2012). Clinical trial groups have created a foundation to collect and share data across institutions. The Children's Oncology Group (COG) is a research consortium that involves nearly 200 treatment facilities to improve the treatment and outcomes of childhood cancers (CureSearch for Children's Cancer, 2012). COG and its affiliated institutions have created scientific evidence that has improved treatment and survival rates. Forty years ago, children with cancer faced a dismal survival rate of 10%. Today, childhood survivors overcome most cancers and can hope to be part of an 80% survival rate (CureSearch for Children's Cancer, 2012).

Treatment plans are determined collaboratively by the primary medical physician, oncologist, and surgeon. Initially, the patient is referred to a pediatric medical oncologist who functions within a children's hospital or large university medical center. The oncology team includes specialists such as pediatric surgeons and pathologists, nurse practitioners (NPs), RNs, child life specialists, art therapists, nutritionists, social workers, and psychologists. The interdisciplinary team is specially trained to meet the needs of both the family and the pediatric patient with cancer.

Family Dynamics and Supportive Care

The blend of clinical nursing principles with family management strategies provides the framework for family-centered care. Family-centered care is an innovative shift to provide medical services and support (Mackay & Gregory, 2011). The interdisciplinary team works collaboratively with the family to make decisions that fit their unique needs. In addition to family-centered care, child life specialists are specially trained to work with children to help prepare and support the child and family during treatment. Supportive care for pediatric patients with cancer is often outlined by segments of the clinical trial, institutional guidelines, and standards from the Association of Pediatric Hematology/Oncology Nurses (Baggott et al., 2011).

The diagnosis of cancer starts a roller coaster of emotions for the child and family. This devastating diagnosis, encompassed with the fear of losing control of the future, begins a life of uncertainty (Wilson & Bryant, 2007). The constant variable for the child and family is often provided by the RN or NP. As part of the healthcare team, these nurses help families navigate the obstacles by providing support and education. Establishing a therapeutic relationship with the patient and family better equips the nurse to advocate on their behalf (Baggott et al., 2011).

Children benefit from maintenance of daily routines in the home and in the hospital. Collaboration with the patient and family to align the treatment regimens with their home routines is essential. The chronologic age does not always equate to the developmental age or emotional stage of the child, especially during a chronic illness such as cancer. As the child grows and enters new developmental stages, adaptations are beneficial with inclusion of new routines and responsibilities.

End-of-Life Issues

Although medical treatment and prognosis have advanced over the past 40 years, childhood cancer still remains a life-threatening disease. When treatment is no longer curative, communication between the multidisciplinary team and the family unit is essential to structure a supportive network and identify strategies for care (National Cancer Institute [NCI], 2013b). When the child is developmentally and medically capable, he or she should be included in discussions about care decisions.

A dilemma occurs when the child, parent, and physicians are not in alignment with the plan of care. The challenge is to balance the underage child's wishes, the parent or legal guardian's plan of care, and the physicians' legal constraints. Some state laws place limitations on the care that can be provided or not provided at end of life (NCI, 2013a). The multidisciplinary team is responsible for being aware of the various state laws as well as institutional policies and procedures to support the family during end-of-life care and decision-making processes (NCI, 2013a).

Surgical Considerations

Surgery for neonates, infants, children, and adolescents is commonly performed for congenital anomalies, traumatic injuries, and acquired diseases and conditions. The pediatric patient presents unique challenges and characteristics, usually related to his or her developmental stage (Warner, 2008). The stages of life and maturation levels are important aspects to assess, as they pose implications for safety, surgical outcomes, disease-free survival, and recovery. Sound knowledge and awareness by all surgical disciplines is critical in the treatment of this vulnerable population entrusted to their care. The following pediatric considerations and characteristics are of high priority in surgery, interventional procedures, and anesthesia services.

Airway and Pulmonary Precautions

Respiratory distress during anesthesia, surgery, and interventional procedures is a continual threat because of the small, funnel-shaped pediatric airways that are easily obstructed by normal secretions, common respiratory disease, and laryngeal sensitivity. Children also have an overall smaller functional pulmonary capacity. Availability of appropriate sizes of all airway equipment is crucial, as is constant awareness of potential changes in respiratory condition (DiFusco, 2011).

Cardiovascular Concerns

Anomalies that were unrecognized at birth may present at the time of surgery, such as persistent transitional circulation, murmurs, decreased cardiac compliance, and parasympathetic hypertonia. In addition, anesthesia-induced vasodilation can potentiate cardiac arrhythmias. Even minimal blood loss may pose critical harm in children whose overall blood volume is small. Therefore, cardiac-specific assessment is important in the preoperative evaluation and postoperative monitoring (Warner, 2008).

Metabolic Implications

Drug uptake, absorption, distribution, and clearance differ among infants, young children, and adolescents due to maturity of liver function, level of basal metabolic rate, total body weight, and extracellular body fluids (DiFusco, 2011). A less mature blood-brain barrier and greater protein binding increases sensitivity to opioids, sedatives, and anesthetics. Drug dosages and administration are specifically scaled to the child's kilogram body weight rather than standard dosing.

Thermal Regulation

The risk of hypothermia in children younger than two years old is increased by immature thermal regulation, a thin adipose layer, and increased ratio of body surface area to weight. Symptoms related to cold may not be evident in this young age group; for example, cold-stressed neonates do not shiver. Increased and persistent cold can lead to acidosis and decreased perfusion. Therefore, providing interventions to maintain warmth is a standard of care (Warner, 2008).

Fluid Management

Children younger than two years old are prone to dehydration because of immature renal function, decreased urine concentration, and insensible fluid loss (DiFusco, 2011). Overall, children have higher fluid requirements than adults. Primary considerations of fluid needs include body weight as well as the length of time without fluid replacement. The best indicators of sufficient fluid intake are urine output and osmolarity as compared to milliliters per kilogram of body weight.

Anesthesia Management

Children require sedation or general anesthesia for surgery and interventional and diagnostic procedures, which include endoscopy, lumbar punctures, percutaneous biopsies, radiation therapy, imaging studies, and eye examinations. Children with chronic diseases such as cancer may be subjected to frequent anesthesia or sedation. Children and parents both share anxiety related to separation from family and friends and fear of pain, procedures, care providers, outcomes, and the unknown. As with any intervention, there are fears of side effects related to the procedure.

Conclusions

Today, pediatric patients with cancer are less likely to undergo debilitating surgical procedures with the advent of multiple neoplastic agents that enable tumor reduction prior to surgery. Cancers that were once treated with surgical removal are now cured with chemotherapy, radiation therapy, and biotherapy. The dramatic progress that has been made in the treatment of pediatric cancers makes long-term survival the expectation for most pediatric patients and families (NCI, 2013a). Nevertheless, childhood cancer survivors face the risk of additional cancers secondary to their primary cancer treatment. Unfortunately, most pediatric survivors experience late side effects from their cancer therapies, which may predispose children and young adults to chronic health conditions and the ultimate risk of premature death secondary to their prior lifesaving cancer treatment. Therefore, pediatric cancer survivors should be followed long-term after their surgical and medical treatment to eliminate or reduce side effects that can mitigate normal development and age-appropriate lifestyle.

References

American Cancer Society. (2014). *Cancer facts and figures 2014.* Retrieved from http://www.cancer.org/research/cancerfactsstatistics/cancerfactsfigures2014/index

Baggott, C., Fochtman, D., Foley, G., & Patterson-Kelly, K. (Eds.). (2011). *Nursing care of children and adolescents with cancer and blood disorders* (4th ed.). Glenview, IL: Association of Pediatric Hematology/Oncology Nurses.

Centers for Disease Control and Prevention. (2013). 10 leading causes of death by age group, United States—2010. Retrieved from http://www.cdc.gov/Injury/wisqars/pdf/10LCD -Age-Grp-US-2010-a.pdf

CureSearch for Children's Cancer. (2012). Previous research: CureSearch to provide $2 million to Children's Oncology Group clinical trials. Retrieved from http://www.curesearch .org/current-research

DiFusco, L.A. (2011). Pediatric surgery. In J.C. Rothrock (Ed.), *Alexander's care of the patient in surgery* (14th ed., pp. 1113–1115). St. Louis, MO: Elsevier Mosby.

Foley, G.V., & Fergusson, J.H. (2011). History, issues, and trends. In N.E. Kline (Ed.), *Essentials of pediatric hematology/oncology nursing: A core curriculum* (4th ed., pp. 2–34). Glenview, IL: Association of Pediatric Hematology/Oncology Nurses.

Mackay, L.J., & Gregory, D. (2011). Exploring family-centered care among pediatric oncology nurses. *Journal of Pediatric Oncology Nursing, 28*, 43–52. doi:10.1177/104345210377179

National Cancer Institute. (2013a). Late effects of treatment for childhood cancer (PDQ®). Retrieved from http://www.cancer.gov/cancertopics/pdq/treatment/lateeffects/Health Professional

National Cancer Institute. (2013b). Pediatric supportive care (PDQ®): End of life. Retrieved from http://www.cancer.gov/cancertopics/pdq/supportivecare/pediatric/healthprofessional/ page4

Rossetto, C. (2008). Surgery. In N.E. Kline (Ed.), *Essentials of pediatric hematology/oncology nursing: A core curriculum* (3rd ed., pp. 92–94). Glenview, IL: Association of Pediatric Hematology/Oncology Nurses.

Warner, B.W. (2008). Pediatric surgery. In C.M. Townsend, R.D. Beauchamp, B.M. Evers, & K.L. Mattox (Eds.), *Sabiston textbook of surgery: The biological basis of modern surgical practice* (18th ed., pp. 2080–2089). Philadelphia, PA: Elsevier Saunders.

Wilson, K., & Bryant, R. (Eds.). (2007). *Foundations of pediatric hematology/oncology nursing: A comprehensive orientation and review course.* Glenview, IL: Association of Pediatric Hematology/Oncology Nurses.

CHAPTER 6

Geriatric Implications in Surgical Oncology

Meghan Routt, RN, MSN, GNP/ANP-BC, AOCNP®

Introduction

More than 55% of cancers are diagnosed in people 65 years old or older; nearly 70% of cancer deaths occur in the same age group (American Cancer Society, 2014). The median age of all cancer diagnoses is 66, whereas the median age of all cancer-related deaths is 72 (Howlader et al., 2013). The term *older adult* has been defined many ways. The population of older adults is heterogeneous, accounting for 101 million people in the United States (U.S. Census Bureau, 2012). Geriatric specialists have divided this population further into three categories: young-old (age 65–74), old (age 75–84), and oldest-old (85 and older). The fastest-growing subgroup of older adults is those aged 85 and older. Chronologic age is not indicative of physiologic age. Physiologic age takes into account functional status, comorbidities, frailty, and the presence of geriatric syndromes (Carreca & Balducci, 2009).

Advanced age in general is associated with inadequate cancer diagnosis and treatment, and this lack of sufficient diagnosis among older adults can translate into shorter survival times (Wedding, Röhrig, Klippstein, Pientka, & Höffken, 2007). Controversy exists among practitioners in regard to older adults and recommended treatment for cancer, including appropriateness for surgery, ability to tolerate chemotherapy, screening and prevention of other cancers, end-of-life care initiation, and participation in clinical trials. As a result, the National Comprehensive Cancer Network (NCCN, 2013) established senior adult oncology recommendations for practitioners, estimating life expectancy based on function and comorbidities. According to the NCCN guidelines, treatment should be avoided if it diminishes an individual's quality of life and offers no significant survival benefit (NCCN, 2013).

Preoperative Assessment

Preservation of function should be the ultimate goal of treating older adult patients with cancer. Function is primarily assessed by activities of daily living (ADL) and instrumental activities of daily living (IADL). The most inclusive tool for evaluating function is the comprehensive geriatric assessment, which incorporates physical activity, comorbidity index, function (ADL, IADL), socioeconomic issues, and the presence of geriatric syndromes (Carreca & Balducci, 2009). A limitation of this assessment tool is the length and time it requires to complete, making it difficult to administer in an office setting.

In oncology, two other tools describe an individual's functional status. The Eastern Cooperative Oncology Group (ECOG) developed a numeric performance scale (0 = fully active, able to carry on all predisease performance without restriction, to 5 = dead) (Oken et al., 1982). It is generally recommended that patients with an ECOG status of 3 or above are not appropriate surgical candidates. The Karnofsky Performance Status is an analog scale (100 = normal, no complaints, to 0 = death) (Karnofsky & Burchenal, 1949). Surgery is not the only modality affected by performance status. Decision making regarding chemotherapy initiation, dose adjustment, and appropriateness for hospice and palliative care also involves use of these scales to guide appropriate treatment.

The International Society of Geriatric Oncology formed a surgical task force to address the inconsistency of preoperative evaluation of older adults and developed a tool to assist surgeons in assessing potential surgical risk in this population. The Preoperative Assessment of Cancer in the Elderly (PACE) tool incorporates the following instruments: mini-mental state inventory, ADL and IADL, geriatric depression scale, Brief Fatigue Inventory (BFI), ECOG performance status, American Society of Anesthesiologists scale, and Satariano's index of comorbidities (Audisio, 2007). NCCN (2013) has adopted this tool and incorporated it into its senior adult oncology guidelines.

The older adult is more likely to suffer from one or more chronic diseases, especially cardiovascular disease, chronic obstructive pulmonary disease, diabetes, and renal impairment. These comorbidities affect not only life expectancy but also how well the patient recovers from surgery.

Postoperative Care

Postoperative management of the older adult population requires careful assessment, especially in regard to pain management. Cancer pain is often inadequately managed and is one of the most frequently reported symptoms in this population (Beck, Towsley, Caserta, Lindau, & Dudley, 2009). Unrelieved pain can lead to depression and sleep and appetite disturbances, as well as an increase in healthcare utilization and cost (Mercadante & Arcuri, 2007). Many factors contribute to poor pain management in older adults. These include clinicians and patients who believe pain is an expected effect of aging. Clinicians struggle with the use of pain scales in patients with cognitive impairment and are concerned with polypharmacy and adverse drug effects in patients with declining organ function (Barford & D'Olimpio, 2008; Mercadante & Arcuri, 2007). Although older adults may be more sensitive to drug side effects, with appropriate treatment they should receive pain relief. Patients undergoing surgery will have pain; therefore, understanding medication management in the older adult is imperative. The American Geriatrics Society (2012) published an updated list of potentially inappropriate medications for use in the older adult, referred to as the Beers Criteria. These criteria serve as guidelines regarding medication usage across all therapeutic classifications. Recommendations for age-adjusted dosing are not available for most analgesics; therefore, many clinicians follow renal impairment recommendations. Nonsteroidal anti-inflammatory drugs (NSAIDs) should be used with caution in older adults because NSAIDs can contribute to renal failure. The most used analgesic in older adults is acetaminophen because it has a greater safety profile and is not associated with adverse renal effects (American Geriatrics Society, 2009). Patient-controlled analgesia is effective for patients with adequate cognitive function and is often the best immediate postoperative pain intervention (Falzone, Hoffmann, & Keita, 2013). Once the patient is able to tolerate a full liquid diet, the transition to oral pain medications can be initiated. When initiating and titrating oral opioids, start low and go slow. Once the patient is on oral pain medications, IV medication should only be used for severe, breakthrough pain.

Geriatric Syndromes

Geriatricians have embraced the term *geriatric syndromes* to highlight unique features of common health conditions in older adults. Often there is not one definite diagnosis but rather a clustering of symptoms that compose the syndrome. The four most often described syndromes include dementia, failure to thrive, delirium, and falls. A multidisciplinary team can help improve the quality of life of cancer survivors by assessing, preventing, and treating these syndromes.

Dementia is defined as an impairment of global intellectual and cognitive function with symptoms of impaired judgment, impaired short- and long-term memory, difficulty with problem solving, personality changes, organization difficulties, and problems with abstract thinking (Knopman et al., 2001). Dementia is characterized by a progressive disease course beginning with mild deficits and can ultimately lead to death. The prevalent types of dementia include Alzheimer dementia, vascular dementia, and dementia with Lewy bodies. Dementia with Lewy bodies has additional symptoms that include alterations in gait and balance, hallucinations, and delusions (Knopman et al., 2001). Cognitive impairment has been associated with poor cancer survival outcomes (Duff, Mold, & Gidron, 2009). When patients are hospitalized or undergo cancer treatments, patients with dementia are more likely to become confused and delirious and are at risk for falls (Lykestos, 2002). Symptoms related to *delirium* include a sudden onset of acute confusion, inattention, acute agitation, acute change in mental status, and thought disorganization (Marcantonio, 2011). Patients who develop delirium have poorer surgical outcomes, including increased risk of death (Ganai, Lee, & Merrill, 2007; Olin et al., 2005). Risk factors for developing delirium include age older than 70–75 years, dementia, frailty, comorbidities, infection, functional disability, history of depression, major cardiac/vascular/abdominal surgery, dehydration, polypharmacy, sensory impairments, and sleep deprivation (Marcantonio, 2012). Older adults are at risk for developing postoperative delirium when emergent or long, complicated surgery is performed (Marcantonio, 2012). Postoperative delirium is present typically on postoperative day 1–2; later-onset delirium is associated with either a major postoperative complication or withdrawal from alcohol or sedatives (Marcantonio, 2012). Treatment of delirium should include systematic assessment of patients, a thorough search for contributing factors, correction of contributing factors, and assurance of patient safety and support through nonpharmacologic methods, although judicious use of antipsychotics has been found to be beneficial in some cases (Young, Murthy, Westby, Akunne, & O'Mahoney, 2010). Resolution of delirium is variable, with half the episodes resolving within two days of onset and one-third persisting until hospital discharge (Marcantonio, 2012).

Conclusions

As the U.S. population continues to grow older, the quality of geriatric cancer care will depend on accurate assessment of risk factors influencing prognosis. Functionality should be preserved at all costs by using interventions that promote independence in ADL (Bellera et al., 2012). A plan of care including collaboration with physical and occupational therapists optimizes functional status. Healthcare professionals have the responsibility of providing ongoing assessment and intervention for geriatric cancer survivors across the cancer care continuum.

References

American Cancer Society. (2014). *Cancer facts and figures 2014*. Retrieved from http://www .cancer.org/research/cancerfactsstatistics/cancerfactsfigures2014/index

American Geriatrics Society. (2009). Pharmacological management of persistent pain in older adults. *Journal of the American Geriatrics Society, 57,* 1331–1346. doi:10.1111/j.1532-5415.2009.0237

American Geriatrics Society. (2012). American Geriatrics Society updated Beers Criteria for potentially inappropriate medication use in the older adult. *Journal of the American Geriatrics Society, 60,* 616–631. doi:10.1111/j.1532-5415.2012.03923.x

Audisio, R.A. (2007). Shall we operate? Preoperative assessment in elderly cancer patients (PACE) can help. A SIOG surgical task force prospective study. *Critical Reviews in Oncology/ Hematology, 65,* 156–163. doi:10.1016/j.critrevonc.2007.11.001

Barford, K.L., & D'Olimpio, J.T. (2008). Symptom management in geriatric oncology: Practical treatment considerations and current challenges. *Current Treatment Options in Oncology, 9,* 204–214. doi:10.1007/s11864-008-0062-4

Beck, S.L., Towsley, G.L., Caserta, M.S., Lindau, K., & Dudley, W.N. (2009). Symptom experiences and quality of life of rural and urban older adult cancer survivors. *Cancer Nursing, 32,* 359–369. doi:10.1097/NCC.0b013e3181a52533

Bellera, C.A., Rainfray, M., Mathoulin-Pelissier, S., Mertens, C., Delva, F., Fonck, M., & Soubeyran, P.L. (2012). Screening older cancer patients: First evaluation of the G-8 geriatric screening tool. *Annals of Oncology, 23,* 2166–2172. doi:10.1093/annonc/mdr587

Carreca, I., & Balducci, L. (2009). Cancer chemotherapy in the older cancer patient. *Urologic Oncology: Seminars and Original Investigations, 27,* 633–642. doi:10.1016/j.urolonc .2009.08.006

Duff, K., Mold, J.W., & Gidron, Y. (2009). Cognitive functioning predicts survival in the elderly. *Journal of Clinical and Experimental Neuropsychology, 31,* 90–95. doi:10.1080/13803390801998664

Falzone, E., Hoffmann, C., & Keita, H. (2013). Postoperative analgesia in elderly patients. *Drugs and Aging, 30,* 81–90. doi:10.1007/s40266-012-0047-7

Ganai, S., Lee, K.F., & Merrill, A. (2007). Adverse outcomes of geriatric patients undergoing abdominal surgery who are at high risk for delirium. *Archives of Surgery, 142,* 1072–1078. doi:10.1001/archsurg.142.11.1072

Howlader, N., Noone, A.M., Krapcho, M., Garshell, J., Neyman, N., Altekruse, S.F., … Cronin, K.A. (Eds.). (2013). *SEER cancer statistics review, 1975–2010* (based on November 2012 SEER data submission). Retrieved from http://seer.cancer.gov/csr/1975_2010/

Karnofsky, D.A., & Burchenal, J.H. (1949). The clinical evaluation of chemotherapeutic agents in cancer. In C.M. MacLeod (Ed.), *Clinical evaluation of chemotherapeutic agents* (pp. 191–205). New York, NY: Columbia University Press.

Knopman, D.S., DeKosky, S.T., Cummings, J.L., Chui, H., Corey-Bloom, J., Relkin, N., … Stevens, J.C. (2001). Practice parameter: Diagnosis of dementia (an evidence-based review). Report of the Quality Standards Subcommittee of the American Academy of Neurologists. *Neurology, 56,* 1143–1153. doi:10.1212/WNL.56.9.1143

Lykestos, C. (2002). Prevalence of neuropsychiatric symptoms in dementia and mild cognitive impairment. *JAMA, 288,* 1475–1483. doi:10.1001/jama.288.12.1475

Marcantonio, E.R. (2011). In the clinic: Delirium. *Annals of Internal Medicine, 154,* ITC6-1–ITC6-15. doi:10.1059/0003-4819-154-11-201106070-01006

Marcantonio, E.R. (2012). Postoperative delirium: A 76-year-old woman with delirium following surgery. *JAMA, 308,* 73–81. doi:10.1001/jama.2012.6857

Mercadante, S., & Arcuri, E. (2007). Pharmacological management of cancer pain in the elderly. *Drugs and Aging, 24,* 761–776.

National Comprehensive Cancer Network. (2013). *NCCN Clinical Practice Guidelines in Oncology: Senior adult oncology* [v.1.2014]. Retrieved from http://www.nccn.org/professionals/physician _gls/pdf/senior.pdf

Oken, M.M., Creech, R.H., Tormey, D.C., Horton, J., Davis, T.E., McFadden, E.T., & Carbone, P.P. (1982). Toxicity and response criteria of the Eastern Cooperative Oncology Group. *American Journal of Clinical Oncology, 5,* 649–655.

Olin, K., Eriksdotter-Jonhagen, M., Jansson, A., Herrington, M.K., Kristiansson, M., & Permert, J. (2005). Post-operative delirium in elderly patients after major abdominal surgery. *British Journal of Surgery, 92,* 1559–1564. doi:10.1002/bjs.5053

U.S. Census Bureau. (2012). State and County QuickFacts, 2012. Retrieved from http://quickfacts.census.gov/qfd/states/00000.html

Wedding, U., Röhrig, B., Klippstein, A., Pientka, L., & Höffken, K. (2007). Age, severe comorbidity and functional impairment independently contribute to poor survival in cancer patients. *Journal of Cancer Research and Clinical Oncology, 133,* 945–950. doi:10.1007/s00432-007 -0233-x

Young, J., Murthy, L., Westby, M., Akunne, A., & O'Mahoney, R. (2010). Diagnosis, prevention and management of delirium: Summary of NICE guidance. *BMJ, 341,* c3704. doi:10.1136/ bmj.c3704

CHAPTER 7

Surgical Care of Head and Neck Cancers

Raymond J. Scarpa, DNP, AOCN®

Introduction

Carcinomas of the head and neck region include anatomic sites from the base of skull to the clavicle such as the lips, oral cavity, pharynx, larynx, neck, nose, paranasal sinuses, and skull base (see Figure 7-1). Malignancies of the salivary, thyroid, and parathyroid glands and skin malignancies on the face and neck can also be included. Squamous cell carcinomas are the most common histopathology and comprise about 90% of all head and neck malignancies (Forastiere et al., 2008).

Cancers of the head and neck can be disfiguring and affect an individual's ability to breathe, eat, and communicate. Surgical intervention remains the cornerstone of treatment, and successful outcomes are influenced by the proficiency and communication of the multidisciplinary team (Carty et al., 2012).

Oral Cavity Cancer

Malignant lesions of the oral cavity include the anterior two-thirds of the tongue, floor of the mouth, buccal mucosa, gingiva, hard and soft palate, retromolar trigone, and lips. To some extent the oral cavity is contiguous with the oropharynx. However, the oral cavity is separated from the oropharynx by the junction of the hard and soft palate, the circumvallate papillae, and the anterior tonsillar pillars. The oropharynx consists of the palatine tonsils, posterior tonsillar pillars, base of the tongue, glossoepiglottic fold, pharyngeal epiglottic fold, valleculae, and oropharyngeal walls (Shariff, 2010).

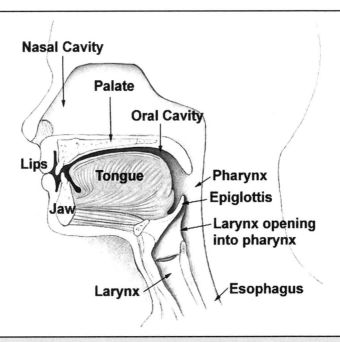

Figure 7-1. Anatomic Structures of the Head and Neck

Note. From "SEER Training Modules: Site-Specific Modules—Head & Neck Cancer," by the National Cancer Institute Surveillance, Epidemiology, and End Results (SEER) Program, n.d. Retrieved from http://training.seer.cancer.gov/head-neck/anatomy/overview.html.

Preprocedure

Following confirmation of malignancy with fine needle aspiration or tissue biopsy, a computed tomography (CT) scan or positron-emission tomography with CT (PET/CT) is obtained to provide clinical data about the size of the primary lesion, depth of invasion, and metastatic disease (Lander, Baloch, McGrath, Loevner, & Mandel, 2012). If extensive reconstruction is anticipated, vascular studies may be ordered to establish the quality and patency of vessels from the donor and recipient sites (Harris et al., 2012). Prophylactic percutaneous endoscopic gastrostomy feeding tube insertion may be planned in anticipation of the need for extended supplementary nutrition (Jack, Dawson, Reilly, & Shoaib, 2011).

Procedure

Treatment of oral cavity carcinomas consists of surgical resection of the primary lesion, with or without neck dissection. Early-stage cancers in the anterior two-thirds of the tongue require a partial glossectomy with 1–2 cm clear margins and will result in minimal speech or swallowing deficits (Forastiere et al., 2008).

Patients with advanced disease pose challenges related to local tumor control, reconstruction of surgical deficits, and maintenance of acceptable functional and cosmetic outcomes (Scarpa, 2009). Advanced lesions may require a total glossectomy, removal of surrounding structures, and extensive reconstruction of muscular, mucosal, dermal, or bone defects. A split-thickness skin graft (STSG) or pedicle tissue/muscle flap is necessary for closure of the surgical site. Donor sites for free flap tissue reconstruction include the radial forearm, the anterior lateral thigh, the scapula, or a fibular osteocutaneous flap to reconstruct the mandible (Ross et al., 2012). Combinations of the various grafts and flaps may be used to obtain optimal function and cosmetic effects. A tracheotomy offers unhindered access to the oral cavity intraoperatively and ensures a patent airway postoperatively until swelling subsides.

Post Procedure

Patients with extensive surgical resections and reconstruction require constant surveillance in the postoperative period with continual observation of flaps for circulatory viability. The arterial blood flow is monitored with a handheld or implantable Doppler ultrasound. The most common cause of flap failure is venous congestion, which is evidenced by bluish discoloration, swelling, and change in capillary refill (Spiegel & Polat, 2007). If this is observed, immediate surgical exploration occurs to remove clots and repair any leaking vessel anastomoses. If surgery is delayed, medicinal leech therapy may be employed to help ensure survival of the flap (Ross et al., 2012). Postoperative anticoagulant therapy with aspirin, heparin, or low-molecular-weight heparin aids in clot prevention. Drains placed in the surgical site prevent fluid buildup and tension on the suture lines; consistency, odor, and amount of drainage must be monitored.

Nutritional support is paramount to adequate wound healing. In addition to IV hydration, a gastric feeding tube may be used postoperatively to ensure adequate caloric intake (Jack et al., 2011). Challenges related to verbal communication are dependent on the degree of postoperative swelling, presence of a tracheotomy, and the extent of surgery. Assurance of ongoing communication with the healthcare team is essential to decrease anxiety and increase independence. Paper and pencil or picture cards are helpful to encourage patients to express themselves. Referral to speech pathology may be beneficial based on the extent of surgery and anticipation of an extended or permanent tracheotomy (Carty et al., 2012).

Laryngeal Cancer

Carcinomas of the larynx typically present with symptoms of voice changes, hoarseness, increasing shortness of breath, or difficulty breathing.

Preprocedure

In select cases, a biopsy of the suspected lesion on the larynx is performed with the patient under anesthesia in the operating room. Direct visualization of the upper aerodigestive tract is accomplished with the use of special ridged endoscopes. The airway can be assessed and the need for a tracheotomy determined. Following confirmation of the malignancy, a PET/CT is obtained to determine the extent of disease and presence of metastatic disease.

Procedure

Surgical management of T1, T2, and some select T3 supraglottic lesions requires a supraglottic laryngectomy, neck dissection, and tracheotomy. It is indicated for lesions that are limited to the epiglottis, infrahyoid and suprahyoid epiglottis, ventricular folds, and aryepiglottic folds. The superior edge of the incision is typically at the level of the hyoid bone. This procedure can be modified to include areas at the base of the tongue, the glottis, and the paraglottic space or extended laterally to include the pyriform sinus and one arytenoid cartilage. The routine supraglottic laryngectomy will remove the hyoid bone, upper half of the thyroid cartilage, epiglottis, false cords, aryepiglottic folds, and ventricle. The patient can be decannulated once the airway is determined to be adequate (Forastiere et al., 2008). This procedure is not indicated when there is fixation or impaired mobility of the true vocal cords, tumor within 5 mm of the anterior commissure, or thyroid cartilage involvement. Patients with chronic pulmonary disease with a forced expiratory volume of less than 50% may not be candidates for this procedure, nor are patients who have chronic swallowing disorders (Mücke et al., 2012). A neck dissection is usually indicated and is the first step in this procedure. It is typically performed on the side that has the majority of the tumor burden or palpable neck disease.

Conventional surgical management for early-stage lesions of the glottis includes a cordectomy, which removes the affected vocal cord. This procedure can be done only when the lesion does not extend to the anterior commissure or arytenoid cartilage. A partial vertical hemilaryngectomy is one of several partial laryngectomy procedures that involve resection of approximately half of the larynx. It is limited to lesions that do not extend to the posterior commissure, arytenoids, or thyroid cartilage (Forastiere et al., 2008).

A CO_2 laser is a novel technique used to perform a transoral endoscopic approach to resecting small lesions on the vocal cords or supraglottis. Robot-assisted surgical resection can also be used, although it is reserved for well-circumscribed lesions in the glottic and supraglottic areas. In studies comparing the two techniques, robot-assisted surgery was not more favorable over the traditional approach as measured by surgical time, cost, and postoperative drainage (Kayhan, Kaya, & Sayin, 2012). Advanced lesions of the larynx require a total laryngectomy, which removes the entire larynx, hyoid bone, and the thyroid and cricoid cartilages. A permanent stoma is created by fastening the trachea to the skin of the anterior neck. Air can no longer enter the upper aerodigestive tract, which results in a loss of smell and taste as well as an inability to sneeze, sniff, or blow the nose (Mücke et al., 2012).

Post Procedure

Postoperative care of the patient following a laryngectomy requires maintenance of an adequate airway, nutritional and emotional support, and a communication plan. The new laryngeal stoma needs vigilant observation, as the suture material, which secures the trachea, acts as a trap for dried mucus and bronchial secretions and may cause the diameter of the stoma to narrow. A laryngectomy tube is placed in the stoma once the patient is fully recovered from the operative procedure. This tube assists in maintaining patency of the airway and diameter of the stoma until the stoma is healed. Humidified oxygen or air is used to decrease the viscosity of secretions and to provide moisture to the air. Upon discharge to home, the use of a cool mist vaporizer or humidified air compressor decreases the viscosity of secretions and allows them to be cleared by coughing. Patients need to be taught how to suction and care for the stoma (Scarpa, 2009).

Patients and family members need assistance with the arduous task of communication. A writing tablet with a pen or pencil and picture boards or cards provide the patient with the means to communicate in the immediate postoperative phase. Referral to speech pathology provides the patient an opportunity to be taught the use of an electrolarynx. This device produces a vibratory sound that when placed on the appropriate area of the neck transmits this sound to the oral cavity and upper pharynx. The sound is converted to words by use of the musculature of the tongue and oral cavity. The speech pathologist can also teach esophageal speech, which enables the patient to swallow and expel air in a controlled burp that vibrates the posterior pharynx. This creates a sound that is converted to words by the musculature and tongue in the oral cavity (Carty et al., 2012).

The speech pathologist can also evaluate the patient for a surgical procedure called a tracheoesophageal puncture (TEP). This procedure will allow for communication without the use of an electrolarynx and is similar to esophageal speech. The surgeon creates a puncture wound on the posterior wall of the trachea within the laryngeal stoma. A catheter is placed into the puncture wound to create a fistula between the esophagus and trachea. Once the fistula is created, a small one-way valve device is placed into the tract. The patient is taught how to get air into the esophagus, cover the stoma, and force the air into the soft tissues of the pharynx, which allows them to vibrate and create a sound that is converted to words (Carty et al., 2012). Routine assessment of the stoma is important to assess the diameter and patency and to rule out any recurrent disease. Suspicious lesions near the stoma need to be biopsied to determine malignancy.

Metastatic Neck Cancer

Preprocedure

A fine needle aspiration of a suspicious lymph node can confirm metastatic neck disease (Lander et al., 2012). A CT or PET/CT scan is used to determine the extent of neck disease and adherence to and encasement of surrounding vessels or other nonlymphatic structures. Surgical management of metastatic disease in the neck is accomplished by a neck dissection.

Procedure

The four types of neck dissections are radical, modified radical, selective, and extended radical neck dissection. The radical neck dissection removes the fascia and all lymphatic structures from level I through level V in the neck, submandibular gland, jugular vein, sternocleidomastoid muscle, and spinal accessory and greater auricular nerves (see Figure 7-2). In the radical neck dissection, the incision begins at the level of the mastoid process and is extended approximately two fingerbreadths below the angle of the mandible to the anterior edge. A second incision is made midpoint to the first incision and extends over the posterior aspect of the sternocleidomastoid muscle in a lazy "S" manner and approaches the midclavicle (Forastiere et al., 2008). The lazy "S" shaped incision is associated with less scar contraction than a straight incision because the tissue within the curves of the "S" shape can stretch. Cosmetic and functional limitations occur from this procedure including a flat cosmetic deformity in the neck caused by the removal of the sternocleidomastoid muscle, limited range of motion, shoulder droop, and atrophy (Mücke et al., 2012).

The modified neck dissection removes all lymphatic structures from levels I through V but preserves one or more of the nonlymphatic structures. The incisions are similar, as are the cosmetic and functional restrictions.

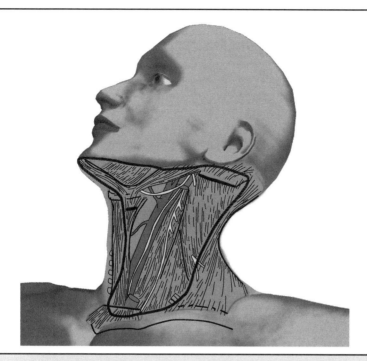

Figure 7-2. Tissue Exposure in a Radical Neck Dissection

Note. Figure courtesy of Raymond J. Scarpa, DNP, AOCN®. Used with permission.

Preservation of the internal jugular vein is an important consideration in order to reduce facial swelling from disrupted lymphatic drainage. If this vessel needs to be sacrificed bilaterally, the procedures should be staged at least one to two weeks apart to allow for the development of collateral circulation (Ross et al., 2012; Spiegel & Polat, 2007).

The selective neck dissection removes lymphatic structures at specified levels in the neck that are associated with the primary tumor. An extended radical neck dissection removes additional lymphatic structures found in the paratrachea, mediastinum, or parapharyngeal regions, as well as nonlymphatic structures such as the carotid artery, vagus nerve, hypoglossal nerve, and overlying skin in the neck (Forastiere et al., 2008).

Post Procedure

Careful assessment of the surgical wound is essential as swelling could be an indication of bleeding and necessitate a return to the operating room. Wound drainage needs to be monitored for consistency, amount, odor, and color. A milky, odorless discharge from the drain especially after ingesting lipids or fats may indicate a chyle leak (Nussenbaum, Liu, & Sinard, 2000). Cloudy discharge with a foul odor may indicate a salivary fistula, which can be confirmed by an amylase test. Healing requires a lengthened time for the drain to be in place, compression, frequent dressing changes to promote granulation to close the fistula, and antibiotic therapy. If this treatment is unsuccessful, surgical repair is indicated (Scarpa, 2009).

Evaluation of the surrounding skin and suture line is important to determine the development of necrosis of the skin flap or infection. Wound healing can be compromised secondary to prior chemotherapy and/or radiation therapy, diabetes, hypertension, peripheral vascular disease, smoking history, or malnutrition. A vacuum-assisted closure (wound VAC) is used to apply negative pressure to the wound, remove excess fluids, and increase blood flow to promote granulation tissue formation. This type of treatment was reported to be successful with chronic diabetes–associated leg wounds but is not as successful with other types of wounds (Xie, McGregor, & Dendukuri, 2010).

Sinonasal Cancer

Although rare, carcinomas of the sinonasal tract can occur in the maxillary, ethmoid, frontal, and sphenoid sinuses. Surgery alone remains the cornerstone for treatment of early-stage T1–T2 maxillary lesions, whereas larger T3–T4 lesions require multimodal therapies (Goldenberg, Tufano, & Goldstein, 2005).

Preprocedure

Diagnostic tests include a CT scan and magnetic resonance imaging; a PET/CT scan is included if metastatic disease is suspected. Biopsy is obtained after radiologic confirmation. This will avoid biopsy of normal dura that may have herniated into a sinus or nasal cavity (creating a cerebrospinal fluid [CSF] leak) or a hypervascular lesion that will cause excessive bleeding in the office setting (Goldenberg et al., 2005).

Procedure

The lateral rhinotomy approach can access the contents of the nasal cavity, paranasal sinuses, and the nasopharynx with an incision from the nostril around the alar groove, along the side of the nose, over the upper lateral cartilage, and around the frontal process of the maxilla to the medial canthus and medial end of the eyebrow. The Weber-Fergusson approach extends the incision to divide the upper lip and includes an incision under the eye for larger tumors. The lateral rhinotomy approach is used for en bloc resections of the ethmoid labyrinth and the wall between the antrum and nasal cavity. It can also be used for resection of tumors that are limited to the anterior nasal cavity, adjacent to the medial third of the maxillary and ethmoid sinuses. Other maxillectomy approaches include the midfacial degloving approach with an incision under the lip and extensive subcutaneous dissection to expose the maxilla without an external incision (Dalgorf & Higgins, 2008; Goldenberg et al., 2005). Extensive tumors that involve the orbital contents may require orbital exenteration. Tumors extending to or through the skull base require a combined maxillectomy and neurosurgical resection, often referred to as a *craniofacial resection* (Goldenberg et al., 2005).

Reconstruction is dependent on the surgical defect. STSG can be used to line the cavity created by a small surgical maxillary resection. A bolster or reinforced nonadherent packing is placed over the STSG to secure it in place. This bolster temporally fills the surgical defect, allowing for intelligible speech and swallowing to occur, and is removed five to seven days postoperatively. Defects of the upper gingiva and hard palate may require a prosthetic device known as a *maxillary obturator* to provide separation of the mouth from the nasal cavity. This improves voice quality and prevents nasal regurgitation of oral intake (Goldenberg et al., 2005).

Larger defects may require microvascular myocutaneous free flaps to fill in the soft tissue defect, especially if the orbital contents or skull base are removed. Additional problems after maxillectomy may include loss of smell and taste, cosmetic facial deformities, foul odor due to crusting of mucus and food, and speech and swallowing difficulties (Dalgorf & Higgins, 2008). Eye symptoms may occur such as diplopia, epiphora, and exophthalmos, especially when the orbital floor and medial wall are resected.

Post Procedure

Coughing or any Valsalva-type maneuvers that will increase intracranial pressure must be avoided to prevent a CSF leak. The head of the bed should be elevated at 30° to avoid intracranial pooling of venous blood and CSF. If a lumbar drain is used, it is clamped on the second or third postoperative day and removed on day 4 if no evidence of a CSF leak is present. Patients are monitored closely for changes in neurologic status (Scarpa, 2009). Sudden changes in mental status may be a sign of pneumocephalus; stat imaging is obtained to observe for presence of air in the cranial cavity. If air is present, patients are returned to the operating room emergently for surgical decompression and repair.

Accidental dislodging of the packing can result in aspiration or choking. Nasal regurgitation of oral intake can occur with an ill-fitting or temporary obturator. A nasogastric feeding tube may be necessary to ensure adequate caloric intake during the postoperative period. Crusted secretions can accumulate within the nasal cavity and lead to persistent nasal congestion and foul odor. Endoscopic nasal debridement may be necessary in the outpatient setting to remove this material.

Thyroid Cancer

Preprocedure

Histologic confirmation of malignancy is accomplished by a fine needle aspiration of the lesion, with or without ultrasound guidance (Lander et al., 2012). Baseline calcium, parathyroid hormone (PTH), and thyroid studies are obtained to confirm values and allow for monitoring of acute changes in the postoperative period. Surgery may be delayed in order to normalize the values with thyroid supplementation. Patients who have had previous bariatric surgery may be at risk for altered absorption of calcium replacement. Hyperthyroid patients with abnormal thyroid levels are at risk for acute hypocalcemia postoperatively (Harris et al., 2012).

Procedure

When atypical cells are noted, a thyroid lobectomy is performed with removal of the designated half of the thyroid. An intraoperative frozen section is performed of the lesion; when the interim pathology indicates a malignancy, a total thyroidectomy is performed. When a partial thyroidectomy is performed and the final pathology indicates a malignancy, the patient must return to the operating room for a second procedure to remove the remaining half of the gland.

Minimally invasive video-assisted thyroidectomy uses an endoscopic approach with magnification. This technique minimizes the size of the incision, identifies nerves and vessels, and attempts to minimize the risk of injury to these structures by allowing for a magnified view. Studies have shown improved swallowing, better voice quality, and less postoperative pain (Sharma & Barr, 2013). It is best used in select cases where the lesion is small and the surgeon is well experienced in endoscopic approaches to this area (Sharma & Barr, 2013).

Bipolar electrocautery has also demonstrated decreased thermal damage to surrounding tissues, nerves, and parathyroid glands and can shorten operative time. Additionally, ultrasonic dissectors decrease thermal injury through generation of ultrasonic motion for coagulation of tissue (Sharma & Barr, 2013).

Post Procedure

Total thyroidectomy patients require close observation in the immediate postoperative period to monitor for bleeding that may present with neck swelling, pain, or symptoms of compromised airway (Sharma & Barr, 2013). The use of drains in thyroid surgery remains controversial. No definitive evidence suggests that drains will prevent hematoma or seroma formation. Nonsuction drains are not recommended because of the risk of infection and need for multiple dressings and tape, which can obscure areas of the neck and any hematoma development (Sharma & Barr, 2013).

Surgical risks in these procedures include damage to the recurrent laryngeal nerve resulting in hoarseness or breathy quality to the voice and damage to or incidental removal of the parathyroid glands. Voice-related symptoms can resolve within six months if the nerve was not transected (Sharma & Barr, 2013).

Hypoparathyroidism may occur after thyroid surgery secondary to compromised parathyroid glands from direct trauma, compromised blood flow, or incidental removal. The four small pea-shaped parathyroid glands are responsible for the production of PTH and the regulation of serum calcium. As PTH level rises, both bone and renal reabsorption of calcium occur. This stimulates the production of vitamin D, which increases serum calcium levels; PTH also increases the renal excretion of phosphorus (Sharma & Barr, 2013). Routine laboratory blood work in the postoperative period is required to monitor calcium and phosphorus levels. Clinical indications of hypocalcemia are the presence of Chvostek or Trousseau signs. Chvostek sign is the presence of facial twitching or contraction when the facial nerve is stimulated by tapping the face near the preauricular area. Trousseau sign is the involuntary contraction of the hand or wrist elicited by inflating a blood pressure cuff on the arm. Oral calcium supplementation is used to replace calcium stores, and IV calcium boluses are administered when immediate replacement is necessary as evidenced by low serum calcium levels and extreme symptoms.

Patients who have undergone removal of the entire thyroid gland should be started on levothyroxine when discharged, although they will need to stop this medication prior to receiving radioactive iodine treatment or radioiodine scanning (Sharma & Barr, 2013). Referral to an endocrinologist is beneficial to monitor the proper thyroid replacement dosing and schedules associated with postoperative radioactive iodine treatment.

Parathyroid Cancer

Parathyroid cancer is extremely rare. It occurs in 1% of individuals diagnosed with hyperparathyroidism. Its incidence is less than 1% with a familial etiology and usually presents with elevated calcium levels of more than 14 mg/dl (Norton, 2001). There is no known medical treatment for this disease. Because of its rarity, controlled trials are difficult to conduct (Kim, 2013).

Preprocedure

Patients present with severe hypercalcemia. Medical management to control this condition is needed preoperatively. Patients undergo diuresis with isotonic saline and furosemide. Bisphosphonates may also be used (Kim, 2013). Patients may present with a palpable mass. A CT scan is useful to determine local invasion or distant metastatic disease. Diagnosis is ascertained by severely elevated calcium and intact PTH levels (Norton, 2001).

Procedure

The goal of surgical intervention is to remove the entire tumor and any surrounding adherent tissue along with the thyroid lobe on the side of the lesion. Any suspicious lymphatic structures should also be removed at the time of surgery (Kim, 2013).

Preservation of the laryngeal nerve should be considered. If a vocal cord was found to be immobile preoperatively, then sacrifice of the nerve is indicated. Removal of both the right and left recurrent laryngeal nerves will require a permanent tracheotomy (Norton, 2001). Once the specimen has been removed, the pathologist can make a definitive diagnosis of carcinoma. Intraoperatively one can have a high suspicion of malignancy based on appearance. A malignant parathyroid gland appears firm and whitish-gray and is diffusely invasive. A nonmalignant lesion such as a parathyroid adenoma usually presents as a reddish-brown mass that is soft, mobile, and noninvasive (Norton, 2001). Pathologic confirmation is made by frequency of mitosis, fibrosis, local invasion, vascular invasion, and nuclear pleomorphism (Norton, 2001).

Post Procedure

Postoperative care is similar to that for patients who underwent thyroid surgery. Hungry bone syndrome may be profound in these patients because of the previous high calcium levels and needs to be monitored (Kim, 2013).

Conclusions

This chapter provides a review of the common surgical procedures in head and neck malignancies. Pre- and postoperative assessment and care are essential to a successful outcome. Challenges regarding functional outcomes, cosmesis, nutritional support, and the ability to interact with the environment can be overwhelming for the patient and family. The multidisciplinary team plays a critical role in attempting to overcome these obstacles. Nurses working with these patients must anticipate these challenges and access available support both in and outside the healthcare system. Optimal outcomes are dependent on evidence-based interventions.

References

Carty, S.E., Doherty, G.M., Inabnet, W.B., Pasieka, J.L., Randolph, G.W., Shaha, A.R., ... Tuttle, R.M. (2012). American Thyroid Association statement on the essential elements of interdisciplinary communication of perioperative information for patients undergoing thyroid cancer surgery. *Thyroid, 22*, 395–399. doi:10.1089/thy.2011.0423

Dalgorf, D., & Higgins, K. (2008). Reconstruction of the midface and maxilla. *Current Opinion in Otolaryngology and Head and Neck Surgery, 16*, 303–311. doi:10.1097/MOO.0b013e328304b426

Forastiere, A.A., Ang, K.K., Brizel, D., Brockstein, B.E., Burtness, B.A., Cmelak, A.J., ... Worden, F. (2008). Head and neck cancers. *Journal of the National Comprehensive Cancer Network, 6*, 646–695. Retrieved from http://www.jnccn.org/content/6/7/646.long

Goldenberg, D., Tufano, R.P., & Goldstein, B.J. (2005). Malignant tumors of the sinonasal tract. *Journal of Postgraduate Medicine, 51*, 35. Retrieved from http://www.jpgmonline.com/text.asp?2005/51/1/35/14541

Harris, R., Ryu, H., Vu, T., Kim, E., Edeiken, B., Grubbs, E.G., & Perrier, N.D. (2012). Modern approach to surgical intervention of the thyroid and parathyroid glands. *Seminars in Ultrasound, CT, and MRI, 33*, 115–122. doi:10.1053/j.sult.2012.01.005

Jack, D.R., Dawson, F.R., Reilly, J.E., & Shoaib, T. (2011). Guideline for prophylactic feeding tube insertion in patients undergoing resection of head and neck cancers. *Journal of Plastic, Reconstructive, and Aesthetic Surgery, 65*, 610–615. doi:10.1016/j.bjps.2011.11.018

Kayhan, F.T., Kaya, K.H., & Sayin, I. (2012). Transoral robotic cordectomy for early glottic carcinoma. *Annals of Otology, Rhinology, and Laryngology, 121*, 497–502.

Kim, L. (2013, September 11). Parathyroid carcinoma treatment and management. Retrieved from http://emedicine.medscape.com/article/280908-treatment

Lander, J.E., Baloch, A.W., McGrath, C., Loevner, L.A., & Mandel, S.J. (2012). Thyroid nodule fine-needle aspiration. *Seminars in Ultrasound, CT, and MRI, 33*, 158–165. doi:10.1053/j.sult.2011.12.002

Mücke, T., Koschinski, J., Wagenpfeil, S., Wolff, K.-D., Kanatas, A., Mitchell, D.A., ... Kesting, M.R. (2012). Functional outcome after different oncological interventions in head and neck cancer patients. *Journal of Cancer Research in Clinical Oncology, 138*, 371–376. doi:10.1007/s00432-011-1106-x

Norton, J.A. (2001). Neoplasms of the endocrine system. In K.I. Bland, J.M. Daly, & C.P. Karakousis (Eds.), *Surgical oncology: Contemporary principles and practice* (pp. 1055–1067). New York, NY: McGraw-Hill.

Nussenbaum, B., Liu, J.H., & Sinard, R.J. (2000). Systematic management of chyle fistula: The Southwestern experience and review of the literature. *Otolaryngology—Head and Neck Surgery, 122,* 31–38.

Ross, G., Yia-Kotola, T.M., Goldstein, D., Zhong, T., Gilbert, R., Irish, J., ... Neiligan, P.C. (2012). Second free flaps in head and neck reconstruction. *Journal of Plastic, Reconstructive, and Aesthetic Surgery, 65,* 1165–1168. doi:10.1016/j.bjps.2012.03.035

Scarpa, R. (2009). Surgical management of head and neck carcinoma. *Seminars in Oncology Nursing, 25,* 175–182. doi:10.1016/j.soncn.2009.05.007

Shariff, S. (2010). *Fundamentals of surgical pathology.* New Delhi, India: Jaypee Brothers Medical Publishers.

Sharma, P.K., & Barr, L.J. (2013, June 17). Complications of thyroid surgery. Retrieved from http://emedicine.medscape.com/article/852184-overview#aw2aab6b4

Spiegel, J.H., & Polat, J.K. (2007). Microvascular flap reconstruction by otolaryngologists: Prevalence, postoperative care, and monitoring techniques. *Laryngoscope, 117,* 485-490. doi:10.1089/MLG.0b013e31802e6366

Xie, X., McGregor, M., & Dendukuri, N. (2010). The clinical effectiveness of negative pressure wound therapy: A systematic review. *Journal of Wound Care, 19,* 490–495.

CHAPTER 8

Surgical Care of Breast Cancer

Joanne L. Lester, PhD, CNP, AOCN®

Introduction

Breast cancer remains the most common cancer diagnosed in women and the second leading cause of cancer deaths in women (American Cancer Society [ACS], 2013). To understand the broad spectrum of breast cancer–related surgery, one must understand the progressive trajectory of breast cancer pathology and the anatomy and physiology of the breast.

Breast cancer diagnoses often are made after a routine screening mammogram or after an individual discovers a lump in the breast. Suddenly, the patient's world is turned upside down because breast cancer has few forewarning symptoms. Patients and families are faced with myriad treatment choices and decisions and feel extreme pressure to rapidly learn the material and make a decision. Nurses who provide care for newly diagnosed patients with breast cancer should empathize with their emotional turmoil and learn the full complement of treatment options, understand the rationale behind choices made, and provide a high level of patience as newly diagnosed patients navigate the educational and decisional byways.

Breast Anatomy

The breasts (see Figure 8-1) are composed of bilateral mammary glands and a large network of lymph nodes (see Figure 8-2) that drain the breast tissue, which includes the axillary, internal, and supra- and infraclavicular nodes. The breast tissue is composed of lobules, the ductal system, and the nipple and areolar complex as well as supportive Cooper ligaments, subcutaneous fat, and glandular and connective tissue. The superficial breast consists of mammary tissue that lies atop the chest wall and pectoralis major and minor muscles and extends vertically from the posterior margin of the clavi-

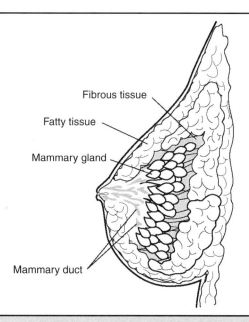

Figure 8-1. Anatomic Representation of the Female Breast

Note. Figure courtesy of The Ohio State University Wexner Medical Center. Used with permission.

cle to the inframammary fold on the chest wall. Horizontally, the superficial breast tissue is present bilaterally from the lateral edge of the sternum to the midaxillary line on the respective side. The normal male breast consists of a nipple, areola, glandular tissue, fat, and skin (National Comprehensive Cancer Network [NCCN], 2013; Zurrida et al., 2011).

Biopsy Techniques

For palpable lesions (see Table 8-1), biopsy options include fine needle aspiration (FNA), core needle biopsy (with or without ultrasound guidance), or incisional or excisional biopsy (Carlson et al., 2011; NCCN, 2013). Open incisional or excisional biopsies should be confined to the second biopsy of the lesion and performed only if more tissue is needed to reexamine a preinvasive condition, such as atypical ductal hyperplasia (ADH), atypical lobular hyperplasia (ALH), or lobular carcinoma in situ (LCIS) (Kounalakis et al., 2011), or to confirm a malignancy when the core biopsy is negative and the clinical suspicion is very high (Carlson et al., 2011; NCCN, 2013; Simpson, Gale, Fulford, Reis-Filho, & Lakhani, 2003).

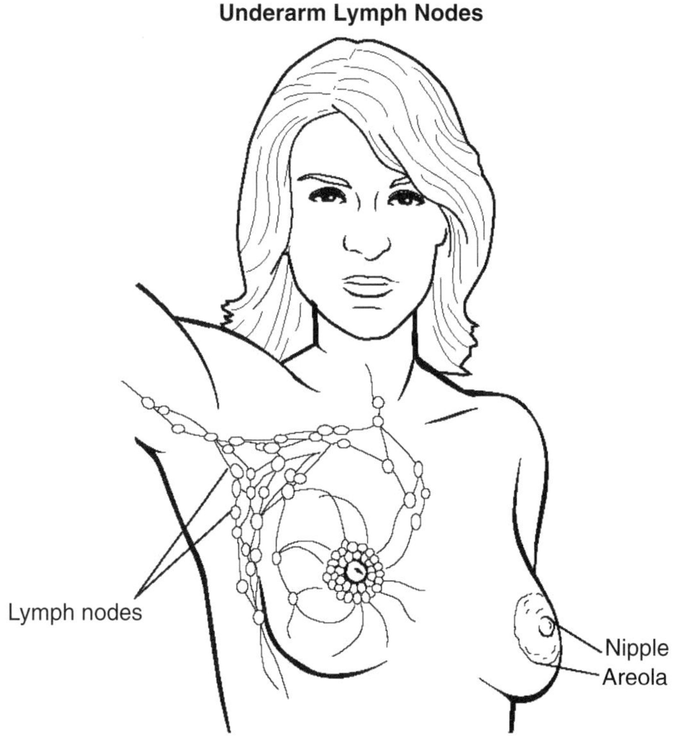

Underarm Lymph Nodes

Lymph nodes

Nipple

Areola

Figure 8-2. Regional Lymph Nodes in the Female Axilla

Note. Figure courtesy of The Ohio State University Wexner Medical Center. Used with permission.

For nonpalpable (see Table 8-1) abnormalities observed on radiographic images, guidance is required to successfully target and biopsy the lesions of concern. When the area of concern revolves around suspicious microcalcifications, a stereotactic core needle biopsy is performed (Simpson et al., 2003). The woman lies prone on the table; the breast of concern drops through an opening in the table and is compressed between two clear Plexiglas plates. A mammographic image confirms the location of the microcalcifications. Several core needle biopsies are obtained and reexamined radiographically to verify that the specimen contains the microcalcifications. A titanium clip is placed in the breast at the point of biopsy; this clip is visible on future radiographic images.

A needle-localization biopsy is performed to locate the area of concern for an excisional biopsy. This operation is performed under local anesthesia, controlled conscious sedation, or general anesthesia, depending on the location of the lesion and a host of other factors.

Table 8-1. Techniques for Biopsies of Palpable and Nonpalpable Lesions

Type of Breast Lesion	Biopsy Recommendation	Expected Outcome
Nonpalpable lesion on mammogram or magnetic resonance imaging	Stereotactic biopsy	Using the stereotactic machine in radiology, tiny slivers of tissue are removed from the lesion. Pathologic data are provided.
	Needle-localization biopsy	Using mammographic or ultrasound guidance, a wire or wires are placed at the site of the lesion; a surgeon makes an incision at the site of wire and follows it down to the lesion. The procedure is used to remove the entire lesion or area if warranted or if stereotactic biopsy indicates atypia or lobular carcinoma in situ. The procedure provides a pathology report of the entire lesion.
Nonpalpable lesion on ultrasound	Ultrasound-guided core biopsy	The lesion is located using ultrasound probe. A core needle biopsy is obtained using a spring-activated core biopsy gun. Slivers of tissue are removed from the lesion. Pathologic data are provided.
Palpable lesion	Fine needle aspiration	A fine needle aspiration is performed using a 21-gauge needle and 12 ml syringe. A cytology report is obtained with "yes" or "no" report of cancer. The procedure is useful to discern solid versus cystic structures.
	Core needle biopsy	A core needle biopsy is obtained using a spring-loaded needle biopsy gun. Slivers of tissue are removed from the lesion. Pathologic data are provided.
	Excisional or incisional biopsy	An incision is made adjacent to the lesion. In an excisional biopsy, the entire lesion is removed; an incisional biopsy obtains a portion of the mass for examination. Excisional biopsy is used to completely remove a benign lesion or to verify findings of malignancy should a core needle biopsy be negative with high clinical suspicion. A full pathologic report is provided.

Note. Based on information from Carlson et al., 2011; Kounalakis et al., 2011; National Comprehensive Cancer Network, 2013; Simpson et al., 2003.

Noninvasive Breast Cancer

High-Risk Markers

ADH, ALH, and LCIS represent a spectrum of ductal and lobular neoplasia that are typically noted as incidental findings on fine needle aspirates, biopsy, or definitive surgery for breast cancer. ADH indicates an increased risk of noninvasive or invasive ductal cancer due to cellular proliferation and abnormal arrangement of the cells. ALH represents cellular proliferation of the lobular cells and may represent tissue of a higher cytologic grade. When ADH or lactate dehydrogenase is identified on a fine needle aspirate or core needle biopsy, an open needle localization biopsy is necessary to target the area and remove surrounding tissue to rule out a higher grade abnormality or malignancy (Kounalakis et al., 2011).

Lobular Carcinoma in Situ

LCIS is an occult finding that is generally not evident on physical examination or in imaging studies. LCIS is often multicentric (50%) and contralateral (30%) and may be linked with mammographic microcalcifications (Kounalakis et al., 2011). If LCIS is incidentally found on surgical biopsy, it is not necessary to clear margins because of its multicentric nature. The remainder of LCIS cells will not turn into an invasive cancer but rather serve to identify the high-risk status. Women older than age 60 diagnosed with LCIS are more likely to develop invasive cancer (25%) versus premenopausal women (8.3%) because of the presence of abnormal proliferation in older, postmenopausal women. Regardless of age, if LCIS is found on core biopsy, a needle-localization excisional biopsy should be performed because 25%–31% of core biopsies contain evidence of ductal carcinoma in situ (DCIS) or invasive cancer (Kounalakis et al., 2011). A review of the biologic characteristics of LCIS and personal and family history may help to determine the threat of invasive disease and the chosen prevention plan with close follow-up, chemoprevention (e.g., tamoxifen), or bilateral mastectomy (Kounalakis et al., 2011).

Ductal Carcinoma in Situ

DCIS is a proliferation of malignant epithelial cells within the breast parenchyma without evidence of invasion across the basement membrane, hence the name *in situ*. DCIS, also known as intraductal carcinoma, is referred to as a stage 0 breast cancer and is the most common noninvasive breast cancer or precancer of the breast (Simpson et al., 2003). These cells are protected by a cellular barrier that does not communicate with lymph and blood vessels; DCIS has no potential to metastasize (Simpson et al., 2003).

Surgical choices for patients with DCIS include lumpectomy or simple or total mastectomy (see Table 8-2). Surgical lumpectomy is aimed at excision of the area of concern with clear margins and is followed by radiation therapy to further reduce the risk that the lesion will recur either as DCIS or invasive cancer (Czyszczon, Roland, & Sahoo, 2012). The selection of a simple or total mastectomy as a treatment modality results in a 90% risk reduction (Czyszczon et al., 2012); radiation therapy is seldom necessary after a mastectomy unless diffuse disease is present at the margins. If the biopsy pathology report indicates the DCIS is high grade, an invasive cancer is more likely to be found in the final pathology specimen (Simpson et al., 2003) and a sentinel lymph node biopsy (SLNB) will often be performed at the same time as the surgical intervention. For low- and medium-grade DCIS, an SLNB is typically not necessary (Kumar, Puri, Gadgil, & Jatoi, 2012).

Table 8-2. Surgical Procedures for Prophylactic Removal of Preinvasive, Noninvasive, and Invasive Breast Cancers

Surgical Procedure	Pathology and Rationale
Lumpectomy	Atypia, lobular carcinoma in situ (LCIS), ductal carcinoma in situ (DCIS)
Lumpectomy, sentinel lymph node biopsy	DCIS high grade, invasive breast cancer
Lumpectomy, axillary node dissection	DCIS high grade, invasive breast cancer with positive sentinel lymph node(s), palpable axillary nodes, or positive biopsy of axillary nodes
Total mastectomy	Widespread DCIS, or patient choice for localized treatment
Total mastectomy with sentinel lymph node biopsy	Widespread high-grade DCIS, invasive breast cancer, or patient choice for localized treatment
Modified radical mastectomy (total mastectomy with axillary node dissection)	DCIS high grade, invasive breast cancer with positive sentinel lymph node(s), palpable axillary nodes, or positive biopsy of axillary nodes
Bilateral total mastectomy	Prophylactic for LCIS, positive genetic findings (e.g., *BRCA1/BRCA2*), strong family history, or patient choice
Radical mastectomy	Rarely done, although may be performed for local control of locally advanced cancer

Note. Based on information from Fisher et al., 2002; Kounalakis et al., 2011; National Comprehensive Cancer Network, 2013; Zurrida et al., 2011.

Invasive Breast Cancer

Invasive breast cancers consist of infiltrating ductal (70%–80%), invasive lobular (8%–10%), and inflammatory (2%) types. Breast cancer can be divided into noninvasive carcinoma such as DCIS (stage 0), operable locoregional disease (clinical stage I, II, and some IIIA), surgically difficult stage IIIA–C, and stage IV, metastatic disease. Systemic neoadjuvant treatment may downgrade stages II–IIIA–C to avail successful surgical treatment (Carlson et al., 2011; NCCN, 2013) with either a lumpectomy or mastectomy. Inflammatory breast cancer is the most virulent type of breast cancer with rapid progression of disease; neoadjuvant chemotherapy followed by surgery and radiation therapy have contributed to improved life expectancy as well as improved locoregional control (Carlson et al., 2011; Dushkin & Cristofanilli, 2011; NCCN, 2013).

Tumor Pathology

Breast cancer treatment consists of local treatment (e.g., surgery, radiation therapy) and systemic therapy (e.g., hormonal therapy, chemotherapy, biologic therapy). Central to breast cancer treatment is the pathologic evaluation of the tumor based on several prognostic and predictive factors: tumor histology, clinical and pathologic tumor characteristics, and stage (Dushkin & Cristofanilli, 2011). The clinical stage is the physical presentation of the breast skin and palpable parenchyma, axilla, supra- and infraclavicular nodes, and information gathered from pretreatment radiographic images and the surgeon, whereas the pathologic stage includes all information provided by the pathologist about the breast and axillary contents. The clinical and pathologic stages do not always match; the clinical stage is important to document when neoadjuvant chemotherapy is administered because successful treatment may downgrade the pathologic stage. The greater of the two stages is considered the patient's stage and level of disease (Carlson et al., 2011; Dushkin & Cristofanilli, 2011).

Serum and Radiographic Workup

Serum and radiologic tests are performed at the time of diagnosis in accordance with the clinical stage of disease and after surgery in accordance with the pathologic stage. In preparation for surgery, serum electrolytes, renal and liver function, alkaline phosphatase, and a complete blood count are obtained (NCCN, 2013). The most important cue is to listen to the patient for new complaints, persistent pain, or a significant loss of energy and order diagnostic studies as indicated. In stage III and inflammatory disease, a metastatic workup is recommended with bone scan, chest and abdominal CT scans, and optional MRI of the head based on presence or absence of symptoms (Carlson et al., 2011; NCCN, 2013). When neoadjuvant chemotherapy is planned, the same laboratory tests are recommended. In addition, a bone scan and CT scan of the chest and abdomen will be obtained, pending clinical stage of disease.

Surgical Management

Evolution of Locoregional Treatment

Surgical treatment of the breast and axilla is termed *locoregional therapy*. Historically, surgical removal of the breast involved a *radical mastectomy*, meaning removal of all breast tissue, overlying skin, and both pectoralis muscles together with complete en bloc removal of axillary lymph nodes (Zurrida et al., 2011). This radical surgery was often necessary because breast cancers presented as locally advanced disease with skin involvement. The Halsted-Meyer theory involved a radical mastectomy with removal of the internal mammary chain because the theory was that even more radical surgery would control the disease. Extended radical mastectomies included the internal mammary chain and possible placement of radiation seeds (Zurrida et al., 2011).

Use of the modified radical mastectomy started in the 1970s with preservation of the pectoralis muscles and internal mammary chain; gradually, the axillary dissection was modified to include level I and II nodes only, unless an advanced cancer required removal of the level III lymph nodes (Zurrida et al., 2011). A *simple mastectomy* was defined as removal of the pectoral fascia en bloc with the breast without removing the lymph nodes. In the early 1970s, Bernard Fisher, MD, initiated an innovative method to treat breast cancer, defined as breast-sparing surgery (Zurrida et al., 2011). The advent of the lumpectomy was a landmark change in the locoregional control of breast cancer. Nearly 30 years later, the lumpectomy with or without SLNB or axillary dissection has demonstrated the same mortality rates as a modified radical mastectomy (Fisher et al., 2002). Radiation therapy accompanies the lumpectomy to complete the treatment of the breast.

Breast-Conserving Surgery

Today, the standard of care is lumpectomy, extended resection with quadrantectomy, or skin-sparing mastectomy, which includes removal of breast tissue, nipple and areolar complex, biopsy scar, and skin overlying the cancer (i.e., if cancer is superficial) with preservation of remaining skin and inframammary fold (Carlson et al., 2011; Fisher et al., 2002; NCCN, 2013).

A few conditions exist in which breast-conserving treatment is contraindicated: history of previous radiation therapy to the chest or breast, current pregnancy, diffuse suspicious-appearing microcalcifications, widespread disease, or positive margins that were not cleared with repeat lumpectomy (Carlson et al., 2011). Breast-conserving treatment may be suboptimal in women with connective tissue disorders that involve the skin (e.g., scleroderma, lupus) or in cases where prophylactic control is indicated, such as prophylactic contralateral mastectomy, positive genetic results, or positive biopsy with LCIS (Carlson et al., 2011).

Studies document that mastectomy with axillary node dissection (AND) is equivalent to lumpectomy plus AND and whole breast radiation therapy for stage I and II disease (Fisher et al., 2002). Risk of local recurrence is decreased if a radiation boost is added at the site of the tumor, which adds to the absolute gain in younger patients because of an anticipated longer life span (Carlson et al., 2011; NCCN, 2013).

Tumor Margins

The goal of negative margins is to decrease the risk of local recurrence of tumor in the breast (Rizzo & Wood, 2011). There is wide speculation about the exact measurements that define a clear margin (e.g., 1–10 mm), but scientists and surgeons universally agree that tumor at the inked margin is unacceptable (Rizzo & Wood, 2011). After breast-conserving surgery, if the pathologist indicates that one or more margins are positive, a re-excision or mastectomy is performed at a future date. A re-excision of margins may be attempted for one or two positive margins, but a mastectomy is most likely indicated when multiple lumpectomy margins are involved by residual tumor (Fisher et al., 2002; NCCN, 2013; Rizzo & Wood, 2011). Although additional surgical interventions may increase the financial and emotional costs, a third attempt to clear specimen margins may occur when mastectomy compromises acceptable physical outcomes for the woman. When mastectomy is inevitable, women should be given the opportunity to explore reconstructive options before surgery.

Mastectomy Options

A simple or total mastectomy is necessary to manage multicentric DCIS, whereas a modified radical mastectomy is indicated for a large invasive tumor, positive margins after lumpectomy, the presence of two invasive carcinomas in separate quadrants, people with contraindications to radiation therapy, or patients who choose mastectomy for their surgical treatment (see Table 8-2) (NCCN, 2013).

A loss of one or both breasts may cause cosmetic, body image, and psychosocial issues for some men and women, which may be partially overcome by reconstructive surgery (Carlson et al., 2011). Breast surgery as performed by oncoplastic surgeons can include immediate or delayed reconstruction of the absent breast(s), augmentation or reduction of the cancerous or contralateral breast, or modification of a lumpectomy scar after the completion of radiation therapy. Multiple options exist for men and women who want to change the appearance of an absent breast or existing breast tissue with the use of surgery, implants, or autologous tissue (Carlson et al., 2011; NCCN, 2013). Reconstruction does not negatively affect local recurrence rate or morbidity and in most cases is a safe option to consider. Patients with underlying diabetes or active tobacco users have increased risks of complications with reconstruction because of compromised vasculature (see Chapter 21).

The concept of total skin-sparing mastectomy (TSSM) may be a feasible option in select patients. A study of 64 breasts in 43 women was conducted prospectively in women with prophylactic mastectomy (n = 29), invasive carcinoma (n = 24), and DCIS (n = 11). Preoperatively a bilateral breast MRI indicated absence of disease within 2 cm of the nipple areolar complex. Postoperative pathology reports indicated occult DCIS in the nipple areolar complex (3%); other complications included implant loss, total skin-sparing skin flap necrosis, and infection. The researchers summarized that total skin-sparing technique is a viable option for cosmesis (Wijayanayagam, Kumar, Foster, & Esserman, 2008). A larger study of 657 breasts in 428 women indicated similar results with postoperative pathology reports of DCIS in nipple tissue (1.7%) and few invasive cancers (1.4%). Again, the researchers concluded that TSSM is an option for certain women (Peled et al., 2012). NCCN (2013), however, continues to recommend complete removal of the nipple areolar complex.

Sentinel Lymph Node Biopsy

SLNB requires an experienced team; otherwise, the patient should be transferred to a facility that is expert in SLNB (NCCN, 2013) as the proficiency lies in how many times the procedure has been done. The SLNB can be performed at the time of the definitive breast surgery or, in the case of neoadjuvant treatment, can be performed alone to determine the true stage of the axilla (NCCN, 2013). The patient should have a clinically negative axilla or FNA negative biopsy of enlarged nodes. The accuracy of SLNB after neoadjuvant chemotherapy remains in question, as well as the optimal timing (Kumar et al., 2012).

A peritumoral injection of technetium-99m (^{99m}Tc) sulfur colloids occurs at least one hour before surgery, followed by a subareolar lymphatic plexus injection of vital blue dye in the operating room with gentle whole breast massage (Fougo et al., 2014). The axilla is surveyed with a gamma probe to find the intensity of radioisotope. Once found, a small incision is made in the axilla to allow the surgeon to search for evidence of the blue dye and an increased auditory sound from the gamma machine. An SLN is identified as a blue node adjacent to a blue lymph channel and a "hot" node per gamma knife. All suspicious axillary nodes (observed or palpated) are removed with assurance that the gamma counts correspond from in vivo to ex vivo (Fougo et al., 2014). After excision, the SLN is taken immediately to pathology. In the case of pathologically positive nodes, the surgeon often proceeds with an AND. Following SLNB, patients should be informed that their urine may be blue, as well as their stools.

Management of the axilla has dramatically changed with the advent of SLNB and its ability to accurately stage the axilla; SLNB has become the standard approach in clinically node-negative disease (Giuliano et al., 2010). SLNB has significantly lowered the rates of axillary complications such as seroma, infection, arm stiffness, pain, paresthesia, and lymphedema as compared to AND. SLNB has increased the findings of minimal nodal disease (e.g., micrometastatic nodal involvement) that previously went undetected with an AND (Bafford, Gadd, Gu, Lipsitz, & Golshan, 2010). Evaluation with hematoxylin and eosin (H & E) staining and cytokeratin immunohistochemistry are performed to assess SLNB, although treatment decisions should only be made on results of H & E staining (Giuliano et al., 2010).

SLNB is not indicated in women undergoing prophylactic mastectomy (Czyszczon et al., 2012) based on a retrospective study of 184 women with 199 prophylactic mastectomies, although it is not uncommon to find occult cancer (n = 12) or noninvasive (n = 10), microinvasive (n = 1), and T1b invasive tumor (n = 1). Of the 199 breasts, 153 underwent SLNB; two breasts had evidence of a positive SLNB (Czyszczon et al., 2012).

Axillary Node Dissection

AND is the removal of levels I and II lymph nodes with dissection and sparing of the axillary vein main trunk, long thoracic nerve, and thoracodorsal neurovascular bundle. Following AND, one suction drain is placed (e.g., Jackson-Pratt or Hemovac). The drain is removed when drainage decreases to 30–40 ml/24-hour period.

The role of AND in treatment decisions is no longer as important, as systemic treatment is based on the presence or absence of nodal disease rather than the number of positive lymph nodes (Wilson, Mattson, & Edge, 2011). The question of the value of AND in locoregional control exists in the prevention of recurrence (Wilson et al., 2011). Recent study findings from the American College of Surgeons Oncology Group (ACOSOG) Z11 trial (Giuliano et al., 2010) found no difference in survival with SLNB versus AND in the presence of positive disease.

Conclusions

Patient preference is the essence of the decision-making process, given that all things are equal between choice of treatment and survival. Psychosocial support is critical throughout the surgical treatment phase of newly diagnosed breast cancer. Pre- and postoperative emotions can be diverse, from a sense of relief to be free of the tumors to feelings of grief or loss of the breast, a symbol of womanhood. Anxiety over proper healing and care of a wound, drainage tube, pain management, and uncertainty of the future are normal, as are concerns about family, personal, and work responsibilities. The nurse must be attentive, actively listen, problem solve with attention to immediate needs, and reassure the patient in order for a successful transition to home.

References

American Cancer Society. (2013). *Breast cancer facts and figures, 2013–2014.* Retrieved from http://www.cancer.org/acs/groups/content/@research/documents/document/acspc-040951.pdf

Bafford, A., Gadd, M., Gu, X., Lipsitz, S., & Golshan, M. (2010). Diminishing morbidity with the increased use of sentinel node biopsy in breast carcinoma. *American Journal of Surgery, 200,* 374–377. doi:10.1016/j.amjsurg.2009.10.012

Carlson, R.W., Allred, D.C., Anderson, B.O., Burstein, H.J., Carter, W.B., Edge, S.B., … Zellers, R. (2011). Invasive breast cancer: Clinical practice guidelines in oncology. *Journal of the National Comprehensive Cancer Network, 9,* 136–222. Retrieved from http://www.jnccn.org/content/9/2/136.long

Czyszczon, I.A., Roland, L., & Sahoo, S. (2012). Routine prophylactic sentinel lymph node biopsy is not indicated in women undergoing prophylactic mastectomy. *Journal of Surgical Oncology, 105,* 651–654. doi:10.1002/jso.23018

Dushkin, H., & Cristofanilli, M. (2011). Inflammatory breast cancer. *Journal of the National Comprehensive Cancer Network, 9,* 233–240. Retrieved from http://www.jnccn.org/content/9/2/233.long

Fisher, B., Anderson, S., Bryant, J., Margolese, R.G., Deutsch, M., Fisher, E.R., … Wolmark, N. (2002). Twenty-year follow-up of a randomized trial comparing total mastectomy, lumpectomy, and lumpectomy plus irradiation for the treatment of invasive breast cancer. *New England Journal of Medicine, 347,* 1233–1241. doi:10.1056/NEJMoa022152

Fougo, J.L., Reis, P., Giesteira, L., Dias, T., Araújo, C., & Dinis-Ribeiro, M. (2014). The impact of the sentinel node on the aesthetic outcome of breast cancer conservative surgery. *Breast Cancer, 21,* 33–39. doi:10.1007/s12282-012-0359-9

Giuliano, A., McCall, L., Beitsch, P., Whitworth, P.W., Blumencranz, P., Leitch, A.M., ... Ballman, K. (2010). Locoregional recurrence after sentinel lymph node dissection with or without axillary dissection in patients with sentinel lymph node metastases: The American College of Surgeons Oncology Group Z0011 randomized trial. *Annals of Surgery, 252,* 426–433. doi:10.1097/SLA.0b013e3181f08f32

Kounalakis, N., Diamond, J., Rusthoven, K., Horn, W., Jindal, S., Wisell, J., ... Borges, V.F. (2011). Diagnosis of invasive lobular carcinoma in a young woman presenting with pleomorphic lobular carcinoma in situ on core biopsy. *Oncology, 25,* 351–356.

Kumar, A., Puri, R., Gadgil, P.V., & Jatoi, I. (2012). Sentinel lymph node biopsy in primary breast cancer: Window to management of the axilla. *World Journal of Surgery, 36,* 1453–1459. doi:10.1007/s00268-012-1635-8

National Comprehensive Cancer Network. (2013). *NCCN Clinical Practice Guidelines in Oncology: Breast cancer* [v.3.2013]. Retrieved from http://www.nccn.org/professionals/physician _gls/pdf/breast.pdf

Peled, A.W., Foster, R.D., Stover, A.C., Itakura, K., Ewing, C.A., Alvarado, M., ... Esserman, L.J. (2012). Outcomes after total skin-sparing mastectomy and immediate reconstruction in 657 breasts. *Annals of Surgical Oncology, 19,* 3402–3409. doi:10.1245/s10434-012-2362-y

Rizzo, M., & Wood, W.C. (2011). The changing field of locoregional treatment for breast cancer. *Oncology, 25,* 813–830.

Simpson, P.T., Gale, T., Fulford, L.G., Reis-Filho, J.S., & Lakhani, S.R. (2003). The diagnosis and management of pre-invasive breast disease: Pathology of atypical lobular hyperplasia and lobular carcinoma in situ. *Breast Cancer Research, 5,* 258–262. doi:10.1186/bcr624

Wijayanayagam, A., Kumar, A.S., Foster, R.D., & Esserman, L.J. (2008). Optimizing the total skin-sparing mastectomy. *Archives of Surgery, 143,* 38–45. doi:10.1001/archsurg.143.1.38

Wilson, J.P., Mattson, D., & Edge, S.B. (2011). Is there a need for axillary dissection in breast cancer? *Journal of the National Comprehensive Cancer Network, 9,* 225–230. Retrieved from http://www.jnccn.org/content/9/2/225.long

Zurrida, S., Bassi, F., Arnone, P., Martella, S., Del Castillo, A., Martini, R.R., ... Caldarella, P. (2011). The changing face of mastectomy (from mutilation to aid to breast reconstruction). *International Journal of Surgical Oncology, 2011,* Article ID 930158. doi:10.1155/2011/980158

CHAPTER 9

Surgical Care of Lung Cancer

Catherine Wickersham, BSN, RN, OCN®

Introduction

Lung cancer continues to be the second most common cancer with the highest associated mortality rate in both men and women (American Cancer Society, 2014). Patients with lung cancer experience significant morbidity and alterations in quality of life secondary to therapeutic interventions or disease progression. These challenges require expert advice and sustained communication and support from nursing staff.

The majority of lung masses are malignant, but benign diagnoses are also considered such as infection, tuberculosis, sarcoidosis, hamartoma, amyloidosis, and granuloma. Lung cancer is classified into two types: small cell (SCLC) and non-small cell lung cancer (NSCLC). NSCLC accounts for 80% of lung cancers; for early-stage patients, surgery is the recommended intervention. The goal of surgery is to prolong and improve quality of life (Denehy, 2008). Multimodality therapy may be recommended for stages IB–IIIA to improve surgical outcomes. For unresectable lung cancers, treatment options include chemotherapy, radiation, targeted agents, or radiofrequency ablation.

SCLC is typically more aggressive at the onset than NSCLC, as the initial presentation is often compromised with metastatic disease. In this setting, treatment typically consists of chemotherapy concurrent with or followed by radiation therapy.

Clinical Presentation

The majority of early-stage lung cancers are asymptomatic, and the diagnosis is reached via an abnormality noted on a routine chest x-ray (CXR). Patients with more advanced disease tend to be symptomatic and experience gradual or rapid decline in functional status (see Table 9-1). Cough is the most common presenting symptom (Beckles, Spiro, Colice, & Rudd, 2003); however, it can be a confounding symptom because of the presence of a chronic cough from chronic obstructive pulmonary disease or tobacco use. Dyspnea often accompanies a cough, which may be caused by an obstructive tumor in the airway (Kvale, 2006). Concomitant cough, dyspnea, fatigue, and weight loss may indicate more severe issues such as pleural effusion, obstructive tumor, or metastatic disease (DiSalvo, Joyce, Tyson, Culkin, & Mackay, 2008).

Chest pain is another common presenting symptom and typically occurs if lymphangitis or tumor has spread into the chest wall. Despite this significant distribution of disease, patients may still be surgical candidates. Pain outside of the chest should prompt suspicion of metastases, for example, to the spine or leg (Aiello-Laws et al., 2009).

Pulmonary Evaluation

Patients are referred to a thoracic surgeon for consideration of resection when pulmonary nodules are visualized on radiologic images. Before surgery, an established diagnosis, disease staging (if malignant), and assessment of overall medical condition are essential. The current staging guidelines include the size of the primary tumor, involvement of lymph nodes, and presence of metastasis (TNM). Patients are considered surgically unresectable if they present with advanced stage IIIB or IV lung cancer with malignant pleural effusion, supraclavicular lymph node involvement, or tumor invading the mediastinal vessels (National Cancer Institute, 2013b). Lung cancer can also metastasize to the distant organs (e.g., other lung, liver, adrenal glands, bones, brain) (National Cancer Institute, 2013a).

Radiographic Evaluation

Computed tomography (CT) scan of the chest is an essential part of the workup for all patients with a thoracic lesion. A CT scan is done to evaluate both the lungs and the mediastinal windows to distinguish the anatomy and locate a pulmonary mass or nodules. Staging of lung cancer involves use of head magnetic resonance imaging (MRI) and positron-emission tomography (PET) scanning. Further staging and diagnostic tests may include a nuclear bone scan or abdominal CT or MRI depending on the patient's symptoms and PET scan results. The use of PET scans increases sensitivity to detect extrathoracic metastases and may reduce the number of futile thoracotomies by catching metastases that other scans missed (Stinchcombe, Bogart, Wigle, & Govindan, 2010). A positive finding on a PET scan may

Table 9-1. Diagnostic Workup of a Newly Diagnosed Lung Cancer

Diagnostic Workup	Description of Examination	Reason for Examination
Clinical Symptoms		
Cough	Chest auscultation with stethoscope	Differentiate new onset of cough, change in character of preexisting cough, or hemoptysis.
Dyspnea	Chest auscultation with stethoscope, pulse oximetry at rest and exertion	Assess for rhonchi, rales, diminished breath sounds, or evidence of pleural effusion.
Chest pain	Assessment of areas of pain with palpation and self-report symptoms	Assess for sternal or lung pain, as well as evidence of metastatic pain.
Fatigue	Assessment of level, frequency, and intensity; observations and self-report	Marked fatigue that is not relieved by rest/sleep is worrisome.
Weight loss	Assessment of previous and current weight; assessment of diet and changes	Weight loss without intent is worrisome for metastatic disease.
Radiology Examinations		
Chest x-ray	Plain film of chest, anterior and posterior; patient stands against x-ray plate in two positions.	Used for initial evaluation of lung symptoms; often mass is obscured by infiltration or pneumonia.
Computed tomography (CT) scan of chest with or without contrast—creates 3-D images	Patient lies flat on table; may receive IV contrast (check creatinine level); with new machines, scan is brief.	To evaluate lungs, mediastinum, and lymph nodes; may obtain abdominal CT if pain, symptoms, or elevated liver function studies.
Magnetic resonance imaging—uses magnets to create 3-D images	May be obtained of head, liver, or other specific anatomic part; patient lies flat on table; scan can take 30–45 minutes per area.	To evaluate for metastatic disease; very sensitive but not always specific.
Nuclear scans such as bone scan or positron-emission tomography (PET) scan	Patient lies on table for 45–60 minutes per scan; will receive radioactive substance several hours prior to scan.	To evaluate for metastatic disease; very sensitive but not always specific.

(Continued on next page)

Table 9-1. Diagnostic Workup of a Newly Diagnosed Lung Cancer (Continued)

Diagnostic Workup	Description of Examination	Reason for Examination
Pathologic Diagnosis		
Fine needle aspiration (FNA)—uses a small-gauge needle with syringe. Can obtain CT-guided biopsy of mass or palpable lymph node (supraclavicular).	Patient sits upright or lies on side on exam table. Local anesthetic injected at site. Pneumothorax is rare.	If tumor is in liver or periphery of lung, tissue may be obtained. FNA only indicates a positive, negative, or nondiagnostic result for cancer.
Core needle biopsy—uses a spring-loaded core needle gun to obtain slivers of tissue	Patient sits upright or lies on side on exam table. Local anesthetic injected at site. Pneumothorax is rare.	If tumor is in liver or periphery of lung, tissue may be obtained. Provides full pathology report.
Bronchoscopy—uses a flexible tube with lighted end or forceps; inserted through mouth or nares	Patient sits or lies, and IV sedation and local anesthetic are provided. Must observe for evidence of pneumothorax.	Provides examination of bronchus and bronchi if not obstructed. Provides for biopsy of mass unless in distal periphery of lung, out of reach of scope.
Endobronchial ultrasound—a bronchoscopy with ultrasound assistance to localize mass	As above; ultrasound is available to aid physician to target mass.	As above.
Mediastinoscopy—uses a scope to biopsy lymph nodes	Patient is in upright position; small incision is made above sternum to allow passage of scope. IV sedation and local anesthetic are provided. Must observe for evidence of pneumothorax.	Used to biopsy lymph nodes associated with lung cancer; helps to stage cancer and guide treatment sequence.
Thoracentesis—uses a long needle to access pleural space. Laboratory tests are used to identify abnormalities in fluid: pH, cell count, glucose, lactate dehydrogenase, total protein, and amylase.	Patient lies over bedside table; performed as outpatient with local anesthetic. Fluid is removed for biopsy as well as relief of effusion. Must observe post-procedure chest x-ray to assess fluid and rule out a pneumothorax.	Obtains pathology report if malignant cells are isolated in pleural fluid. Lack of positive findings does not equal lack of metastatic disease in pleura.

(Continued on next page)

Table 9-1. Diagnostic Workup of a Newly Diagnosed Lung Cancer
(Continued)

Diagnostic Workup	Description of Examination	Reason for Examination
Wedge biopsy—performed when additional tissue is needed for diagnosis or when other tests fail to diagnose lung cancer in presence of positive signs and symptoms.	Performed under anesthesia with patient on side. Must observe for pneumothorax with post-procedure chest x-ray. Can be done through muscle-sparing thoracotomy or video-assisted thoracoscopic surgery.	Provides wedge of tissue for affirmative diagnosis of lung cancer; provides enough tissue for full analysis. At times, the lesion proves to be benign, although may be completely removed at time of surgery.

be suggestive of a malignancy or inflammation. PET scans are very sensitive but not always specific for malignancy. Up to 35% of nodes considered positive on PET scan do not contain metastasis on node dissection (McKenna, 2007), thereby creating a false positive with impaired specificity. In a separate study, 15%–26% of patients who have a negative mediastinum on PET have pathologic N2 disease at time of resection (Farjah, Lou, Sima, Rusch, & Rizk, 2013). MRI of the brain is obtained based on the presence of any neurologic symptoms or the diagnostic stage of the tumor.

Pathologic Diagnosis

The approach to cytologic or tissue biopsy is variable and dependent on the location of the tumor and possible sites of metastatic disease. The pathologic diagnosis may be obtained by thoracentesis, bronchoscopy, fine needle aspiration (FNA), or endobronchial ultrasound (EBUS) (Wagner et al., 2011).

Bronchoscopy can be performed to obtain tissue and to look at the anatomy in preparation for a more extensive surgical procedure. A flexible bronchoscope is inserted into the nares or through the mouth; biopsies are obtained if the mass is in or in close proximity to the airway. Pulmonary resections routinely begin with bronchoscopy to position the double-lumen tube and determine the endobronchial extent of tumor.

Mediastinoscopy involves a small incision above the collarbone; a scope is inserted to facilitate a biopsy of the mediastinal lymph nodes. In the advent of an abnormal PET scan, biopsy of mediastinal lymph nodes should occur before surgery when possible (Yasufuku, 2013). EBUS is an ultrasound-guided bronchoscopy to biopsy either the lymph nodes or lung nodules. A minimum of three aspirates with separate needles for each biopsy optimizes the diagnostic yield and prevention of cross-contamination (Rusch et al., 2011). EBUS–transbronchial needle aspiration (EBUS-TBNA) or endoscopic ultrasound-guided FNA (EUS-FNA) may be preferred procedures over mediastinoscopy to biopsy lymph nodes with the benefit of ultrasound guidance (Yasufuku, 2013).

Pleural fluid may accumulate secondary to metastatic disease of the pleura. Thoracentesis is an outpatient procedure that removes this fluid with the insertion of a needle into the pleural cavity (see Figure 9-1). Laboratory tests (e.g., fluid pH, cell count, glucose, lactate dehydrogenase, total protein and amylase) of the aspirated fluid can aid in the evaluation and staging of the cancer (Heffner & Klein, 2008) and guide subsequent treatment. Not all effusions are malignant; other causes could be trauma to the chest, pneumonia, or congestive heart failure.

Preoperative Tests

Preoperative pulmonary and cardiac function studies are performed to evaluate the patient's ability to tolerate general anesthesia and surgery.

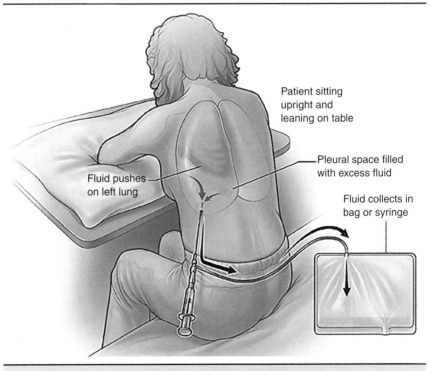

Patient sitting upright and leaning on table

Pleural space filled with excess fluid

Fluid pushes on left lung

Fluid collects in bag or syringe

Figure 9-1. Thoracentesis

Note. From "What to Expect During Thoracentesis," by the National Heart, Lung, and Blood Institute, 2012. Retrieved from http://www.nhlbi.nih.gov/health/health-topics/topics/thor/during.html.

These tests include pulse oximetry and pulmonary function tests. The pulse oximetry is intended to measure the effect of exertion on oxygenation and should be obtained at baseline and after the patient climbs a full flight of stairs. A pulmonary perfusion scan may be necessary to determine if the patient has adequate lung function to sustain ventilation after a pulmonary resection. Surgical candidates should have adequate pulmonary function to tolerate the recommended resection. A stress test is recommended to evaluate cardiac function based on the patient's age and medical and smoking history and the extent of planned surgery. If the stress test is abnormal, a cardiac catheterization may be indicated to rule out concomitant coronary artery disease, which is common in long-term smokers. In addition, maximal oxygen consumption (VO_2 max) is decisive when cardiopulmonary reserve is compromised by concomitant disease (Rocco et al., 2013).

Surgery

Surgery provides the most promise of a cure in patients with NSCLC and is performed in early localized malignancies. Surgery may be performed in patients with SCLC after chemotherapy administration if the disease remains localized. The effectiveness of surgery depends on the stage and histology of the tumor. With the use of radiographic images, the patient will be evaluated preoperatively for the proximity of the tumor to the pericardium, pulmonary vessels, chest wall, and bronchi to prevent intraoperative complications. The surgeon and patient will discuss the location, size, and number of lesions and the surgical options available.

The nursing plan of care for these patients, family members, and caregivers begins preoperatively with education about exercise, deep breathing, smoking cessation, and preparation for the postoperative period. Preoperatively, the nurse needs to assess the patient's pain; smoking, alcohol, and substance abuse history; daily exercise level; and current respiratory status. The use of tobacco can have negative outcomes for those undergoing surgery for lung cancer, even in the absence of chronic lung disease (Cooley, Sipples, Murphy, & Sarna, 2008). Antiplatelet drugs and aspirin are typically stopped 5–10 days prior to surgery; however, controversy exists regarding whether a patient could continue taking 81 mg of aspirin until the day before surgery.

Perioperative Care

The patient is positioned supine for the bronchoscopy and then placed in the lateral decubitus position for surgery. Precautions are taken to prevent pressure sores and nerve compression in all extremities. Precise positioning of the endotracheal tube is important so that the contralateral lung can be fully and adequately ventilated and to allow egress of air from the lung undergoing the surgery. Fluid management is imperative, especially in patients undergoing a complete lung resection, because acute respiratory distress syndrome (ARDS) can occur with fluid overload. Antibiotic prophylaxis is is recommended in patients undergoing pulmonary resection because it is considered a *clean-contaminated operation* in which bacterial contamination may occur during the opening of the bronchial tree (Schussler et al., 2008). Nurses and the surgical team need to closely monitor fluids, oxygenation, hemodynamics, monitors, IV and arterial lines, and ventilation to maximize patient outcomes.

Surgical Management

Surgical approaches for removal of abnormal lung masses or lymph nodes are thoracotomy, video-assisted thoracoscopic surgery (VATS), or robotic approach. Thoracotomy has been the gold standard, but more recently, VATS, a less invasive surgical technique, has gained acceptance (Taoli, Lee, Lesser, & Flores, 2013). The VATS approach emerged in the early 1990s and is used for surgical biopsy, wedge resection, segmentectomy, or lobectomy. VATS is a minimally invasive surgery in which one to three small, 2–4 cm incisions are made in order to visualize the lung and enable biopsy or resection. During VATS, if uncontrolled bleeding occurs or the entire tumor cannot be successfully resected, conversion to a full thoracotomy is an option.

The robotic approach is similar to VATS, in that the same three incisions are used. Controversy exists about the benefits of robotic surgery versus the VATS procedure because robotic surgery is typically more time consuming and cumbersome and the surgeon is separated from the patient. The procedure appears to have no clear-cut advantages over VATS, although one institution's study (Jang, Lee, Park, & Zo, 2011) noted that blood loss was less and was well controlled with the robotic approach, patients were discharged from the hospital at earlier intervals (6 vs. 9 days, $p < 0.001$), and patient-reported complaints of pain and fatigue were reduced.

Surgical Procedures

The wedge resection, segmentectomy, and lobectomy are surgical procedures that may be performed a through a muscle-sparing thoracotomy, VATS, or robotic approach. A wedge resection removes a small portion of the lung regardless of anatomic boundaries, whereas a segmentectomy removes a designated portion of the lobe with the intent of clean margins around the tumor (Rami-Porta & Tsuboi, 2009). The removal of an entire lobe of the lung continues to be the standard surgical resection for early-stage lung cancers, as the local recurrence rate for a lobectomy is lower compared to wedge or segmentectomy resection for stage IA cancers (Rami-Porta & Tsuboi, 2009). Five-year survival after lobectomy for pathologic stage I NSCLC ranges from 43% to 65%, depending on whether the patient has stage IA or IB disease and on the location of the tumor (Ou, Zell, Ziogas, & Anton-Culver, 2007). Regardless of the surgical approach, patients who have undergone a thoracotomy can have acute detrimental effects on spirometry that persist for up to 8–12 weeks postoperatively, with a 35% drop in a functional residual capacity on postoperative day 1 (Ferguson, 2008). Sarna et al.'s (2008) results indicated that post-thoracotomy symptoms decreased at four months, but some symptoms still persisted. Fatigue, dyspnea, cough, pain, and lack of appetite were the main symptoms (Sarna et al., 2008). Pain and impairment of functional health status can persist for six months after lung resection (Handy et al., 2002).

Pneumonectomy refers to removal of the entire lung, which is necessary in approximately 10% of lung cancer resections (Rami-Porta & Tsuboi, 2009). This operation is associated with significantly higher operative mortality and morbidity with worse functional outcomes and deterioration of cardiopulmonary function over time (Deslauriers et al., 2011).

Surgical Management of Metastatic Disease

Many malignancies spread to the lungs either by direct extension or through the lymph or hematologic systems. Over the past 100 years, pulmonary metastasectomy has developed into an acceptable treatment modality for a select group of patients with specific malignancies who have lung metastases, such as sarcoma, melanoma, and colon, breast, kidney, and germ cell cancers (Predina et al., 2011). The goal is to improve the patient's survival by the resection of either solitary or multiple nodules in one or both lungs.

Palliative Resection

Palliative resections may be performed to improve quality of life through control of hemoptysis, pain secondary to tumor invasion, empyema, or malignant pleural effusion. Recurrent malignant pleural effusion may require a tunneled pleural catheter designed to allow long-term intermittent drainage (Chee & Tremblay, 2011).

A *pleurodesis* is a procedure that is done at bedside or in the operating room and is intended to avoid relapse of malignant pleural effusion or pneumothorax. If it is performed at the bedside, a sclerosing agent is instilled into a chest tube, which is subsequently clamped; the patient assumes four distinct positions over one to two hours to circulate the fluid around in the pleural space. The agent acts as an irritant to create an inflammatory fibrotic response that obliterates the space and creates an extensive adhesion of the visceral and parietal pleura (Rodriguez-Panadero & Montes-Worboys, 2012). Talc, bleomycin, and tetracyclines are the most frequently used sclerosants (Shaw & Agarwal, 2009). Nurses should monitor the patient for pain, fever, and respiratory distress.

Postoperative Management

The complete surgical pathology report provides the final information about tumor type, nodal status, margins, and presence or absence of vascular invasion. Findings from molecular studies demonstrate promise in those patients with epidermal growth factor receptor (EGFR) or v-Ki-ras2 Kirsten rat sarcoma viral oncogene homolog (KRAS), a targeted oncogene, accompanied by a new anaplastic lymphoma kinase (ALK) fusion protein (Chaft et al., 2012). These targeted agents enable the oncologist to personalize the patient's treatment to the genetic characteristics of the tumor. Often nurses must help interpret the physician's conversations and further explain the pathologic findings to the patient. Therefore, it is necessary for the surgical oncology nurse to have a basic understanding of cytology, pathology, and genomics as related to patient care. Knowledge of the disease, potential complications, and surgical procedures is vital in the postoperative management of the patient who has had surgery for lung cancer. Nurses play a crucial role in the postoperative setting by educating the patient about daily expectations and initiation of discharge teaching. Post-procedure patient care may include administration of oxygen, care of urinary and via IV catheters and chest tubes, and use of pneumatic compression boots. Pain medication is administered either through an epidural catheter or IV patient-controlled analgesia. Aggressive pulmonary toileting begins immediately by the nurse and includes coughing, deep breathing, incentive spirometry, chest physiotherapy, postural drainage, and early ambulation. Early mobilization improves the quality of the postoperative course (Kanedea, Saito, Okamoto, Maniwa, & Imamura, 2007). Daily review of CXRs and hematologic status and frequent assessment of vital signs, intake, and both urinary and chest tube output are closely monitored. Chest tubes re-expand the lung and evacuate fluid and air and are placed on water seal unless there is an air leak, in which case suction may be used. Patients with a persistent air leak may be discharged from the hospital with a collection device with a one-way valve that allows drainage but prevents air and fluid from entering the pleural cavity. Effective pain measures are crucial for the patient to continue to conduct daily pulmonary toileting. Patients receiving pain medications need to be closely monitored for common side effects such as constipation, nausea, and sedation.

Despite improved surgical techniques, postoperative complications still are routine occurrences. The identification of early warning signs can lead to prompt interventions and improved outcomes. Smoking-associated complications included surgical site infection, cardiovascular complications (e.g., myocardial infarction, cardiac arrest, stroke), and pulmonary complications (e.g., pneumonia, failure to wean, re-intubation) (Singh et al., 2013). Nosocomial pneumonia is a prominent risk for morbidity and mortality after thoracotomy. Implementation of early ambulation and pulmonary toileting can minimize the risk of pneumonia.

As the number of patients older than age 70 continues to increase, thoracic surgeons will face the challenge of performing surgery on patients who could benefit from preoperative optimization in an effort to minimize postoperative complications (Hollings et al., 2010). Ongoing assessments for fever, hypoxemia, atelectasis, pain, arrhythmia, and wound infection along with assessment for evidence of air leak, subcutaneous air, myocardial infarction, aspiration, urinary tract infection, *Clostridium difficile*, stroke, and bleeding are paramount to recovery. Venous thromboembolism prophylaxis is imperative to prevent thrombosis. Acute lung injury and ARDS remain significant sources of morbidity and mortality after pulmonary resection for lung cancer (Alam et al., 2007). In addition, regardless of surgical approach, atrial fibrillation after lobectomy occurs with equal frequency (Amar et al., 2000). Despite improvements in surgical and anesthetic techniques, postoperative complications remain prevalent, and it is essential to recognize the warning signs early.

Conclusions

Thoracic surgery poses many risk factors to peri- and postoperative lung function. Preoperative assessment is essential to aid patients in the acceptance of the diagnosis and recommended treatment. Oncology nurses need to remain current on patient care, clinical trials, and new surgical procedures. Nurses can affect patient outcomes with continuing education and research that examines challenges with quality of life, outcomes, and cost-benefit analyses. Many nursing research opportunities are available related to symptom cluster management and the role of rehabilitation across the lung cancer continuum.

Nurses need to understand the biology of the various types of lung cancer, current treatment modalities, and rehabilitation. These patients are physically and psychologically challenged with multiple symptoms both at diagnosis and in postoperative recovery. The surgical management of patients who undergo a lung resection requires meticulous nursing care. These efforts will contribute to improved treatment outcomes and influence individuals to make appropriate lifestyle choices to reduce their risks of developing a malignancy.

References

Aiello-Laws, L., Reynolds, J., Deizer, N., Peterson, M., Ameringer, S., & Bakitas, M. (2009). Putting evidence into practice: What are the pharmacologic interventions for nociceptive and neuropathic cancer pain in adults? *Clinical Journal of Oncology Nursing, 13,* 649–655. doi:10.1188/09.CJON.649-655

Alam, N., Park, B., Wilton, A., Seshan, V., Bains, M., Downey, R.J., ... Amar, D. (2007). Incidence and risk factors for lung injury after lung cancer resection. *Annals of Thoracic Surgery, 84,* 1085–1091. doi:10.1007/s00595-006-3264-z

Amar, D., Roistacher, N., Rusch, V.W., Leung, D.H.Y., Ginsburg, I., Zhang, H., ... Ginsberg, R.J. (2000). Effects of diltiazem prophylaxis on the incidence and clinical outcome of atrial arrhythmias after thoracic surgery. *Journal of Thoracic and Cardiovascular Surgery, 120,* 790–798. doi:10.1067/mtc.2000.109538

American Cancer Society. (2014). *Cancer facts and figures 2014.* Retrieved from http://www.cancer.org/research/cancerfactsstatistics/cancerfactsfigures2014/index

Beckles, M.A., Spiro, S.G., Colice, G.L., & Rudd, R.M. (2003). Initial evaluation of the patient with lung cancer. Symptoms, signs, laboratory tests, and paraneoplastic syndromes. *Chest, 123*(Suppl. 1), 97S–104S. doi:10.1378/chest.123.1_suppl.97S

Chaft, J.E., Arcila, M.E., Paik, P.K., Lau, C., Riely, G.J., Pietanza, M.C., ... Kris, M.G. (2012). Coexistence of PIK3CA and other oncogene mutations in lung adenocarcinoma—Rationale for comprehensive mutation profiling. *Molecular Cancer Therapeutics, 11,* 485–491. doi:10.1158/1535-7163.MCT-11-0692

Chee, A., & Tremblay, A. (2011). The use of tunneled pleural catheters in the treatment of pleural effusions. *Current Opinion in Pulmonary Medicine, 17,* 237–241. doi:10.1097/MCP.0b013e3283463dac

Cooley, M., Sipples, R.L., Murphy, M., & Sarna, L. (2008). Smoking cessation and lung cancer: Oncology nurses can make a difference. *Seminars in Oncology Nursing, 24,* 16–26. doi:10.1016/j.soncn.2007.11.008

Denehy, L. (2008). Physiotherapy and thoracic surgery: Thinking beyond usual practice. *Physiotherapy Research International, 13,* 69–74. doi:10.1002/pri.404

Deslauriers, J., Ugalde, P., Miro, S., Deslauriers, D.R., Ferland, S., Bergeron, S., ... Provencher, S. (2011). Long-term physiological consequences of pneumonectomy. *Seminars in Thoracic Cardiovascular Surgery, 23,* 196–202. doi:10.1053/j.semtcvs.2011.10.008

DiSalvo, W., Joyce, M., Tyson, L., Culkin, A., & Mackay, K. (2008). Putting evidence into practice: Evidence-based interventions for cancer-related dyspnea. *Clinical Journal of Oncology Nursing, 12,* 341–352. doi:10.1188/08.CJON.341-352

Farjah, F., Lou, F., Sima, C., Rusch, V.W., & Rizk, N.P. (2013). A prediction model for pathologic N2 disease in lung cancer patients with a negative mediastinum by positron emission tomography. *Journal of Thoracic Oncology, 8,* 1170–1180. doi:10.1097/JTO.0b013e3182992421

Ferguson, M.K. (2008). Preoperative assessment of the thoracic surgical patient. In G.A. Patterson, J.D. Cooper, A.E. Deslauriers, M.R. Lertu, J.D. Luketich, & T. Rice (Eds.), *Pearson's thoracic and esophageal surgery* (3rd ed., pp. 9–18). Philadelphia, PA: Elsevier Churchill Livingstone.

Handy, J.R., Jr., Asaph, J.W., Skokan, L., Reed, C.E., Koh, S., Brooks, G., ... Silvestri, G.A. (2002). What happens to patients undergoing lung cancer surgery? *Chest, 122,* 21–30. doi:10.1378/chest.122.1.21

Heffner, J.E., & Klein, J.S. (2008). Recent advances in the diagnosis and management of malignant pleural effusions. *Mayo Clinic Proceedings, 83,* 235–250. doi:10.4065/83.2.235

Hollings, D., Higgins, R.S., Penfield, F., Warren, W.H., Liptay, M.J., Basu, S., & Kim, A.W. (2010). Age is a strong risk factor for atrial fibrillation after pulmonary lobectomy. *American Journal of Surgery, 199,* 558–561. doi:10.1016/j.amjsurg.2009.11.006

Jang, H.J., Lee, H.S., Park, S.Y., & Zo, J.I. (2011). Comparison of the early robot-assisted lobectomy experience to video-assisted thoracic surgery lobectomy for lung cancer: A single-institution case series matching study. *Innovations, 6,* 305–310. doi:10.1097/IMI.0b013e3182378b4c

Kanedea, H., Saito, Y., Okamoto, M., Maniwa, T., & Imamura, H. (2007). Early postoperative mobilization with walking at 4 hours after lobectomy in lung cancer patients. *General Thoracic and Cardiovascular Surgery, 55,* 493–498. doi:10.1007/s11748-007-0169-8

Kvale, P.A. (2006). Chronic cough due to lung tumors: ACCP evidence-based clinical practice guidelines. *Chest, 129*(Suppl. 1), 147S–153S. doi:10.1378/chest.129.1_suppl.147S

McKenna, R.J. (2007). Surgical management of primary lung cancer. *Seminars in Oncology, 34,* 250–255.

National Cancer Institute. (2013a, March 28). Fact sheet: Metastatic cancer. Retrieved from http://www.cancer.gov/cancertopics/factsheet/Sites-Types/metastatic

National Cancer Institute. (2013b, May 30). Non-small cell lung cancer treatment (PDQ®) [Health professional version]. Retrieved from http://www.cancer.gov/cancertopics/pdq/treatment/non-small-cell-lung/healthprofessional

Ou, S.H., Zell, J.A., Ziogas, A., & Anton-Culver, H. (2007). Prognostic factors for survival of stage I non-small cell lung cancer patients: A population-based analysis of 19,702 stage I patients in the California Cancer Registry from 1989 to 2003. *Cancer, 110,* 1532–1541. doi:10.1002/cncr.22938

Predina, J.D., Puc, M.M., Bergey, M.R., Sonnad, S.S., Kucharczuk, J.D., Staddon, A., … Shrager, J.B. (2011). Improved survival after pulmonary metastasectomy for soft tissue sarcoma. *Journal of Thoracic Oncology, 6,* 913–919. doi:10.1097/JTO.0b013e3182106f5c

Rami-Porta, R., & Tsuboi, M. (2009). Sublobar resection for lung cancer. *European Respiratory Journal, 33,* 426–435. doi:10.1183/09031936.00099808

Rocco, G., Gatani, T., DiMaio, M., Meoli, I., La Rocca, A., Martucci, N., … Stefanelli, F. (2013). The impact of decreasing cutoff values for maximal oxygen consumption (VO[2] max) in the decision-making process for candidates to lung cancer surgery. *Journal of Thoracic Disease, 5,* 12–18. doi:10.3978/j.issn.2072-1439.2012.12.04

Rodriguez-Panadero, F., & Montes-Worboys, A. (2012). Mechanisms of pleurodesis. *Respiration, 83,* 91–98. doi:10.1159/000335419

Rusch, V.W., Hawes, D., Decker, P.A., Martin, S.E., Abati, A., Landreneau, R.J., … Cote, R.J. (2011). Occult metastasis in lymph nodes predict survival in resectable non-small cell lung cancer: Report of the ACOSOG Z0040 Trial. *Journal of Clinical Oncology, 29,* 4313–4319. doi:10.1200/JCO.2011.35.2500

Sarna, L., Cooley, M., Brown, J., Chernecky, C., Elashoff, D., & Kotlerman, J. (2008). Symptom severity 1 to 4 months after thoracotomy for lung cancer. *American Journal of Critical Care, 17,* 455–467. Retrieved from http://ajcc.aacnjournals.org/content/17/5/455.long

Schussler, O., Dermine, H., Alifano, M., Casetta, A., Coignard, S., Roche, N., … Regnard, J.F. (2008). Should we change antibiotic prophylaxis for lung surgery? Postoperative pneumonia is the critical issue. *Annals of Thoracic Surgery, 86,* 1727–1733. doi:10.1016/j.athoracsur.2008.08.005

Shaw, P.H.S., & Agarwal, R. (2009). Pleurodesis for malignant pleural effusions. *Cochrane Database of Systematic Reviews, 2009*(1). doi:10.1002/14651858.CD002916.pub2

Singh, J., Hawn, M., Campagna, E., Henderson, W., Richman, J., & Houston, T. (2013). Mediation of smoking-associated postoperative mortality by perioperative complications in veterans undergoing elective surgery: Data from Veterans Affairs Surgical Quality Improvement Program. *BMJ Open, 3*(4). doi:10.1136/bmjopen-2012-002157

Stinchcombe, T.E., Bogart, J., Wigle, D.A., & Govindan, R. (2010). Annual review of advances in lung cancer clinical research: A report for the year 2009. *Journal of Thoracic Oncology, 5,* 935–939. doi:10.1097/JTO.0b013e3181e3a2e6

Taoli, E., Lee, D.S., Lesser, M., & Flores, R. (2013). Long-term survival in video-assisted thoracoscopic lobectomy vs. open lobectomy in lung-cancer patients: A meta-analysis. *European Journal of Cardio-Thoracic Surgery, 44,* 591–597. doi:10.1093/ejcts/ezt051

Wagner, J.M., Hinshaw, J.L., Lubner, M., Robbins, J.B., Kim, D.H., Pickhardt, P.J., & Lee, F.T. (2011). CT-guided lung biopsies: Pleural blood patching reduces the rate of chest tube placement for postbiopsy pneumothorax. *American Journal of Roentgenology, 197*, 783–788. doi:10.2214/AJR.10.6324

Yasufuku, K. (2013). Relevance of endoscopic ultrasonography and endobronchial ultrasonography to thoracic surgeons. *Thoracic Surgery Clinics, 23*, 199–210. doi:10.1016/j.thorsurg.2013.01.016

CHAPTER 10

Surgical Care of Upper Gastrointestinal Cancers

Lisa Parks, MS, RN, CNP

Introduction

The gastrointestinal (GI) tract includes organs found from the mouth to the anus (see Figure 10-1). This tract is often divided into upper and lower segments; the upper GI tract includes the organs found from the mouth to the ileum. Discussion within this chapter will include cancers that affect the upper GI tract: esophageal, gastric, pancreatic, and gallbladder cancers and cholangiocarcinomas.

Esophageal Cancer

Esophageal cancer is the eighth most common cancer in the world (Ajani et al., 2011). Squamous cell carcinoma is the cell type in 90%–95% of esophageal cancers worldwide; however, adenocarcinoma is the pathology in 50%–80% of esophageal cancers in the United States (Ajani et al., 2011; Kleinberg & Forastiere, 2007).

Squamous cell carcinoma arises from the epithelial cells that line the upper two-thirds of the esophagus. Adenocarcinoma is found in the lower one-third of the esophagus in close proximity to the esophagogastric junction. Risk factors for adenocarcinoma include tobacco use, obesity, high body mass index, chronic gastroesophageal reflux, and a personal history of Barrett's esophagus (Ajani et al., 2011; Baker, Wooten, & Malloy, 2011).

Signs and symptoms of esophageal cancer include dysphagia (difficulty swallowing), odynophagia (painful swallowing), weight loss due to poor nutrition, and reduced appetite. Late-stage symptoms include sternal or epigastric burning pain worsened by swallowing any form of food, nausea and

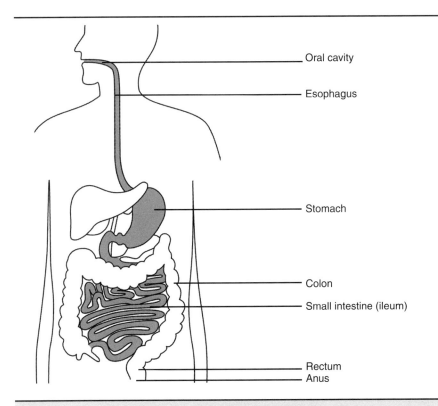

Figure 10-1. The Digestive System

Note. Public domain image from Wikimedia Commons. Retrieved from http://commons.wikimedia.org/wiki/ File:Upper_gastrointestinal_tract.svg.

vomiting due to tumor disruption of normal peristalsis, hematemesis due to bleeding of the tumor's surface, and pneumonia caused by food aspiration (Baker et al., 2011).

Evaluation for cancer involves esophagogastroduodenoscopy (EGD) with biopsy, which is the gold standard. Computed tomography (CT) scan of the chest, abdomen, and pelvis, positron-emission tomography/CT (PET/CT) scan, and esophageal endoscopic ultrasound (EUS) can provide staging information in regard to the level of tumor invasion and lymph node involvement. Barium swallow study may also be useful (Ajani et al., 2011).

Cancer staging is determined by hypoechoic expansion of the esophageal wall layers. Expansion of layers 1–3 corresponds with infiltration of the superficial and deep mucosa plus submucosa. Localized tumor without infiltration of the muscularis propria is indicative of T1 disease. Penetration of the muscularis propria correlates with T2 disease. Expansion beyond the smooth outer border of the muscularis propria to the adventitia is T3 disease. Loss of bright tissue planes between the area of tumor and surrounding tissue (trachea, aorta, or liver) correlates with infiltration of tumor into surrounding organs and is classified as T4 disease (Tangoku, Yamamoto, Furukita, Goto, & Morimoto, 2012; Yoshinaga, Oda, Nonaka, Kushima, & Saito, 2012). Clinical nodal status can be estimated after staging scans, whereas pathologic nodal status is determined after surgical resection. Prognosis for patients with locally advanced esophageal cancer is poor. The age of the patient, the stage of cancer at diagnosis, and the location of the tumor are predictors of survival (Sweed, Edmonson, & Cohen, 2009).

Surgical Management

The most commonly performed surgical procedure for esophageal cancer is the Ivor Lewis esophagectomy. The incision is transthoracic through a right thoracotomy. The esophagus is dissected and removed; the stomach is pulled into the thorax through the esophageal hiatus to create an anastomosis between the distal end of the esophagus and the stomach fundus (Ajani et al., 2011; Sweed et al., 2009). An alternative procedure is called a colonic interposition, where a piece of bowel is used to replace the esophagus when it is removed (Gunner, Gilshtein, Kakiashvili, & Kluger, 2013) (see Figure 10-2).

Postoperative Care

Pain management is essential to prevent atelectasis and complications related to immobility secondary to the thoracotomy incision. Epidural analgesia is often used while anastomoses are healing and the patient is cleared for an oral diet. Hypotension may be a side effect of the epidural anesthesia. IV narcotics may be used for breakthrough pain.

Respiratory care is essential because patients are prone to acute respiratory distress syndrome (ARDS) due to disruption of the mediastinal lymphatics, which drain the pulmonary interstitial fluid. Although mechanisms that lead to development of ARDS are not fully understood, one theory includes initiation of a generalized systemic inflammatory response. Aggressive pulmonary toilet with incentive spirometry every hour while the patient is awake is imperative. Patients may require percussion and postural drainage and nebulizer treatments to prevent atelectasis and pneumonia. Day 1 postoperative ambulation is vital and assists with ventilation and prevention of thrombotic events (Guyatt et al., 2012).

Patients will have chest tubes that require diligent care. Postoperative day 1 chest tube drainage should average 100–200 ml/hour (Mackenzie, Pollewell, & Billingsley, 2004; Sweed et al., 2009). Drainage should decrease over time and change from bloody to serosanguinous a few hours postoperatively. Chest tubes should be stripped every two hours to maintain patency; drainage

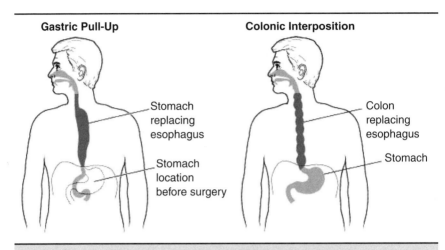

Figure 10-2. Types of Esophagogastrectomy

Note. Figure courtesy of The Ohio State University Wexner Medical Center. Used with permission.

should be serially recorded on the container. A chyle leak (fluid leak from the lymphatic vasculature) is noted as milky drainage from the chest tube and results from injury to the thoracic duct during surgery. Fluid may be tested for triglycerides to verify chyle; a level of 1.2 mm/L or greater is considered diagnostically positive (Logue & Griffin, 2011). The thorax should be palpated to assess for subcutaneous emphysema, which may indicate an air leak.

Fluid resuscitation with isotonic sodium chloride solution or lactated Ringer's solution at a rate of 100–200 ml/hour should run for 12–16 hours postoperatively (Logue & Griffin, 2011). This ensures adequate circulating volume and blood supply to the anastomoses. Major fluid shifts may occur after surgery, which require additional IV fluid boluses. Crystalloids and blood products may be used to restore circulating volume. Patients should be placed on a heparin product to prevent thromboembolic events. Foley catheter should be discontinued as soon as the epidural is removed to avoid urinary tract infections (Logue & Griffin, 2011; Sweed et al., 2009).

Patients are restricted from oral intake for five to seven days after surgery to prevent anastomotic leak or fistula formation. Bowel decompression is maintained with a nasogastric tube connected to low wall suction. Oral medications are crushed and placed down the nasogastric tube, not swallowed, until oral intake is cleared by a swallow study or upper GI fluoroscopy. Patients may be started on jejunostomy tube feedings two to three days postoperatively. The nutritional goal is more than 1,500 kcal/day. Prior to discharge, patients will be instructed to eat six to eight small meals a day; if unable to eat adequately by mouth, patients will require education on jejunostomy tube feeding administion and care. Patients should also be instruct-ed to refrain from consuming hot or cold beverages and spicy foods to avoid irritation of the surgical sites. Because the lower esophageal sphincter is sac-rificed during the surgery, patients are instructed to always maintain at least a 30° head elevation (Logue & Griffin, 2011).

Gastric Cancer

The incidence of gastric cancer has declined globally since World War II and is one of the least common cancers in North America. However, world-wide it is the fourth most common cancer (Ajani et al., 2010). Gastric cancer is often diagnosed at a late stage because symptoms are often mistaken for gastroenteritis or gastric ulcer. Early symptoms may include indigestion or a burning sensation, early satiety, loss of appetite, and abdominal discomfort. Symptoms may progress to weakness and fatigue. Stomach bloating may oc-cur, especially after meals. Late-stage disease symptoms may include upper abdominal pain, nausea and vomiting, diarrhea or constipation, weight loss, bleeding, and dysphagia (Shah & Kelsen, 2010).

Several risk factors may lead to adenocarcinoma of the stomach. Proxi-mal gastric cancer (gastric cardia and gastroesophageal junction) can be ini-tiated through chronic inflammation caused by *Helicobacter pylori*. The pro-gression of disease is through chronic atrophic gastritis and reduced acid production, which leads to intestinal metaplasia and dysplasia. Tobacco use, high salt intake, and alcohol abuse also are risk factors. A mutation or epi-genetic silencing of the E-cadherin gene leads to a predisposition for hered-itary gastric cancer (Shah & Kelsen, 2010).

Cancers that originate in the glandular tissue of the stomach are classi-fied as adenocarcinomas. Brinton disease, a rare type of gastric cancer, orig-inates in the glandular tissue lining the stomach. Diffuse proliferation of the connective tissue occurs, termed as *gastric linitis plastica*, which results in tis-sue thickening with restriction and rigidity. The stomach has restricted ex-pansion to oral intake, which results in poor nutrition. This disease spreads rapidly and metastasizes to other organs and lymph nodes. Prognosis is very poor and treatment options are limited (Maduekwe & Yoon, 2011).

GI stromal tumors (GISTs) are rare mesenchymal neoplasms of the GI tract (Efron & Lillemoe, 2005). These tumors develop from the interstitial lining and are innervated cells associated with the Auerbach plexus (Deme-tri et al., 2010) and express c-kit (CD-117) (Barnes & Reinke, 2011). Tumor characteristics are predictive of the aggressiveness of disease and include a mitotic rate of greater than 5^{10} and tumors larger than 5–10 cm; small bowel GISTs are more aggressive (Raut, 2010). Clinical evaluation of gastric cancer is accomplished with EGD with biopsies, EUS to assess tumor depth, upper

GI series, CT of the abdomen and pelvis to determine invasion into adjacent tissues or the spread to local lymph nodes, and PET/CT scan.

Gastric staging requires at least 15 lymph nodes in the pathologic sample. Stage 0 is limited to the inner lining of the stomach and is treatable by endoscopic mucosal resection. Stage I disease penetrates the second and third layers of the stomach (stage IA) or to the second layer plus nearby lymph nodes (stage IB). Stage II involves penetration of the second layers and more distant lymph nodes, to the third layer and nearby lymph nodes, or to all four layers but not the lymph nodes. Stage III gastric cancer involves penetration of the third layer and distant lymph nodes or penetration of the fourth layer and nearby tissues or distant lymph nodes. Stage IV gastric cancer has spread to nearby tissues and distant lymph nodes or metastasized to an organ (Ajani et al., 2010).

Surgical Management

Treatment includes surgical control, colonic stents if necessary, and chemotherapy. The goal of therapy is to control disease progression. Approximately 50% of patients present with advanced disease and have a poor prognosis; 70%–80% of patients have involvement of the regional lymph nodes on initial presentation (Ajani et al., 2010). The primary goal of surgery is a complete gastric resection with negative surgical margins or R0 resection (Callister & Gunderson, 2010). This outcome is achieved 50% of the time. Subtotal gastrectomy is the preferred approach for distal gastric cancer. Proximal and total gastrectomies are indicated for proximal gastric cancer. These procedures are all associated with postoperative nutritional impairment (Colavelli et al., 2010).

Postoperative Care

Postoperative complications include anastomotic leaks. Patients should be monitored for back pain, left shoulder pain, pelvic pain, substernal pressure, hiccups, restlessness, tachycardia, and low urine output (Barth & Jenson, 2006). Approximately five days postoperatively, patients will undergo a swallow study to exclude anastomotic leak. With a normal swallow study, patients will be advanced to a clear liquid diet. They are progressed to a postgastrectomy diet, which consists of small, frequent meals. For patients with an anastomotic leak, jejunostomy enteral feedings, if a jejunostomy was placed at the time of gastrectomy, may be initiated. Otherwise, a central line is placed and the patient is started on total parenteral nutrition. A repeat swallow study is performed a week after the previous study.

Postgastrectomy patients are at high risk for venous thromboembolism and pulmonary embolism. Postoperative care includes early ambulation, sequential compression stockings, and prophylactic anticoagulation therapy

(Barth & Jenson, 2006). Dehydration and third spacing of fluids may manifest as decreased urine output, tachycardia, and hypotension. Patients with a history of pulmonary edema and heart failure can experience exacerbations with fluid supplementation and should be monitored closely.

The most common long-term side effect of the surgical procedure is delayed gastric emptying, commonly known as *dumping syndrome*. Prokinetic agents such as metoclopramide are prescribed, yet are often ineffective. Antibiotics such as erythromycin and azithromycin may be prescribed for their side effect of increased GI motility. Vomiting and diarrhea may occur for up to 12 months following gastrectomy in nearly 50% of patients despite interventions. Patients who undergo a gastrectomy experience nutritional side effects, including malabsorption of protein, vitamin deficiencies, and loss of absorption sites for iron, calcium, and vitamin B_{12}. Patients will require monthly vitamin B_{12} injections over their lifetime (Baker et al., 2011).

Pancreatic Cancer

Pancreatic cancer accounts for only 3% of all new cancer diagnoses (Bratton & Kurtin, 2010). Ductal adenocarcinoma is the cell type in 90% of pancreatic cancers; the remaining are islet cell cancers. The peak age of occurrence is 70–80 years old. A higher incidence of pancreatic cancer is reported in African Americans than in other populations. Five-year survival following resection for node-negative disease is 25%–30%. Risk factors for pancreatic cancer include cigarette smoking and increased body mass index. Also, 5%–10% of patients have a familial pancreatic cancer gene mutation of *CDKN2A*, *BRCA2*, and *PALB2* (Bratton & Kurtin, 2010). A sudden onset of type 2 diabetes in people older than age 50 may be linked to a new diagnosis of pancreatic cancer.

Symptoms of pancreatic cancer include weight loss, jaundice, floating stools, abdominal pain, dyspepsia, and nausea. Tumors of the body and tail of the pancreas present with advanced symptoms late in the disease course. Median survival of patients who have had the tumor resected is 15–19 months (Daniel & Kurtin, 2011). Pancreatic cancer is clinically evaluated by various methods. CA 19-9 is a pancreatic cancer tumor marker; any elevation may indicate carcinoma. Spiral CT scan with pancreatic protocol is useful in that it shows the highest contrast enhancement during the late arterial phase and assesses the degree of vascular invasion of the tumor.

As biliary obstruction and jaundice are often the first symptoms, the goal is preoperative biliary drainage to alleviate pruritus and prevent cholangitis. The desired outcome is decreased morbidity with improvements in liver function prior to surgery. Biliary stents are placed by endoscopic retrograde cholangiopancreatography or percutaneous cholangiogram.

The Whipple procedure (see Figure 10-3) is the most common surgical procedure performed for pancreatic cancer. This procedure involves removal of the gallbladder, common bile duct, head of the pancreas, and a portion of the duodenum (Wang et al., 2008). After the surgery, patients typically experience an ileus of the bowel and delayed gastric emptying. Prokinetic agents such as metoclopramide and antibiotics such as erythromycin or azithromycin may be used to increase GI motility (Daniel & Kurtin, 2011). A nasogastric tube is used in the immediate postoperative period. Prolonged delayed gastric emptying may require gastrostomy tube placement intraoperatively or by endoscopy (Tani et al., 2006). These patients become endocrine deficient, are treated like type 2 diabetics, and require referral to endocrinology for long-term management (Bratton & Kurtin, 2010). Exocrine insufficiency leads to postprandial diarrhea and malnutrition due to lack of fat absorption and weight loss. Pancreatic enzymes are administered before meals to assist in fat absorption. Medications are administered to control diarrhea, such as loperamide, diphenoxylate, tincture of opium, codeine, and cholestyramine resin. Opioids are also used for the beneficial side effect of constipation. Because of the gastrojejunostomy, biliary reflux is a lifelong concern with symptoms of chronic acid reflux and nausea with bilious emesis. Patients require lifetime acid suppression

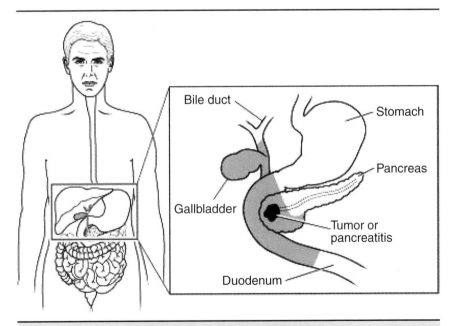

Figure 10-3. The Whipple Procedure

Note. Figure courtesy of The Ohio State University Wexner Medical Center. Used with permission.

with a proton pump inhibitor to prevent ulceration and subsequent perforation. Antiemetics may be used to control the nausea (Keim, Klar, Poll, & Schoenberg, 2009). One in four patients who undergo resection will not recover from the surgery to allow administration of systemic chemotherapy.

Cholangiocarcinoma

Cholangiocarcinoma is rare and refers to intrahepatic, perihilar, and distal extrahepatic tumors of the bile ducts. Fifty to sixty percent of tumors are perihilar (involving the bifurcation of the ducts) and are referred to as *Klatskin tumors*. Most patients with cholangiocarcinoma are older than 65 years of age. Risk factors for this cancer include choledochal cysts, chronic biliary irritation, primary sclerosing cholangitis, and ulcerative colitis (Hiriat, Laurent, & Blanc, 2011; Skipworth et al., 2011). Five-year survival in these patients is less than 5%. These tumors are usually diagnosed at an advanced stage and are aggressive in nature. Ninety percent of these tumors are adenocarcinomas. Symptoms mimic biliary colic or chronic cholecystitis with painless jaundice and abdominal pain. Pruritus and weight loss occur with jaundice; fever may indicate cholangitis. Stools appear gray or clay colored and urine is cola colored (Benson et al., 2009; Pack, O'Connor, & O'Hagan, 2001).

Evaluation of cholangiocarcinoma is through CT scan of the abdomen, pelvis, and chest. Patients who present with jaundice are evaluated through magnetic resonance cholangiopancreatography and liver function tests. Cholangiography is another method to visualize the biliary tree, which is completed by percutaneous injection of dye (Benson et al., 2009; Pack et al., 2001). Surgery is the only curative modality and involves a cholecystectomy, en bloc hepatic resection, and lymphadenectomy with or without bile duct excision and biliary reconstruction. Tumor encasement of the hepatic artery or portal vein, liver metastasis, and lymphadenopathy are all contraindications to surgery (Skipworth et al., 2011).

Postoperative care is similar to that for patients undergoing a Whipple procedure.

Conclusions

Considerable advances have been made in the treatment of cancers of the upper GI tract. The National Comprehensive Cancer Network (NCCN, 2013a, 2013b) provides an evidence-based systematic approach to the management of these cancers. NCCN recommends that patients participate in well-designed clinical trials to enable further advances in cancer treatment.

Nurses need to be aware of changes in cancer therapy and postsurgical care in order to provide optimal patient care.

References

Ajani, J.A., Barthel, J.S., Bekaii-Saab, T., Bentrem, D.J., D'Amico, T.A., Das, P., ... Yang, G. (2010). Gastric cancer. *Journal of the National Comprehensive Cancer Network, 8,* 378–409.

Ajani, J.A., Barthel, J.S., Bentrem, D.J., D'Amico, T.A., Das, P., Denlinger, C., ... Wright, C.D. (2011). Esophageal and esophagogastric junction cancers. *Journal of the National Comprehensive Cancer Network, 9,* 830–887.

Baker, A., Wooten, L., & Malloy, M. (2011). Nutritional considerations after gastrectomy and esophagectomy for malignancy. *Current Treatment Options in Oncology, 12,* 85–95. doi:10.1007/s11864-010-0134-0

Barnes, T., & Reinke, D. (2011). Practical management of imatinib in gastrointestinal stromal tumors. *Clinical Journal of Oncology Nursing, 15,* 533–545. doi:10.1188/11.CJON.533-545

Barth, M.M., & Jenson, C.E. (2006). Postoperative nursing care of gastric bypass patients. *American Journal of Critical Care, 15,* 378–387.

Benson, A.B., III, Abrams, T.A., Ben-Josef, E., Bloomston, P.M., Botha, J.F., Clary, B.M., ... Zhu, A.X. (2009). Hepatobiliary cancers. *Journal of the National Comprehensive Cancer Network, 7,* 350–391.

Bratton, M., & Kurtin, S.E. (2010). Collaborative approach to managing a 59-year-old woman with stage IIB pancreatic cancer and diabetes? *Journal of the Advanced Practitioner in Oncology, 1,* 257–265.

Callister, M.D., & Gunderson, L.L. (2010). Advancements in radiation techniques for gastric cancer. *Journal of the National Comprehensive Cancer Network, 8,* 428–436.

Colavelli, C., Pastore, M., Morenghi, E., Coladonato, M., Tronconi, C., Rimassa, L., ... Cozzaglio, L. (2010). Nutritional and digestive effects of gastrectomy for gastric cancer. *Nutritional Therapy and Metabolism, 28,* 129–136. Retrieved from http://air.unimi.it/bitstream/2434/165030/2/129-136_NT%26M_09_00040_Colavelli.pdf

Daniel, S., & Kurtin, S. (2011). Pancreatic cancer? *Journal of the Advanced Practitioner in Oncology, 2,* 141–155.

Demetri, G.D., von Mehren, M., Antonescu, C.R., DeMatteo, R.P., Ganjoo, K.N., Maki, R.G., ... Wayne, J.D. (2010). NCCN Task Force report: Update on the management of patients with gastrointestinal stromal tumors. *Journal of the National Comprehensive Cancer Network, 5,* S1–S41. Retrieved from http://www.jnccn.org/content/8/Suppl_2/S-1.long

Efron, D.T., & Lillemoe, K.D. (2005). The current management of gastrointestinal stromal tumors. *Advances in Surgery, 39,* 193–221.

Grunner, S., Gilshtein, H., Kakiashvili, E., & Kluger, Y. (2013). Adenocarcinoma in colonic interposition. *Case Reports in Oncology, 6,* 186–188. doi:10.1159/000350743

Guyatt, G., Eikelboom, J., Gould, M., Garcia, D., Crowther, M., Murad, H., ... American College of Chest Physicians. (2012). Approach to outcome measurement in the prevention of thrombosis in surgical and medical patients: Antithrombotic therapy and prevention of thrombosis, 9th ed: American College of Chest Physicians evidence-based clinical practice guidelines. *Chest, 141,* 185S–194S. doi:10.1378/chest.11-2289

Hiriat, J.-B., Laurent, C., & Blanc, J.-F. (2011). Perihilar cholangiocarcinoma, the need for a new staging system. *Clinics and Research in Hepatology and Gastroenterology, 35,* 697–698. doi:10.1016/j.clinre.2011.06.004

Keim, V., Klar, E., Poll, M., & Schoenberg, M.H. (2009). Postoperative care following pancreatic surgery. *Deutsches Ärzteblatt International, 106,* 789–794. doi:10.3238/arztebl.2009.0789

Kleinberg, L., & Forastiere, A.A. (2007). Chemoradiation in the management of esophageal cancer. *Journal of Clinical Oncology, 25,* 4110–4117.

Logue, B., & Griffin, S. (2011). Road map to esophagectomy for nurses. *Critical Care Nurse, 31,* 69–85. doi:10.4037/ccn2011426

Mackenzie, D.J., Pollewell, P.K., & Billingsley, K.G. (2004). Care of patients after esophagectomy. *Critical Care Nurse, 24,* 16–29.

Maduekwe, U.N., & Yoon, S.S. (2011). An evidence-based review of the surgical treatment of gastric adenocarcinoma. *Journal of Gastrointestinal Surgery, 15,* 730–741. doi:10.1007/s11605-011-1477-y

National Comprehensive Cancer Network. (2013a). *NCCN Clinical Practice Guidelines in Oncology: Esophageal and esophagogastric junction cancers (excluding the proximal 5 cm of the stomach)* [v.2.2013]. Retrieved from http://www.nccn.org/professionals/physician_gls/pdf/esophageal.pdf

National Comprehensive Cancer Network. (2013b). *NCCN Clinical Practice Guidelines in Oncology: Gastric cancer (including cancer in the proximal 5 cm of the stomach)* [v.2.2013]. Retrieved from http://www.nccn.org/professionals/physician_gls/pdf/gastric.pdf

Pack, D.A., O'Connor, K., & O'Hagan, K. (2001). Cholangiocarcinoma: A nursing perspective. *Clinical Journal of Oncology Nursing, 5,* 141–146.

Raut, C.P. (2010). Gastrointestinal stromal tumors: What oncologists need to know about the treatment of localized and advanced disease. *Clinical Oncology News, 5*(1). Retrieved from http://www.clinicaloncology.com/ViewArticle.aspx?d_id=157&a_id=14467

Shah, M.A., & Kelsen, D.P. (2010). Gastric cancer: A primer on the epidemiology and biology of the disease and an overview of the medical management of advanced disease. *Journal of the National Comprehensive Cancer Network, 8,* 437–447.

Skipworth, J.R.A., Damink, S.W.M.O., Olde, M., Imber, C., Bridgewater, J., Pereira, S.P., & Malagó, M. (2011). Surgical, neo-adjuvant and adjuvant management strategies in biliary tract cancer. *Alimentary Pharmacology and Therapeutics, 34,* 1063–1078. doi:10.1111/j.1365-2036.2011.04851.x

Sweed, M., Edmonson, D., & Cohen, S. (2009). Tumors of the esophagus, gastroesophageal junction, and stomach. *Seminars in Oncology Nursing, 25,* 1–15. doi:10.1016/j.soncn.2008.10.005

Tangoku, A., Yamamoto, Y., Furukita, Y., Goto, M., & Morimoto, M. (2012). The new era of staging as a key for an appropriate treatment for esophageal cancer. *Annals of Thoracic and Cardiovascular Surgery, 18,* 190–199. doi:10.5761/acts.ra.12.01926

Tani, M., Terasawa, H., Kawai, M., Ina, S., Hirono, S., Uchiyama, K., & Yamaue, H. (2006). Improvement of delayed gastric emptying in pylorus-preserving pancreaticoduodenectomy. *Annals of Surgery, 243,* 316–320. doi:10.1097/01.sla.0000201479.84934.ca

Wang, C., Wu, H., Xiong, J., Zhou, F., Tao, J., Liu, T., & Gou, S. (2008). Pancreaticoduodenectomy with vascular resection for local advanced pancreatic head cancer: A single center retrospective study. *Journal of Gastrointestinal Surgery, 12,* 2183–2190. doi:10.1007/s11605-008-0621-9

Yoshinaga, S., Oda, I., Nonaka, S., Kushima, R., & Saito, Y. (2012). Endoscopic ultrasound using ultrasound probes for the diagnosis of early esophageal and gastric cancers. *World Journal of Gastrointestinal Endoscopy, 4,* 218–226. doi:10.4253/wjge.v4.i6.218

CHAPTER 11

Surgical Care of Lower Gastrointestinal Cancers

Lynne Brophy, RN-BC, MSN, AOCN®

Introduction

The lower gastrointestinal (GI) tract contains organs from the cecum to the anus. The entire GI tract is responsible for ingestion, secretion, mixing and movement, digestion, absorption of nutrients, and defecation (Smith, 2011); the lower GI tract completes the digestion process. The large intestine reabsorbs water and electrolytes and ultimately forms fecal material. The absorbed nutrients are used to form B complex vitamins and synthesize vitamin K for the clotting pathway. The muscles within the large intestine, rectum, and anus expel waste in the form of fecal material.

Surgery is the primary treatment for cancers diagnosed within or adjacent to the lower GI tract. Leakage of intestinal contents at the time of or after surgery can cause infection or damage adjacent structures. Therefore, measures must be taken before, during, and after surgery to prevent infection and tissue damage (Smith, 2011).

Colorectal Cancer

Screening

Colorectal cancer screening is an effective means to decrease morbidity and mortality from the disease. Mandel et al. (1993) noted a positive effect on mortality rates related to colorectal cancer when annual fecal occult blood screening was performed. Patients with a positive fecal occult blood test (FOBT) underwent colonoscopy, and over a period of 13 years, a 33% reduction in mortality occurred.

The evidence supports the use of FOBT, sigmoidoscopy, and colonoscopy at age- and risk-appropriate intervals as methods to provide screening and early detection to reduce the mortality from colorectal cancer (U.S. Preventive Services Task Force, 2008). The National Comprehensive Cancer Network (NCCN) provides screening and treatment guidelines for colon (2013a) and rectal (2013b) cancers. Despite clear indications that colorectal screening saves lives, the Centers for Disease Control and Prevention has estimated that only 65% of the eligible U.S. population is appropriately screened for colorectal cancer (Richardson, Tai, Rim, Joseph, & Plescia, 2011).

Diagnosis

The diagnosis of colorectal cancers can occur in a number of ways, although colonoscopy is a key procedure used to examine approximately 60 cm of the lower intestinal tract. Primary sporadic colon cancers usually occur in the left side of the colon, whereas inherited colon cancers typically occur in the right side. Symptoms related to sporadic colon cancers differ somewhat from the symptomatology of inherited colon cancers (Bhankamkar, Crane, Rodriguez-Bigas, Kopetz, & Eng, 2011). Presenting symptoms of left-sided colon cancers include vomiting, abdominal distention, or other signs of bowel obstruction; constipation or small-diameter (e.g., caliber) stools; or fecal impaction (Bhankamkar et al., 2011). Right-sided colon cancers may also present with symptoms of bowel obstruction, but often patients report abdominal pain with bleeding in the form of melena, hematochezia, positive FOBT, or microcytic anemia (Bhankamkar et al., 2011). Patients with metastatic colorectal disease at the time of initial diagnosis often report weight loss, decreased appetite, fatigue, and other generalized symptoms (Bhankamkar et al., 2011). These symptoms are often attributed to aging or other conditions, which may delay a timely diagnosis.

The only serum tumor marker recommended for routine use in the diagnosis, surveillance, and treatment of colorectal cancer is the carcinoembryonic antigen (CEA). CEA is a glycoprotein found in the embryonic endodermal epithelium. Elevated CEA levels may be present in colorectal cancer but can also be found in breast, lung, pancreatic, ovarian, prostate, and hepatocellular cancers. Therefore, it is paramount to determine the primary site and type of cancer when an elevated CEA level is noted (Meric-Bernstam & Pollock, 2010).

Surgical Management

Surgery is the primary treatment modality for colorectal cancer. The aim of surgery is complete resection of the tumor mass, related lymph nodes, and adjacent surfaces or organs that may be affected (Bisanz et al., 2008).

Removal of a large bowel segment involves complete removal of the tumor with a large section of disease-free bowel (e.g., colon or rectum) on either end of the malignant lesion. The two ends are then reconnected or anastomosed to attach the bowel loops back together. After surgery, it is hoped that the anastomosed segment of bowel will work in tandem with remaining bowel loops to return bowel function to normal (Bisanz et al., 2008). This goal is dependent on preexisting conditions, history of other bowel pathology, postoperative course, and overall health of the patient. Surgical resections are described by anatomic site of resection. Examples of surgical resection of the bowel are demonstrated in Figure 11-1.

Comprehensive Preoperative Evaluation

A thorough physical assessment and patient and family history are essential to comprehensive preoperative care. This process may be initiated days to weeks before elective surgery, which offers the surgical team an opportunity to plan the surgery, provide anesthesia clearance, and avoid toxicity caused by possible diminished organ function. With a preliminary pathologic diagnosis of colorectal cancer, staging scans are obtained and include abdominal and chest computed tomography (CT), magnetic resonance imaging, or positron emission tomography (PET) scans. Laboratory testing may include complete blood count with differential, serum electrolytes, platelet count, coagulation studies, liver function tests, kidney function tests, pancreatic function tests, tests related to nutritional status, and tumor markers.

When significant anemia (e.g., hemoglobin less than 8.5 g/dl), thrombocytopenia (e.g., platelet count less than $50,000/mm^3$), or abnormal coagulation (e.g., increased prothrombin time and international normalized ratio) exist prior to surgery, blood products or coagulant agents may be administered

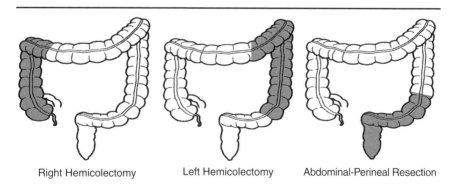

Right Hemicolectomy   Left Hemicolectomy   Abdominal-Perineal Resection

Shaded area indicates section being surgically removed.

Figure 11-1. Examples of Surgical Resection of the Bowel

Note. Figure courtesy of The Ohio State University Wexner Medical Center. Used with permission.

to correct significant deficiencies that may compromise surgical outcomes (Smith, 2011).

Patient Education

The nurse can be especially helpful to the patient and family by providing teaching about the surgical procedure. Information about skin preparation before surgery, bowel preparation, activities on the day of surgery, pulmonary toilet, deep vein thrombosis preventive measures, symptom management, care of tubes and drains, diet, and potential activity restrictions after hospital discharge such as lifting, working, and driving should be discussed. When an ostomy is anticipated, the nurse should consult with the wound, ostomy, and continence nurse to provide additional education and guidance and to mark the ostomy site if the patient's condition allows. Additional supportive care and psychological interventions can be provided to the patient and family to augment education and improve outcomes.

Day of Surgery

On the day of surgery, the patient is evaluated through a focused nursing assessment and anesthesia evaluation. The nurse works as a member of the multidisciplinary team to explain the preoperative tasks and experiences such as IV catheter insertion, skin preparation, and positioning. The wound, ostomy, and continence nurse is consulted to mark any potential ostomy sites if not completed prior to the day of surgery. The patient education completed previously in regard to immediate postoperative care is again reviewed with the patient and family.

Positioning

Proper patient positioning is important not only to ease the surgical approach but also in preventing skin breakdown or hospital-acquired pressure ulcers during the operative procedure. Before positioning, the nurse should determine whether the patient has any preexisting conditions that would necessitate the need for modifications. A thorough skin examination (e.g., Braden scoring) should be completed and documented to determine the patient's risk for pressure ulcer development. If the Braden score is indicative of high risk for pressure ulcer development, the nurse should consider applying padding to pressure points or using devices to reduce pressure. The specialized foam mattress overlays are superior over standard operating table mattresses and can be effective in the reduction of postoperative pressure ulcers (Nixon, McElvenny, Mason, Brown, & Bond, 1998). Other studies have also supported the efficacy of a thick, dense sheepskin as an operating table overlay to reduce the incidence of postoperative pressure ulcers (Reddy, Gill, & Rochon, 2006).

Once the patient has been moved to the operating room and anesthesia has been induced, a urinary catheter and nasogastric tube may be placed.

For most colorectal procedures, the patient is placed in a supine position with feet secured to the table. The patient's arms are placed on padded boards that are at a less than 90° angle to the body with palms up. This position prevents stretching of the brachial plexus nerve. In cases where access to the rectum is needed for the surgery, the patient may be placed in a modified lithotomy position with the legs in stirrups (Davies & Nelson, 2007). When a patient is in stirrups, it is important to monitor circulation by checking peripheral pulses at hourly intervals during the procedure. If the abdominal organs need to be displaced during the operation, the patient may be placed in the Trendelenburg position for a period of time to offset the effects of gravity. For a left hemicolectomy, the patient may be placed in a modified lithotomy position with arms at the side (Davies & Nelson, 2007). If the surgeon needs to approach the abdomen through the thorax, the patient will be moved to a side-lying or lateral position (Smith, 2011).

Postoperative Care

Postoperative nursing care after lower GI tract surgery focuses on the return of bowel function, fluid and electrolyte balance, pulmonary toilet, management of pain and nausea, prevention of deep vein thrombosis, early identification of complications, and ostomy education, if applicable. The number of postoperative days required for return of bowel function varies based on multiple factors. Recovery time is affected by the type of procedure, amount of bowel manipulation, type and length of anesthesia, pain management techniques, and overall health and nutrition of the patient. Early ambulation, use of sequential compression for the lower legs, and aggressive pulmonary toilet may prevent postoperative pneumonia, atelectasis, and thromboembolic events.

Often, bowel function returns within three to five days after an open or laparoscopic procedure (Smith, 2011). Stomach motility returns within 24–48 hours, but the large bowel does not usually resume function for 48–72 hours. Bowel sounds may be heard in the upper abdominal quadrants when stomach motility returns. The key sign of return of full bowel function is passage of flatus or stool (Bisanz et al., 2008).

Oral feedings are resumed after GI motility returns. Feeding usually begins with ice chips and progresses to clear liquids, full liquids, then a soft or regular diet. The patient may experience nausea during the process of resumption of oral feeding. Often, the diet is advanced at each meal if nausea does not occur and the patient tolerates the meal. Evidence has emerged that oral food intake or gum chewing as early as 4–12 hours after surgery may trick the gut into a return to normal motility earlier after surgery (Bisanz et al., 2008). Studies of early feeding resulted in more rapid return of bowel function, shorter length of stay, and fewer complications during and after the hospital stay (Han-Geurts et al., 2007; Lassen et al., 2008). Another body of research examined the use of gum chewing as a method to encourage early return of peristalsis (Asao et al., 2002; Schuster, Grewel, Greaney, & Waxman, 2006).

For the patient with colorectal cancer, postoperative bowel habits are dependent upon the amount and location of bowel resection and the potential function that is lost with resection. The nurse should understand the impact of the specific resection, dietary adjustments, and medication changes to aid the patient in an optimal recovery. Discharge teaching should include diet, activity, incision care, drain or ostomy care as indicated, and medication updates.

Primary or Metastatic Liver Cancer

Primary or metastatic liver cancer is often diagnosed when a CT scan is performed to monitor existing cirrhosis or hepatomegaly as noted on routine physical examination. At the time of presentation, the patient may report abdominal pain, ankle swelling, abdominal bloating, increased girth, or pruritus. The patient may also be diagnosed in the midst of diagnostic testing for a GI bleed. However, 24% of people with liver cancer are asymptomatic at the time of diagnosis (Carr, 2012). Primary liver cancer occurs most frequently in White men who have a history of cirrhosis (Carr, 2012). Common serum laboratory findings at the time of diagnosis are elevated liver function studies and anemia. Tumor markers for primary liver cancer include alpha-fetoprotein and des-gamma-carboxy prothrombin. Tumor markers for metastatic liver cancer are those reflective of the primary cancer (e.g., CEA for colorectal cancer).

Surgical Management

Hepatic surgery is approached to achieve one or more goals: (a) anatomic resection to remove tumor present along the portal vein, (b) enucleation to remove benign lesions that presumably have not invaded adjacent tissues, and (c) nonanatomic approach to remove a tumor or debulk a large tumor with limited chance of clean margins (Neil, 2011). The patient undergoing liver surgery may be placed in the supine or mid-Trendelenburg position for the approach of a right subcostal incision.

If metastatic disease is limited to the liver, hepatic resection may be considered. An adequate amount of viable liver must remain after completion of the surgical procedure (Reddy, Pawlik, & Zorzi, 2007). Bleeding is a major risk factor during hepatic resection because of the vascularity of the liver; therefore, blood products are placed on hold prior to surgery. When resection of liver metastasis is not possible, chemoembolization, ablative techniques, and conformal beam radiation therapy may be alternatives to surgical excision (Reddy et al., 2007).

Postoperative Care

Detailed handoff communication after surgery is extremely important and includes the type of surgical procedure performed, length of anesthesia, estimated blood loss, lowest mean arterial pressure or systolic blood pressure, lowest heart rate, any changes in cardiac rhythm during the procedure or in the postanesthesia care unit (PACU), length of time in the PACU, special positioning methods, and any new abnormal skin finding from assessment after completion of the surgical procedure that may indicate pressure ulcer risk, development, or symptoms (Gawande, Kwaan, Regenbogen, Lipsitz, & Zinner, 2007).

The return of bowel function after a liver resection is more expedient than with a colon or rectal resection, as the bowel is minimally manipulated and does not have an intestinal anastomosis. Postoperative challenges include symptoms related to inadequate liver function such as confusion secondary to electrolyte imbalance or hepatic encephalopathy, abdominal ascites formation, or anasarca. The nurse must discern potential complications, ensure patient safety, and teach the patient and caregivers to recognize concerns and understand symptom management, diet, activity and incision care prior to discharge.

Palliative Measures

Palliative measures, both surgical and interventional, may be used to provide increased comfort for the patient who suffers with complications of colorectal or hepatocellular cancer. A diverting colostomy or partial tumor debulking may be performed to bypass an unresectable colorectal cancer. After surgery, the consistency of the stool is dependent on the amount of bowel removed. Typically, the patient's stool will be soft, unformed and paste-like, or liquid, and the frequency of bowel movements can be unpredictable (Monahan, Neighbors, & Green, 2011). Patients who suffer from partial bowel obstruction may be candidates for endoscopic placement of a metal stent to open the bowel (Blanke & Faigel, 2012).

Temporary implantable closed drainage devices may be placed to drain ascites due to metastatic disease. Patients with these types of catheters must be taught site care, dressing changes, and how to drain the catheter before discharge. These palliative measures often provide excellent pain and symptom control and allow the patient to remain at home with family.

Conclusions

Patients and families who face a diagnosis of colorectal cancer, with or without hepatic involvement, have few choices for treatment, as surgery is the primary intervention. Although progress has been made in the type of surgical procedure, approach, technique, and patient outcomes, cancer-related colorectal surgery can have a negative effect on survivors as basic functions of the human anatomy and physiology are permanently altered. Nurses are essential to provide informed education for patients, family members, and caregivers and to provide psychological support to those in need.

References

Asao, T., Kuwano, H., Nakamura, J., Morinaga, N., Hirayama, I., & Ide, M. (2002). Gum chewing enhances early recovery from postoperative ileus after laparoscopic colectomy. *Journal of the American College of Surgeons, 195*, 30–32.

Bhankamkar, N., Crane, C.H., Rodriguez-Bigas, M., Kopetz, S., & Eng, C. (2011). Colorectal cancer. In H.M. Kantarjian, R.A. Wolff, & C.A. Koller (Eds.), *The MD Anderson manual of medical oncology* (2nd ed.). Retrieved from http://www.accessmedicine.com/content.aspx?aID=8306534

Bisanz, A., Palmer, J.L., Reddy, S., Cloutier, L., Dixon, T., Cohen, M.Z., & Bruera, E. (2008). Characterizing postoperative paralytic ileus as evidence for future research and clinical practice. *Gastroenterology Nursing, 31*, 336–344. doi:10.1097/01.SGA.0000338278.40412.df

Blanke, C.D., & Faigel, D.O. (2012). Neoplasms of the small and large intestine. In L. Goldman & A.I. Schafer (Eds.), *Goldman's Cecil medicine* (24th ed.). Retrieved from http://www.nursingconsult.com/nursing/books/978-1-4377-1604-7

Carr, B.I. (2012). Tumors of the liver and biliary tree. In D.L. Longo, A.S. Fauci, D.L. Kasper, S.L. Hauser, J.L. Jameson, & J. Loscalzo (Eds.), *Harrison's principles of internal medicine* (18th ed., pp. 777–785). New York, NY: McGraw-Hill.

Davies, M.M., & Nelson, H. (2007). Small bowel/colon resection. In *Maingot's abdominal operations* (11th ed.). Retrieved from http://www.accesssurgery.com/content.aspx?aID=130603

Gawande, A.A., Kwaan, M.R., Regenbogen, S.E., Lipsitz, S.A., & Zinner, M.J. (2007). An Apgar score for surgery. *Journal of the American College of Surgeons, 204*, 201–208. doi:10.1016/j.jamcollsurg.2006.11.011

Han-Geurts, I.J., Hop, W.C., Kok, N.F., Lim, A., Brouwer, K.J., & Jeekel, J. (2007). Randomised clinical trial of the impact of early enteral feeding postoperative ileus and recovery. *British Journal of Surgery, 94*, 555–561. doi:10.1002/bjs.5753

Lassen, K., Kjaeve, J., Fetveit, T., Trano, G., Sigurdsson, H.K., Horn, A., & Revhaug, A. (2008). Allowing normal food at will after major upper gastrointestinal surgery does not increase morbidity: A randomized multicenter trial. *Annals of Surgery, 247*, 721–729. doi:10.1097/SLA.0b013e31815cca68

Mandel, J.S., Bond, J.H., Church, T.R., Snover, D.C., Bradley, M., Schuman, L.M., & Ederer, F. (1993). Reducing mortality from colorectal cancer by screening for fecal occult blood. *New England Journal of Medicine, 328*, 1365–1371. doi:10.1056/NEJM199305133281901

Meric-Bernstam, F., & Pollock, R.E. (2010). Oncology. In F.C. Brunicardi, D.K. Anderson, T.R. Billiar, D.L. Dunn, J.G. Hunter, J.B. Matthews, & R.E. Pollock (Eds.), *Schwartz's principles of surgery* (9th ed.). Retrieved from http://www.accessmedicine.com/content. aspx?aID=5021163

Monahan, F.D., Neighbors, M., & Green, C.J. (2011). *Swearingen's manual of medical-surgical nursing: A care planning resource.* Retrieved from http://www.nursingconsult.com/nursing/ books/978-0-323-07254-0

National Comprehensive Cancer Network. (2013a). *NCCN Clinical Practice Guidelines in Oncology: Colon cancer* [v.1.2014]. Retrieved from http://www.nccn.org/professionals/physician _gls/pdf/colon.pdf

National Comprehensive Cancer Network. (2013b). *NCCN Clinical Practice Guidelines in Oncology: Rectal cancer* [v.1.2014]. Retrieved from http://www.nccn.org/professionals/physician _gls/pdf/rectal.pdf

Neil, J. (2011). Surgery of the liver, biliary tract, pancreas, and spleen. In J.C. Rothrock (Ed.), *Care of the patient in surgery* (14th ed., pp. 357–395). St. Louis, MO: Elsevier Mosby.

Nixon, J., McElvenny, D., Mason, S., Brown, J., & Bond, S. (1998). A sequential randomised controlled trial comparing a dry visco-elastic polymer pad and standard operating table mattress in the prevention of post-operative pressure sores. *International Journal of Nursing Studies, 35,* 193–203.

Reddy, M., Gill, S.S., & Rochon, P.A. (2006). Preventing pressure ulcers: A systematic review. *JAMA, 296,* 974–984. doi:10.1001/jama.296.8.974

Reddy, S.K., Pawlik, T.M., & Zorzi, D. (2007). Simultaneous resections of colorectal cancer and synchronous liver metastases: A multi-institutional analysis. *Annals of Surgical Oncology, 14,* 3481–3491.

Richardson, L.C., Tai, E., Rim, S.H., Joseph, D., & Plescia, M. (2011). Vital signs: Colorectal cancer screening, incidence, and mortality—United States, 2002–2010. *Morbidity and Mortality Weekly Report, 60*(26). Retrieved from http://www.cdc.gov/mmwr/preview/mmwrhtml/ mm6026a4.htm?s_cid=mm6026a4_w

Schuster, R., Grewel, N., Greaney, G.C., & Waxman, K. (2006). Gum chewing reduces ileus after elective open sigmoid colectomy. *Archives of Surgery, 141,* 174–176. doi:10.1001/ archsurg.141.2.174

Smith, C.E. (2011). Gastrointestinal surgery. In J.C. Rothrock (Ed.), *Care of the patient in surgery* (14th ed., pp. 295–356). St. Louis, MO: Elsevier Mosby.

U.S. Preventive Services Task Force. (2008, October). Screening for colorectal cancer. Retrieved from http://www.uspreventiveservicestaskforce.org/uspstf/uspscolo.htm

CHAPTER 12

Surgical Care of Cancers of the Female Pelvis

Frances Cartwright-Alcarese, PhD, RN-BC, AOCN®

Introduction

This chapter discusses the surgical management of cancers of the female reproductive system, which includes the vulva, vagina, cervix, corpus uteri, ovaries, and fallopian tubes. It is organized by a discussion of the anatomy of each organ, common presenting signs and symptoms, diagnostic and staging procedures, tumor histology, prognostic and treatment indicators, and surgical treatment options. A discussion of optimal treatment options that are consistent with both the goals of surgery (e.g., staging, curative, control, palliation) and the patient's quality of life, personal priorities, and risks and benefits is essential. Ideally, each case is reviewed by a multidisciplinary team with a multimodality approach to treatment with surgery, radiation therapy (RT), and chemotherapy as necessary to optimally manage the cancer. A discussion of chemotherapy and RT is beyond the scope of this chapter; for a comprehensive discussion of these topics see the National Comprehensive Cancer Network (NCCN) guidelines (www.nccn .org/professionals/physician_gls/f_guidelines.asp). The content of this chapter is a synthesis of many authors who have provided information based on the outcomes of clinical trials and their expert review of these topics.

Anatomy and Physiology

A thorough understanding of the normal anatomy and physiology of the female reproductive system augments understanding of how surgical treatment options can affect the physical and psychosocial aspects of care and, more specifically, how surgical outcomes will affect the patient's quality of life and personal priorities. Figure 12-1 is a detailed illustration of the female pelvic floor that shows the anatomy of the female pelvis. Radiographic images of tumor growth patterns are available from other sources and will add clarity to this text (Bickley & Szilagyi, 2007; Cartwright-Alcarese & O'Sullivan, 2010; Lee, Oliva, Hahn, & Russell, 2011).

Diagnostic Tests

Several tests and procedures are used to diagnose gynecologic cancers and include but are not limited to the following.

- Colposcopy uses a magnifying lens to enhance examination and biopsy of the vagina and cervix.
- Cystoscopy and proctoscopy use small scopes to view urogenital and rectal structures.
- Computed tomography (CT) scan uses x-ray to produces two-dimensional images.
- Positron-emission tomography (PET) scan uses nuclear energy and produces three-dimensional images.
- Ultrasound uses high-frequency sound waves to produce precise images of involved structures.

Several biopsy techniques are used to diagnose gynecologic cancers such as fine needle aspiration, core needle biopsy, and incisional or excisional biopsies. Accurate diagnosis and staging of gynecologic cancers are essen-

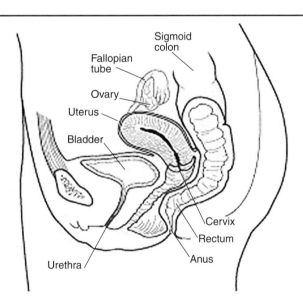

Figure 12-1. Female Pelvic Anatomy

Note. Figure courtesy of The Ohio State University Wexner Medical Center. Used with permission.

tial to the determination of the most effective multimodal-therapy treatment plan. The 2009 International Federation of Gynecology and Obstetrics (FIGO) definitions and staging system are used by the NCCN (2013a) panel, and the staging system is approved by the American Joint Committee on Cancer (AJCC) (Edge et al., 2010; Pecorelli, Zigliani, & Odicino, 2009). Gynecologic cancers spread via direct extension into surrounding structures and through the lymphatic system to local, regional, and distant sites. A thorough understanding of the lymphatic system is essential to ensure adequate surgical dissection and staging of gynecologic cancers.

Vulvar Cancer

Anatomy and Presentation

The term *vulva* refers to the external structures that are visible in the perineal region (see Figure 12-2) and extend anatomically to the symphysis pubis (anterior), buttocks (posterior), and thighs (lateral) (Aikins-Murphy, 1990). The vulva includes the mons pubis, labia minora, labia majora, clitoris, vaginal vestibule, and perineal body. Cancers of the vulva present with vulvar inflammation, growths, itching, and pain in the early stages, with bleeding and discharge in later stages.

Diagnostic and Staging Procedures

Biopsy of the lesions and evaluation of lymph node involvement is obtained with colposcopy, cystoscopy, and proctoscopy. Staging is based on the revised FIGO staging for carcinoma of the vulva (Edge et al., 2010; Hacker, 2009). Squamous cell carcinoma is the most common histologic type; verrucous carcinoma, Paget disease, adenocarcinoma, basal cell carcinoma, and Bartholin gland carcinoma are all less common histologic types.

Tumor size and lymph node status are the most important prognostic indicators in vulvar cancers. Common sites of malignancy include direct extension of adjacent structures such as femoral, inguinal, and iliac lymph nodes. Distant metastasis can occur in both regional and distant organs.

Surgical Management

Surgery alone is considered curative when the tumor can be completely excised with wide negative margins (see Figure 12-3). Stage IA disease requires wide local excision; stages IB and II require radical excision/vulvectomy and nodal dissection. Stages III and IV require more extensive sur-

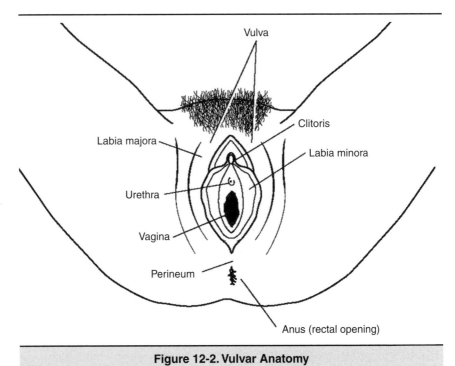

Figure 12-2. Vulvar Anatomy

Note. Figure courtesy of The Ohio State University Wexner Medical Center. Used with permission.

gery with systemic therapy. Tantipalakorn, Robertson, Marsden, Gebski, and Hacker (2009) reported no significant difference in recurrence rates, time to recurrence, or survival for patients with stages I and II squamous cell vulvar cancer. Vulvar-conserving surgery may be an option for even large tumors.

Vaginal Cancer

Anatomy and Presentation

The vagina is a flexible, elastic opening that extends from the cervix to the vulva. The upper part of the vagina surrounds the cervix. This pouch-like space, which is a shallow recess around the cervix, is called the *fornix*. The vagina is divided by the cervix into the posterior and anterior fornices and the lateral fornices (Cartwright-Alcarese & O'Sullivan, 2010). The presentation of vaginal cancer may be asymptomatic in its early stages, and a watery vaginal discharge and unexplained vaginal bleeding are common in the

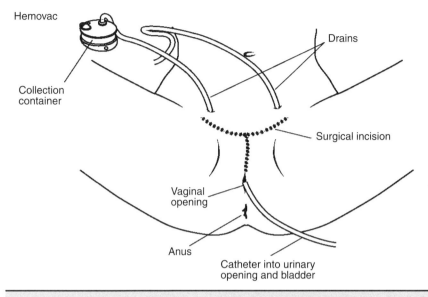

Hemovac

Drains

Collection container

Surgical incision

Vaginal opening

Anus

Catheter into urinary opening and bladder

Figure 12-3. Postvulvectomy Wound and Drain Care

Note. Figure courtesy of The Ohio State University Wexner Medical Center. Used with permission.

invasive stage. Painful urination, pelvic pain, and constipation can occur in late-stage disease.

Diagnostic and Staging Procedures

Staging is based on the FIGO staging for carcinoma of the vagina (Edge et al., 2010; Hacker, 2009) and includes biopsy of the lesion, cystoscopy, proctoscopy, and CT of the abdomen and pelvis. Squamous cell carcinoma is the most common histologic type; occasionally adenocarcinoma, melanoma, and clear cell cancers originate in the vagina. Local extension of the tumor can occur, as well as metastatic disease in regional lymph nodes.

Surgical Management

Complete excision of the tumor with wide negative margins, plus a vaginectomy and hysterectomy followed by RT is a common treatment plan for early-stage disease. In advanced vaginal cancer, a pelvic exenteration (see Figure 12-4) may be performed with curative intent. This includes removal of the cervix, uterus, bladder, rectum, and part of the colon. Reconstructive surgery can restore anatomy and function; therefore, a referral should

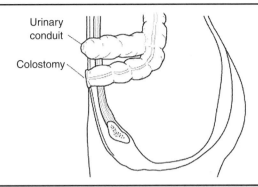

Urinary
conduit

Colostomy

Figure 12-4. After Pelvic Exenteration

Note. Figure courtesy of The Ohio State University Wexner Medical Center. Used with permission.

be made to a reconstructive surgeon who has experience with these procedures. Surgery may not be an option in later-stage cancer because the bladder and rectum are close in proximity to the vagina. RT alone may be recommended.

Cervical Cancer

Anatomy and Presentation

The cervical canal (see Figure 12-1) extends from the isthmus to the vagina. The transformation zone or squamo-columnar junction is the point at which the columnar epithelium of the cervix meets the squamous epithelium of the vagina. This is a site of continuous cell renewal and, thus, a common site of cancer. Cervical cancer may occur along the lining of the vagina or in the canal (Cartwright-Alcarese & O'Sullivan, 2010).

Cervical carcinoma is often asymptomatic. Once cancerous cells invade nearby tissue, abnormal vaginal bleeding occurs and is the most common presenting symptom.

Diagnostic and Staging Procedures

While routine screening with the Papanicolaou (Pap) smear can prevent cancer by identifying the presence of cancer-causing human papillomavirus, it can also detect cancer in its earliest stage (American

Cancer Society, 2013). NCCN (2013a) recommends a cone biopsy to accurately determine the presence of microinvasive or invasive disease. Once cervical cancer is diagnosed, further diagnostic testing with surgical staging should be performed (NCCN, 2013a). Moore (2008) reported that although the outcomes of randomized clinical trials demonstrated surgical staging to be more accurate, radiographic diagnostic and staging procedures may still be very effective. Surgical staging may detect microscopic nodal disease that cannot be detected with radiologic imaging.

Laparoscopic and robotic approaches for staging and treatment planning show promise for decreased hospital length of stay, reduced morbidity, and more rapid recovery (Lowe et al., 2009; NCCN, 2013a), although long-term data are not available to compare these methods with traditional surgical staging. Investigators who evaluated PET/CT scans in early-stage cervical carcinoma reported that they may be useful to correct false negatives (Yu et al., 2011). The role of sentinel lymph node biopsy is not yet validated with cervical cancer and should be used in a clinical trial setting only. The most common histologic types of cervical cancer include cervical intraepithelial neoplasia, squamous cell carcinoma in situ, invasive squamous cell carcinoma, and invasive adenocarcinoma. Lymph node involvement is the strongest prognostic and treatment indicator (Forner & Lampe, 2011; NCCN, 2013a). Serum tumor markers may provide important information regarding lymph node status. For example, both P16INK4A overexpression and fluorescence in situ hybridization (known as FISH) markers predict lymph node metastasis in cervical carcinomas (Huang & Lee, 2012; Wangsa et al., 2009). Common sites of metastases in cervical cancer include direct extension into the parametrium, vagina, lower uterine segment, abdomen, lymph nodes, lung, liver, and bone.

Surgical Management

In nonivasive cervical cancer, an extrafacial hysterectomy is recommended. However, observation is an option for patients who have negative margins on cone biopsy. If lymphovascular invasion is present, a modified hysterectomy or trachelectomy is recommended. Although only low-level evidence is available, NCCN (2013d) recommends a pelvic lymph node dissection when lymphovascular invasion is present. Ideally, this approach should be conducted in a clinical trial. In stage I–II invasive cervical cancer, a radical hysterectomy or radical trachelectomy with pelvic lymph node dissection and para-aortic lymph node sampling is recommended. In stage II–IVA, a radical hysterectomy is recommended, and nodal status determines the need for additional surgical treatment, systemic therapy, and RT (Reynolds et al., 2010).

Endometrial Cancer

Anatomy and Presentation

Endometrial cancer, also termed *uterine cancer*, is the most common gynecologic malignancy (American Cancer Society, 2014). The uterus is a hollow, flattened, pear-shaped, fibromuscular organ that is composed of two parts: (a) body or corpus, which is the superior, thick-walled portion, and (b) cervix, the lower portion that extends into the vagina. These two parts are joined together by the isthmus, which is the narrowed part of the corpus. The fundus is the convex upper portion of the uterus where the fallopian tubes are suspended (Cartwright-Alcarese & O'Sullivan, 2010).

Endometrial cancer is often localized when diagnosed, as postmenopausal women present with symptoms of irregular vaginal bleeding. Nevertheless, the mortality rate for African Americans exceeds that for Caucasians (five-year survival of 61% versus 84%) (American Cancer Society, 2014), which may be related to an increased rate of advanced-stage cancers, high-risk histologies (i.e., serous tumors), and inadequate staging.

Diagnostic and Staging Procedures

In addition to routine evaluation and workup, genetic counseling may be indicated (NCCN, 2013d). The College of American Pathologists protocol for endometrial carcinoma was revised in February 2011 and includes the FIGO/AJCC staging update. In a woman with unexplained bleeding, a negative endometrial biopsy must be followed by a fractional dilation and curettage (NCCN, 2013d). For unexplained persistent bleeding, a hysteroscopy is indicated to detect lesions (e.g., polyps, cancer).

The NCCN (2013d) guidelines organize endometrial cancer into three categories to determine treatment: (a) disease limited to the uterus, (b) suspected or gross cervical involvement, and (c) suspected extrauterine disease. For all stages, pathologic and prognostic data from surgical staging are used to determine treatment options. The most common histologic types of endometrial cancer include epithelial carcinoma, uterine papillary serous carcinoma, clear cell carcinoma, or carcinosarcoma, which is also known as *malignant mixed Müllerian tumor*. Common sites of invasive endometrial cancers include local extension and distal intra-abdominal sites, distant organs, and lymph nodes.

Surgical Management

In disease limited to the uterus, surgical management includes peritoneal lavage for cytology and total hysterectomy/bilateral salpingo-oophorectomy (TH/BSO) with dissection of pelvic and para-aortic lymph nodes.

In suspected or gross cervical involvement, a radical hysterectomy is recommended with BSO, cytology with peritoneal lavage, and dissection of pelvic and para-aortic lymph nodes.

In suspected extrauterine disease with intra-abdominal involvement (e.g., ascites; omental, nodal, ovarian, or peritoneal involvement), surgical intervention includes TH/BSO, cytology with peritoneal lavage, pelvic and para-aortic lymph node dissection, and surgical debulking as warranted. The surgical goal is to remove all measurable disease. Patients with unresectable extrauterine pelvic disease (e.g., vaginal, bladder, bowel/rectal, or parametrial involvement) are typically treated with external beam RT or brachytherapy with or without chemotherapy, followed by reevaluation of tailored surgery. For extra-abdominal disease (e.g., liver involvement), palliative TH/BSO with or without chemotherapy, RT, and hormonal therapy may be considered (NCCN, 2013d).

In lieu of aforementioned surgeries, laparoscopic pelvic and para-aortic lymphadenectomy in association with total laparoscopic hysterectomy may be efficacious, with several caveats (Barnett et al., 2011; NCCN, 2013d). As previously discussed, patients who undergo procedures that are contrary to traditional standards need to be followed in a clinical trial.

Ovarian, Fallopian Tube, and Primary Peritoneal Cancers

Anatomy and Presentation

The two ovaries are almond-shape structures located near the lateral walls of the pelvic cavity, one on each side. The two fallopian tubes, also called *oviducts* or *uterine tubes*, each measure about 8–12.5 cm in length and 1 cm in width. They are located on each side of the uterus just below the fundus. The infundibulum is the fringed funnel-shaped end that curves up and over the two ovaries (Cartwright-Alcarese & O'Sullivan, 2010).

Presenting symptoms for ovarian cancer include a collection of symptoms such as palpable pelvic mass, ascites, abdominal distention, bloating, pelvic or abdominal pain, difficulty eating, early satiety, urinary urgency or frequency, change in bowel habits, and unexplained weight loss (American Cancer Society, 2014; Redman, Duffy, Bromham, & Francis, 2011).

Diagnostic and Staging Procedures

Diagnostic procedures include an abdominal/pelvic examination, gastrointestinal evaluation if clinically indicated, ultrasound and abdominal/pelvic CT scan, and chest imaging, as well as tests to evaluate serum CA 125, HE4, or other tumors markers as clinically indicated. The PET/CT scan has demonstrated its accuracy to diagnose primary and recurrent ovarian cancer with lesions greater than 1 cm; false positives are a limitation (Prakash, Cronin, & Blake, 2010). The common sites of metastasis include local extension to adjacent organs, the peritoneal cavity, lymph nodes, and, less commonly, distant organs. Genetic and family risk history should be evaluated (NCCN, 2013b).

Surgical Management

Laparotomy/hysterectomy with comprehensive staging is recommended for patients with early-stage disease. Unilateral salpingo-oophorectomy for patients who desire to preserve fertility may be considered in select patients (NCCN, 2013c). Cytoreductive surgery is the goal for clinical stages II, III, and IV. The surgical management of patients with ovarian cancer is extensive and includes a comprehensive and meticulous inspection of the peritoneum with excision of all suspicious disease. It is essential to quantify the extent of initial and residual disease with aspiration of ascites, peritoneal lavage for cytologic examinations, and biopsies of the peritoneal surface or adhesions suspicious for harbored metastasis from the entire surgical region. For stage II–IV disease, omentectomy and aortic lymph node dissection are also recommended.

NCCN (2013c) recommends that primary peritoneal and fallopian tube cancers be treated in the same manner as ovarian cancer with extensive surgical clearance of disease. In general, the goal of surgery for ovarian, fallopian tube, or primary peritoneal cancer is to establish the extent of disease and to cytoreduce the tumor burden to less than 1 cm or to completely remove all disease (NCCN, 2013c). Aspiration of ascites or peritoneal lavage, excision or biopsy of any suspicious sites, hysterectomy, bilateral salpingectomy, and bilateral oophorectomy is recommended with removal of encapsulated masses intact. NCCN (2013c) recommends that the following procedures be considered for optimal surgical cytoreduction in all stages of disease: bowel resection, cholecystectomy, diaphragm stripping, distal pancreatectomy, partial cystectomy, partial gastrectomy, partial hepatectomy, splenectomy, radial pelvic dissection, and ureterocystostomy.

For patients with advanced disease, ancillary palliative surgical procedures include insertion of a gastrostomy tube, indwelling peritoneal or pleural catheter, intestinal stents, ureteral stents/nephrostomy, or vascular access device, as well as paracentesis, surgical relief of intestinal obstruction, thoracentesis/pleurodesis, and video-assisted thoracoscopy.

Conclusions

Ideally, all patients with gynecologic cancers should be managed in a clinical trial setting. Oncology nurses support patients using a multidisciplinary approach, which ensures access to resources that address all aspects of care, including physical, functional, psychological, social, cultural, spiritual, and financial. Patients with gynecologic cancer who undergo surgery may experience distress associated with alterations in appearance, functional status, sexuality, and fertility. Nursing knowledge of the surgical management of gynecologic cancers and an understanding of the perception of symptom experience throughout the plan of care is essential. Resources can be directed toward the causes of distress, symptom management, and education to promote optimal recovery and health during this challenging time in a woman's life. The NCCN guidelines for supportive care and the Oncology Nursing Society Putting Evidence Into Practice resources (Eaton & Tipton, 2009) provide evidence-based education and interventions to address distress and symptoms commonly associated with cancer and its sequelae.

References

Aikins-Murphy, P. (1990). Anatomy and physiology of the female reproductive system. In R. Lichtman & S. Papera (Eds.), *Gynecology: Well-woman care* (pp. 3–17). East Norwalk, CT: Appleton and Lange.

American Cancer Society. (2014). *Cancer facts and figures 2014.* Retrieved from http://www.cancer.org/research/cancerfactsstatistics/cancerfactsfigures2014/index

Barnett, J.C., Havrilesky, L.J., Bondurant, A.E., Fleming, N.D., Lee, P.S., Secord, A.A., ... Valea, F.A. (2011). Adverse events associated with laparaocopy vs laparotomy in the treatment of endometrial cancer. *American Journal of Obstetrics and Gynecology, 205,* e1–e6. doi:10.1016/j.ajog.2011.03.012

Bickley, L.S., & Szilagyi, P.G. (2007). *Bates' guide to physical examination and history taking* (9th ed.). Philadelphia, PA: Lippincott Williams & Wilkins.

Cartwright-Alcarese, F., & O'Sullivan, J. (2010). Anatomy, physiology, and pathophysiology. In L. Almadrones-Cassidy (Ed.), *Site-specific cancers series: Gynecologic cancers* (pp. 3–15). Pittsburgh, PA: Oncology Nursing Society.

Eaton, L.H., & Tipton, J.M. (Eds.). (2009). *Putting evidence into practice: Improving oncology patient outcomes.* Pittsburgh, PA: Oncology Nursing Society.

Edge, S.B., Byrd, D.R., Compton, C.C., Fritz, A.G., Greene, F.L., & Trotti, A., III. (Eds.). (2010). *AJCC cancer staging manual* (7th ed.). New York, NY: Springer.

Forner, D.M., & Lampe, B. (2011). Exenteration as a primary treatment for locally advanced cervical cancer. *American Journal of Obstetrics and Gynecology, 205,* e1–e6. doi:10.1016/j.ajog.2011.03.057

Hacker, N.F. (2009). Revised FIGO staging for carcinoma of the vulva. *International Journal of Gynecology and Obstetrics, 105,* 105–106. doi:10.1016/j.ijgo.2009.02.011

Huang, L.W., & Lee, C.C. (2012). P16INK4A overexpression predicts lymph node metastasis in cervical carcinomas. *Journal of Clinical Pathology, 65,* 117–121. doi:10.1136/jclinpath-2011-200362

Lee, S.I., Oliva, E., Hahn, P.F., & Russell, A.H. (2011). Malignant tumors of the female pelvic floor: Imaging features that determine therapy: Pictorial review. *American Journal of Roentgenology, 196,* S15–S23. doi:10.2214/AJR.09.7209

Lowe, M.P., Johnson, P.R., Kamelle, S.A., Kumar, S., Chamberlain, D.H., & Tillmanns, T.D. (2009). A multi-institutional experience with robotic-assisted hysterectomy with staging for endometrial cancer. *Obstetrics and Gynecology, 114,* 236–243. doi:10.1097/AOG.0b013e3181af2a74

Moore, D.H. (2008). Surgical staging and cervical cancer: After 30 years, have we reached a conclusion? *Cancer, 112,* 1874–1876. doi:10.1002/cncr.23386

National Comprehensive Cancer Network. (2013a). *NCCN Clinical Practice Guidelines in Oncology: Cervical cancer* [v.3.2013]. Retrieved from http://www.nccn.org/professionals/physician_gls/pdf/cervical.pdf

National Comprehensive Cancer Network. (2013b). *NCCN Clinical Practice Guidelines in Oncology: Genetic/familial high-risk assessment: Breast and ovarian* [v.4.2013]. Retrieved from http://www.nccn.org/professionals/physician_gls/f_guidelines.asp#genetic/familial

National Comprehensive Cancer Network. (2013c). *NCCN Clinical Practice Guidelines in Oncology: Ovarian cancer including fallopian tube cancer and primary peritoneal cancer* [v.2.2013]. Retrieved from http://www.nccn.org/professionals/physician_gls/pdf/ovarian.pdf

National Comprehensive Cancer Network. (2013d). *NCCN Clinical Practice Guidelines in Oncology: Uterine neoplasms* [v.1.2013]. Retrieved from http://www.nccn.org/professionals/physician_gls/pdf/uterine.pdf

Pecorelli, S., Zigliani, L., & Odicino, F. (2009). Revised FIGO staging for carcinoma of the cervix. *International Journal of Gynecology and Obstetrics, 105,* 107–108. doi:10.1016/j.ijgo.2009.02.012

Prakash, P., Cronin, C.G., & Blake, M.A. (2010). Role of PT/CT in ovarian cancer. *American Journal of Radiology, 194,* W464–W470.

Redman, C., Duffy, S., Bromham, N., & Francis, K. (2011). Recognition and initial management of ovarian cancer: Summary of NICE guidance. *BMJ, 342,* 1–4. doi:10.1136/bmj.d2073

Reynolds, E.A., Tierney, K., Keeney, G.L., Felix, J.C., Weaver, A.L., Roman, L.D., & Cilby, W.A. (2010). Analysis of outcomes of microinvasive adenocarcinoma of the uterine cervix by treatment type. *Obstetrics and Gynecology, 116,* 1150–1157. doi:10.1097/AOG.0b013e3181f74062

Tantipalakorn, C., Robertson, G., Marsden, D.E., Gebski, V., & Hacker N.F. (2009). Outcome and patterns of recurrence for International Federation of Gynecology and Obstetrics (FIGO) stages I and II squamous cell vulvar cancer. *Obstetrics and Gynecology, 113,* 895–901. doi:10.1097/AOG.0b013e31819b413f

Wangsa, D., Heselmeyer-Haddad, K., Ried, P., Eriksson, E., Schagger, A.A., Morrison, L.E., … Lundqvist, E.A. (2009). Fluorescence in situ hybridization markers for prediction of cervical lymph node metastases. *American Journal of Pathology, 175,* 2637–2645. doi:10.2353/ajpath.2009.090289

Yu, L., Jia, C., Wang, X., Lu, P., Tian, M., Wang, W., & Lou, G. (2011). Evaluation of ^{18}F-FDG PET/CT in early-stage cervical carcinoma. *American Journal of Medicine and Science, 341,* 96–100. doi:10.1097/MAJ.0b013e3181f48df6

CHAPTER 13

Surgical Care of Cancers of the Male Pelvis and Urologic Cancers

Joanne L. Lester, PhD, CNP, AOCN®

Introduction

Male primary pelvic cancers consist of internal and external reproductive cancer sites, including the urinary tract (i.e., bladder, kidney, ureter, and urethra), rectum, and anus. Internal male reproductive cancers are limited to the prostate; external reproductive cancers include penile and testicular cancers. The male anatomy has multiple structures in close proximity with an extensive nodal component that is opportune for regional metastasis, as well as distal metastasis through hematopoietic and lymphocytic channels (see Figure 13-1). Surgical techniques and the frequency and volume of specialized techniques are important outcome variables for male pelvic cancers. The National Comprehensive Cancer Network (NCCN) provides detailed algorithms that describe evidence-based interventions for the treatment of these cancers.

Penile Cancer

Penile cancer is a relatively rare cancer (Clark et al., 2013; Siegel, Ma, Zou, & Jemal, 2014) that presents as an ulcerated lesion on the penile skin or as a mass on or within the organ. Lesions can originate under the foreskin and may present as a festering, infected wound (Held-Warmkessel, 2012). Associated urinary symptoms are rare unless more extensive disease is found with tumor encroachment of the internal uri-

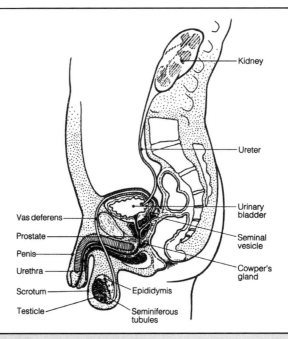

Figure 13-1. Male Pelvic Anatomy

Note. Figure courtesy of the National Cancer Institute.

nary structures. At presentation, a thorough physical examination is indicated to identify the lesion or mass of origin; examination of the scrotum is essential to determine direct extension of disease. The clinical stage of disease is based on the size of the lesion, pathology results, radiographic evaluation, and palpation of surrounding structures with biopsies as needed.

Biopsy

Tissue biopsy is essential to the differential diagnosis between primary penile cancer and lesions secondary to sexually transmitted diseases. An incisional wedge biopsy is recommended (Held-Warmkessel, 2012) because a small superficial biopsy may not provide enough cells for a definitive diagnosis. Enlarged or palpable lymphadenopathy at diagnosis may reflect infected, reactive, or metastatic lymph nodes. Palpable lymph nodes can be assessed with fine needle aspiration (Ercole, Pow-Sang, & Spiess, 2011); core needle biopsy should be performed with caution because structures within the pelvis may be accidentally punctured by the spring-regulated needle. Ultrasound guidance may aid the surgeon is isolating the lymph nodes in question and prevent disruption of underlying structures. Lymph node status remains the most important prognostic factor (Clark et al., 2013).

Surgical Management

Similar to other solid tumor therapies, the recommended treatment of penile cancer is based on signs and symptoms, pathology results, and the clinical stage of disease. Eradication of in situ disease can be accomplished through surgical excision, laser therapy, or topical chemotherapeutic agents (Held-Warmkessel, 2012). Mohs micrographic surgery may be effective treatment for small low-grade lesions with suture closure or by secondary intent wound healing (Wells & Taylor, 2010).

Invasive disease findings require local control and consideration of regional and distal involvement. Surgical interventions include partial or full organ removal (e.g., penectomy) and sampling or removal of the affected pelvic lymph nodes. Distal lesions may be controlled with circumcision and glans-sparing surgical resection to preserve the overall organ (Held-Warmkessel, 2012), whereas medial lesions require resection of most of the penis in an attempt to provide local disease control.

Evaluation of the nodal system is essential to disease management of primary penile cancer. The level of lymph node involvement is predictive of disease management and survival status (Ercole et al., 2011). Sentinel lymph node biopsy can be used to identify and remove the first draining nodes of the primary lesion with potential preservation of remaining nodes. Ipsilateral or bilateral pelvic and inguinal lymphadenectomy may be performed depending on the clinical stage of disease as determined by physical and radiographic evaluation.

Side Effects of Penile Surgery

Despite attempts to preserve the overall organ, patients who undergo surgical resection for penile cancer may experience side effects that compromise their physical and emotional healing. Sexual and urinary function may be altered depending on the extent of surgery and degree of healing. Compromised wound healing is common because of the organ location, warm and moist healing conditions, and involvement of eroded skin surfaces. Side effects after bilateral pelvic or inguinal nodal dissections include wound infection or dehiscence, lymphocele, hematoma, lymphedema, and deep vein thrombosis (Ercole et al., 2011). Alterations in body image are also common depending on the extent of surgical resection, degree of healing, perceived image of the penis, and level of sexual functioning. Patients who undergo inguinal or pelvic lymph node dissection can be challenged with the side effects of lymphedema with ipsilateral, contralateral, or bilateral leg swelling and pain. Once lymphedema has been identified, interventions to control the lymphedema and education for patients with self-management techniques are essential.

Prostate Cancer

Prostate cancer affects the male reproductive gland that is anatomically located in the pelvis below the bladder and in front of the rectum. The urethra goes through the prostate gland from the bladder to the penis. An enlarged prostate gland can negatively affect the urinary system and cause infection, pain, and erectile dysfunction. Prostate cancer is common in older men and is more common in African American men than White men in the United States. From 2005–2009, African American men had a 63% higher incidence of prostate cancer than Caucasian men (DeSantis, Naishadham, & Jemal, 2013).

Surgical Management

Robotic-assisted laparoscopy is often used for prostate surgery because of the movement abilities and agility of the machine's instruments. Men undergoing a robotic prostatectomy experience less blood loss, decreased pain, decreased hospital stay, reduced recovery time, and greater satisfaction as compared to men who underwent traditional open surgery. In addition, they have five small port holes rather than the 7-inch abdominal incision required for open surgery (Chitlik, 2011).

The treatment of prostate cancer has been variable over the past several years with treatment options including close observation, radiation therapy, brachytherapy, cryotherapy, prostatectomy, radical prostatectomy, bilateral orchiectomy, and systemic treatment with hormonal therapy. Treatment recommendations are based on the patient's age, projected size of the tumor, potential lymph node involvement, pathology, grade (e.g., Gleason score), and metastatic potential.

Positioning is important when preparing for a radical prostatectomy, for which the total time under anesthesia is longer than for a standard open approach. The goals of positioning are to enable excellent access for the surgical team and to prevent obstacles to a successful surgery such as peripheral, brachial plexus, or ulnar nerve injury or alterations to skin integrity (Chitlik, 2011).

After surgery, patients go home with a urinary catheter; therefore, family and patient education includes catheter care. The urine may remain pink-tinged for weeks during the healing process. Patients can experience blood clots after surgery, so education also should include how to recognize them and when to call the physician or go to the emergency department for intervention.

Side Effects of Prostate Surgery

Erectile dysfunction (ED) is a common side effect of prostate surgery regardless of the surgical approach. ED can be caused by an assortment of changes, including damage to the neurovascular bundle branches, corporal smooth muscle damage, and penile hypoxia. The recovery of erectile function can be affected by age, erectile hemodynamic changes, and neurovascular branch preservation (Mirza, Griebling, & Kazer, 2011). It is important to assess presurgical erectile function to ascertain changes since surgery. ED can also occur after radiation therapy based on penile blood flow secondary to occlusive vascular disease, arterial dysfunction, and erectile hemodynamics (Mirza et al., 2011).

Urinary incontinence is also a common side effect of prostate surgery. The most common type is stress incontinence, which occurs when the bladder neck has lost outlet resistance. Urge urinary incontinence is prevalent because the bladder detrusor muscle involuntarily contracts during filling. When the bladder does not completely empty, men can experience overflow incontinence secondary to bladder contractures or urethral stricture. Men can also experience mixed incontinence with more than one specific type (Mirza et al., 2011).

Testicular Cancer

Testicular cancer forms in tissues of one or both testicles and most commonly occurs in young or middle-aged men, although is a relatively uncommon cancer (Siegel et al., 2014). Most testicular cancers arise from germ cells and are thus referred to as *malignant germ cell tumors*.

Surgical Management

The standard surgical treatment for testicular cancer includes unilateral or bilateral orchiectomy with unilateral or bilateral retroperitoneal lymph node dissection as primary treatment and secondary treatment following neoadjuvant chemotherapy (NCCN, 2013; Viatori, 2012). Nerve-sparing techniques are used when this approach does not interfere with resection of potential or evident disease (NCCN, 2013). In the neoadjuvant setting, it is recommended that patients undergo surgery at a comprehensive cancer center with a high volume of surgeries to maximize outcomes. Completeness of resection remains an important predictive variable of future disease-related outcomes (NCCN, 2013).

Side Effects of Testicular Surgery

The potential side effects of testicular surgery are directly related to the level of treatment recommended (e.g., chemotherapy, radiation therapy, surgery), the pathologic extent of disease, and the extent of individual treatments. In regard to surgery, an orchiectomy can have a negative impact on fertility regardless of whether a unilateral or bilateral orchiectomy is performed. All patients with testicular cancer should be given the option for sperm banking before any treatment begins to ensure viability of their sperm for future use. In addition, the absence of one or both testicles, potential or real ED, and potential life changes may cause significant psychological distress. Nurses should screen for distress and assess for difficulties or expressed changes in self-image, depression, frustration, and alterations in sexual dysfunction (Moore, Higgins, & Sharek, 2012).

Urinary Tract and Urothelial Cancers

Urinary tract and urothelial cancers are not limited to males, although they occur twice as often in men than women (Siegel et al., 2014). Cancers such as bladder, renal, ureter, and urethral may be some of the most preventable cancers, as nearly 80% are related to tobacco use, including secondary smoke exposure. American Indians and Alaska Natives are among the highest racial/ethnic group in the United States to be affected (Siegel et al., 2014). Of additional concern is the potential for a second primary malignancy (16%) that may involve another urothelial structure within five years of the initial diagnosis (Pruthi, Nugent, Czaykowski, & Demers, 2013) or cancers of the lung or breast.

Bladder Cancer

Bladder cancers most commonly occur in the inner tissues that line the bladder and present with painless hematuria. Cellular types of bladder cancer include transitional cell, squamous cell, and adenocarcinoma). Treatment may differ based on the origin of the cancer and the depth of invasion into surrounding tissues and layers of the bladder. People with bladder cancer may undergo cystoscopies every three months for surveillance, which is an examination of the bladder through the urethra using a lighted scope. Treatment for noninvasive bladder cancer may be limited to close surveillance or local chemotherapy instillations.

Surgical Management

Invasive bladder cancer that penetrates through the muscular layers is treated by a radical cystectomy (Tyler, 2012). The surgical procedure may differ between men and women based on regional genital organs that may also be affected. In men, the surgery typically involves a radical cystectomy, prostatectomy, and lymphadenectomy; in women, a pelvic exenteration may occur with a cystectomy, lymphadenectomy, hysterectomy, bilateral salpingo-oophorectomy, and removal of vaginal tissue (Tyler, 2012) because local control of the disease is of prime importance.

After a cystectomy, urinary function must be restored with one of several urinary diversion procedures, such as incontinent cutaneous diversion or ileal conduit, continent cutaneous diversion, bladder reconstruction, or neobladder (see Figures 13-2–13-4) with orthotopic reconstruction (Lester, 2012). Differences in the reconstruction are based on the extent of cancer surgery, history of previous abdominal surgeries, patient preference, and remaining anatomic structure. Reconstruction can include an external stoma with bag (e.g., incontinent cutaneous diversion, or Bricker ileal conduit), stoma with one-way valve for self-catheterization (e.g., continent diversion, or Indiana pouch), reservoir inside the pelvis connected to the urethra for natural voiding (e.g., neobladder), indwelling catheter from the renal pelvis to an external bag (e.g., nephrostomy), or ureteral stoma with bag (e.g., ureterostomy) (Lester, 2012; Tyler, 2012).

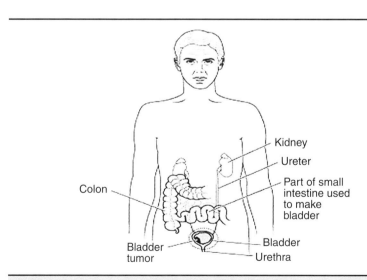

Figure 13-2. Ileal Conduit

Note. Figure courtesy of The Ohio State University Wexner Medical Center. Used with permission.

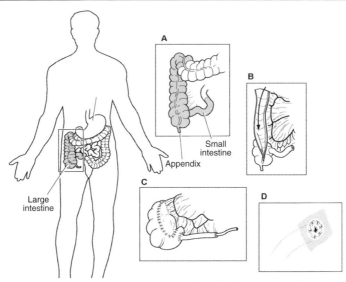

A: The shaded area is removed to make a pouch. B and C: The bowel will be cut open, folded and then stitched. D: A pouch is created from the large intestine to store urine. A valve at the junction of the large and small intestines keeps urine from flowing out of the pouch. The end of the small intestine is brought out to the abdominal wall to make a stoma, through which a catheter is placed to drain the pouch.

Figure 13-3. Continent Urinary Diversion

Note. Figure courtesy of The Ohio State University Wexner Medical Center. Used with permission.

Renal Cancer

Renal cancers affect the kidney and ureteral structures, specifically the renal pelvis and ureter. The mainstay of surgery for these cancers has been the radical nephrectomy with removal of the entire kidney along with the hilar vessels as indicated. In small tumors, treatment options include radical nephrectomy, partial nephrectomy, ablation, and surveillance (Yang, Villalta, Meng, & Whitson, 2012). The overall goal of surgery is to preserve renal and cardiovascular integrity and decrease early mortality using nephron-sparing treatments. Patients undergoing a radical nephrectomy increase their risk of future chronic kidney disease by 25% (Weight et al., 2010).

The surgical treatment of renal cell carcinoma includes radical nephrectomy or partial nephrectomy with noninvasive approaches, such as laparoscopy and robotic procedures, or the traditional open abdominal surgery (Lucas, Mellon, Erntsberger, & Sundaram, 2012). Preoperative data such as previous history of renal cancer surgery, solitary kidneys, or metastatic

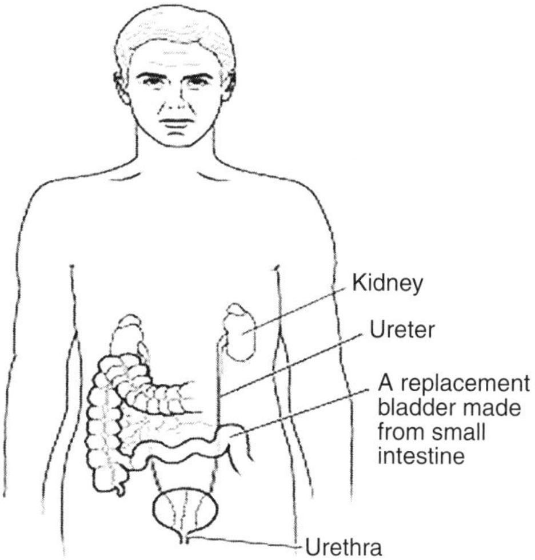

Figure 13-4. Neobladder

Note. Figure courtesy of The Ohio State University Wexner Medical Center. Used with permission.

disease are important considerations for surgical decision making, as well as age, sex, race, glomerular filtration rate, comorbidities, and body mass index. The open approach involves greater blood loss and longer hospital stay time, although it is a faster surgery with less ischemia to any remaining kidney. The robotic approach is a longer surgery; however, it is associated with less morbidity, less blood loss, and a shorter hospital stay (Lucas et al., 2012).

Conclusions

Cancers of the male pelvis and urologic cancers are often complex with multiple physical and psychosocial alterations. Issues related to urinary, genital, and sexual function are of prime concern to most patients and may lead to suboptimal treatment decisions. Ongoing discussion with the patient and family is important in order to identify barriers to comprehension about the disease and personal goals and objectives to disease management.

Early rehabilitation with attention to survivorship issues may enhance patient and caregiver acknowledgment of physical or psychosocial alterations and ensure mutual communication and support. Timely referral to institutional or community resources may advance physical recovery, improve function, and increase ongoing dialogue. Nurses can facilitate communication between the physician and patient and the caregiver and patient and can provide resources to the patient and family, offering an integral measure of support for patients who may struggle with changes in their anatomy and bodily function.

References

Chitlik, A. (2011). Safe positioning for robotic-assisted laparoscopic prostatectomy. *AORN Journal, 94*, 37–45. doi:10.1016/j.aorn.2011.02.012

Clark, P.E., Spiess, P.E., Agarwal, N., Biagioli, M.C., Eisenberger, M.A., Greenberg R.E., ... Ho, M. (2013). Penile cancer. *Journal of the National Comprehensive Cancer Network, 11*, 594–615.

DeSantis, C., Naishadham, D., & Jemal, A. (2013). Cancer statistics for African Americans, 2013. *CA: A Cancer Journal for Clinicians, 63*, 151–166. doi:10.3322/caac.21173

Ercole, C.D., Pow-Sang, J.M., & Spiess, P.E. (2011). Update in the surgical principles and therapeutic outcomes of inguinal lymph node dissection for penile cancer. *Urologic Oncology: Seminars and Original Investigations, 31*, 505–516. doi:10.1016/j.urolonc.2011.02.020

Held-Warmkessel, J. (2012). Penile cancer. *Seminars in Oncology Nursing, 28*, 190–201. doi:10.1016/j.soncn.2012.05.008

Lester, J. (2012). Restoring and maintaining urinary function. *Seminars in Oncology Nursing, 28*, 163–169. doi:10.1016/j.soncn.2012.05.005

Lucas, S.M., Mellon, M.J., Erntsberger, L., & Sundaram, C.P. (2012). A comparison of robotic, laparoscopic and open partial nephrectomy. *Journal of the Society of Laparoendoscopic Surgeons, 16*, 581–587. doi:10.4293/108680812X13462882737177

Mirza, M., Griebling, T.L., & Kazer, M.W. (2011). Erectile dysfunction and urinary incontinence after prostate cancer treatment. *Seminars in Oncology Nursing, 27*, 278–298. doi:10.1016/j.soncn.2011.07.006

Moore, A., Higgins, A., & Sharek, D. (2012). Barriers and facilitators for oncology nurses discussing sexual issues with men diagnosed with testicular cancer. *European Journal of Oncology Nursing, 17*, 416–422. doi:10.1016/j.ejon.2012.11.008

National Comprehensive Cancer Network. (2013). *NCCN Clinical Practice Guidelines in Oncology: Testicular cancer* [v.1.2013]. Retrieved from http://www.nccn.org/professionals/physician _gls/pdf/testicular.pdf

Pruthi, D.K., Nugent, Z., Czaykowski, P., & Demers, A.A. (2013). Urothelial cancer and the diagnosis of subsequent malignancies. *Canadian Urological Association Journal, 7*, E57–E64. doi:10.5489/cuaj.234

Siegel, R., Ma, J., Zou, Z., & Jemal, A. (2014). Cancer statistics, 2014. *CA: A Cancer Journal for Clinicians, 64*, 9–29. doi:10.3322/caac.21208

Tyler, A. (2012). Urothelial cancers: Ureter, renal pelvis, and bladder. *Seminars in Oncology Nursing, 28*, 154–162.

Viatori, M. (2012). Testicular cancer. *Seminars in Oncology Nursing, 28*, 180–189. doi:10.1016/j.soncn.2012.05.007

Weight, C.J., Larson, B.T., Fergany, A.F., Gao, T., Lane, B.R., Campbell, S.C., ... Novick, A.C. (2010). Nephrectomy induced chronic renal insufficiency is associated with increased risk of cardiovascular death and death from any cause in patients with localized cT1b renal masses. *Journal of Urology, 183*, 1317–1323. doi:10.1016/j.juro.2009.12.030

Wells, M.J., & Taylor, R.S. (2010). Mohs micrographic surgery for penoscrotal malignancy. *Urologic Clinics of North America, 37,* 403–409. doi:10.1016/j.ucl.2010.04.012

Yang, G., Villalta, J.D., Meng, M.V., & Whitson, J.M. (2012). Evolving practice patterns for the management of small renal masses in the USA. *BJU International, 110,* 1156–1162. doi:10.1111/j.1464-410X.2012.10969,10987.x

CHAPTER 14

Surgical Care of Skin Cancer

Kathleen E. Morton, MSN, RN, and Catherine L. Levy, MS, RN

Introduction

The three primary histologic types or classifications for skin cancer tumors are basal cell carcinoma (BCC), squamous cell carcinoma (SCC), and cutaneous malignant melanoma. Although each tumor has its defective cell of origin located somewhere within the skin, each type also has an independent trajectory for treatment and potential for metastasis that defines its natural history and malignant potential.

Basal and Squamous Cell Carcinomas

BCC is the most common form of cancer worldwide. Of the 2.2 million new cases of skin cancer diagnosed in the United States each year, 80% are BCC (Netscher et al., 2011). These lesions typically penetrate the deepest layer of the epidermis and are commonly found on the head and neck areas of the body, areas highly exposed to ultraviolet radiation. Additional common sites of occurrence include other sun-exposed parts of the body such as the scalp, back, and shoulders. BCC can appear as shiny or translucent bumps on the skin that are white, pink, or red in color, or it may simply appear as a reddish patch of skin. A common first sign of BCC is a persistent, nonhealing sore on the skin. This sore may bleed, ooze, crust, or remain unhealed for weeks. BCCs tend to be slow growing and rarely metastasize to surrounding tissues and organs.

SCC is the second most common form of skin cancer with more than 250,000 new cases diagnosed each year. SCC risk factors include chronic sun exposure and immunosuppression, and it is particularly common among solid-organ transplant recipients (Netscher et al., 2011). SCCs have premalignant precursors and an in situ variant that arises from epithelial cells. They typically appear as a slow-growing round or scaly ulcer or a skin plaque that is red to brown in color. SCC is not limited to sun-exposed areas; it can occur in mucous membranes and genitalia and has the potential to metastasize via the lymphatic and hematopoietic systems. Perineurial invasion is a poor prognostic sign and is associated with both recurrence and metastasis (Tufaro et al., 2011).

Preprocedure

Surgical management for primary skin cancer varies significantly based on the malignant potential and anatomic location of the lesion. Well-demarcated BCCs with circumscribed pathology can be surgically managed by curettage, electrodessication and curettage, cryosurgery, or surgical excision. When clear pathologic margins are obtained, the cure rate is very high. Lesions with ill-defined edges may require more extensive surgery, typically Mohs micrographic procedure. In patients with multiple BCC lesions, electrodessication and curettage may be a more reasonable procedure. Typically, sentinel lymph node dissection is not indicated for BCC and SCC; however, in larger lesions with a high metastatic potential, it may be included depending on the anatomic area of the lesion (Netscher et al., 2011).

Procedure

Electrodessication and curettage for well-circumscribed, low-risk lesions compares favorably to excisional biopsy in regard to five-year local recurrence rates (Netscher et al., 2011). Confirmative diagnosis may still be obtained from residual material, although it is difficult to determine whether margins are positive or negative for tumor. Surgical excision can be accomplished with local anesthetic to the skin. The margin size is based on the primary lesion. For example, BCC requires a 2 mm margin for 1 cm lesions and margins of 3–5 mm with extension into the subcutaneous fat for lesions between 1 cm and 2 cm; for lesions larger than 2 cm, margins as wide as 10 mm may be necessary for local control (Netscher et al., 2011). Frozen sections are not typically performed for these excisions because of expense and time. Therefore, if the pathology report indicates positive margins, a reexcision must be performed. The exception may be for BCC and SCC lesions that are larger than 2 cm, especially if skin grafting is part of the surgery (Netscher et al., 2011).

Mohs Micrographic Surgery

Mohs surgery is a very precise procedure that attempts to remove a minimal amount of healthy tissue while removing thin layers of affected tissue. Mohs is indicated for BCC and SCC lesions that are greater than 2 cm, recurrent lesions, lesions with indistinct margins, and lesions in cosmetically sensitive regions such as around the eyes, ears, nose, or mouth. Mohs surgery is contraindicated in recurrent tumors within surgical scars (Netscher et al., 2011).

Mohs micrographic surgery removes layers of skin through a series of excisions. After each excision, tissue is frozen and the lateral and deep margins are mapped and stained for immediate examination under a microscope. Once skin layers are found to be disease free, the surgery is complete. The precision of this procedure allows the surgeon to remove all visible areas of cancer as well as irregular skin layers not visible to the naked eye. In the case of a non-Mohs surgery, a simple excision may require a second procedure to obtain clear margins. The ideal situation to prevent a second surgical procedure utilizes Mohs surgery to preserve tissue in facial lesions and reduce the overall amount of tissue removed while avoiding a skin graft (Viola et al., 2012). The patient must be sterilely prepped for the procedure for several hours, which will require him or her to remain in one position for an extended period of time. The duration of the procedure depends on the location and depth of the lesion.

Melanoma

Of the common skin cancers, melanoma is the histology with a metastatic potential that can cause premature death in younger people. Melanoma is often referred to as *cutaneous malignant melanoma* and has several morphologic subtypes, including rapid radial growth, superficial spreading, lentigo maligna, acral lentiginous, and other unclassified lesions. Other forms of melanoma include ocular melanoma, which arises within the eye, and mucosal melanoma, which commonly arises within the intestine or the vulva. Vertical growth of the lesion determines tumor depth and is one of the prognostic indicators. Breslow thickness measures the epidermal basement membrane to the deepest melanoma cells; the Clark level is the thickness of the lesion both above and below the skin's surface (Netscher et al., 2011).

Subungual and acral lentiginous melanoma occurs on the palms of the hands and soles of the feet and under the nail beds of the fingers and toes. The lesions are more common in dark-pigmented, non-Caucasian populations; 35%–60% of lesions occur in Americans of color as compared to 3% in Caucasians. At least 25% of patients present with clinically positive lymph nodes or metastatic disease; computed tomography or positron-emission tomography scans are often ordered preoperatively to determine the presence of metastatic disease (Woods, Bacon, Ballard, & Beech, 2012).

Melanoma is staged based on the pathologic assessment of the primary tumor. The American Joint Committee on Cancer (AJCC) Melanoma Staging Committee has gradually changed the staging of melanoma. Currently, prognosis and metastatic potential are based on tumor size, ulceration, and mitotic rate (Dickson & Gershenwald, 2011). Tumor size is designated as thin (less than 1 mm), intermediate (1–4 mm), and thick (greater than 4 mm). Ulceration of the skin related to the primary tumor is also assessed and defined as the lack of intact dermis overlying the lesion. This finding signifies a more aggressive tumor phenotype with a higher likelihood of metastasis (Dickson & Gershenwald, 2011). The primary tumor mitotic rate represents a new change in the AJCC staging. The hot spot or area of most mitotic figures is examined. This criterion replaces the Clark level of invasion and is used to determine if sentinel lymph node biopsy is warranted in T1b or higher lesions. In addition to the aforementioned criteria, variables such as age, gender, primary tumor site, extent of microscopic tumor burden, and number of sites of distant metastasis have prognostic relevance (Dickson & Gershenwald, 2011). Biomarkers are also used to determine the use of targeted agents (McGuire, Disa, Lee, Busam, & Nehal, 2012).

Surgical Management

Surgery is a primary treatment for melanoma, although consideration is given to positivity of regional lymph nodes and the presence of metastatic disease. For local control of lesions, wide excisions seek clear margins of 5 cm. If regional lymph nodes are positive or evidence of metastatic disease is present, it is unlikely that wide margins (e.g., 5 cm) will improve local control or survival.

The type of incision used is dependent on the location of the lesion. For lesions on long bone extremities, a longitudinal elliptical incision is typically used. Lesions on the trunk are generally made congruent to the muscle group, as improved healing will occur through primary intention. Lesions on the scalp, face, and neck may require a split-thickness skin graft (STSG) or a rotational flap to prevent dimpling or puckering at the operative site. Lesions that traverse joints or bending junctions may require a STSG to provide extra tissue for healing and prevent joint restriction after healing is complete.

Sentinel Lymph Node Biopsy

The most important prognostic factor in melanoma staging is the presence or absence of lymph node metastasis. Sentinel lymph node biopsy is used to stage melanoma through detection of micrometastatic disease in the associated lymph node basin. Patients with lesions with a Breslow thickness of greater than 1 mm or tumors smaller than 1 mm with an associated Clark level IV or V should undergo a sentinel lymph node biopsy. Current recommendation is to offer sentinel lymph node biopsy in patients with a thin (1

mm or less) melanoma if the primary tumor mitotic rate is 1 mitosis/mm²
or greater (Dickson & Gershenwald, 2011).

The standard method of sentinel node biopsy for melanoma includes injection of blue dye at the site of the lesion just before surgery, although some
surgeons also add radioactive technetium and perform lymphoscintigraphy
several hours before surgery. A small incision is made at the nodal bed (e.g.,
typically the axilla, popliteal region, groin, occipitus) to remove the nodes
that exhibit uptake of the blue dye and technetium (i.e., the sentinel node).
If the sentinel lymph node is positive, a lymph node dissection may be performed at that time (National Cancer Institute, 2011).

Postoperative Care

Wound care will vary depending on the size and location of the surgical site. If the surgery requires a large resection or lymph node dissection,
a closed suction drain may be placed to decrease the risk of hematoma or
seroma development. In extremity and trunk excisions, preoperative activities can be gradually resumed as tolerated. For patients who have had a
lymph node dissection, passive range-of-motion exercises are recommended to minimize restricted mobility of the extremity. Lifting is restricted to 10
pounds until the incisions are healed.

Sutures or staples are used to close the wound. Closures on incisions of
the extremities and back are typically left in place for two weeks because of
the relatively thin skin and movement associated with these areas. Sutures
on the face are typically left in place for approximately five days because of
the high vasculature associated with the face and also to minimize scarring.
Sutures in all other locations are left in place for 7–10 days.

If an STSG has been used, the donor site will appear as a partial thickness
"scrape" of the skin. A nonadherent or gauze dressing is typically placed over
the donor site to provide moisture and protection. Gradually the donor site
will heal through secondary intention, although it may take several weeks.
This is the most bothersome site for the patient, but moisture improves the
tension of the skin during the healing process. The skin graft is sutured using
a bolster dressing over the graft that remains in place for five to seven days to
minimize shearing or shifting of the graft. It is important to keep this dressing
intact; knowledge of how the graft was created allows the surgical team to remove the first dressing and replace it as necessary (Dunn, Ignotz, Mole, Cockwill, & Smith, 2011).

Surgical Management of Local Recurrent Disease

When recurrent disease is isolated to a limb, a repeat excision or perfusion with melphalan may be an option. Isolated limb perfusion is a surgical
therapy in which blood flow to the affected limb is isolated from the rest of

the body with the use of a tourniquet on the affected extremity. Venotomy and arteriotomy catheters are inserted into the main artery and vein of the limb to create a circuit that allows for infusion and removal of a high dose of chemotherapy with a bypass machine (Neto et al., 2012). This high dose of chemotherapy would be toxic if given systemically.

Hyperthermic limb infusion is a less invasive surgical procedure that utilizes small catheters in the affected limb's main artery and vein. These catheters are inserted percutaneously and a tourniquet is applied. A high dose of chemotherapy is infused and removed via a syringe, thus sparing the rest of the body from the cytotoxic drugs. Hyperthermic limb infusion is less invasive by avoiding the extracorporeal circulation with the bypass machine. Attention to first- or second-time use, as well as body surface mass, may decrease limb complications (Neto et al., 2012).

Conclusions

Nursing considerations for skin cancer will vary based on tumor histology and may include teaching of the diagnosis, causative factors, and guidelines for surgical management. BCCs, SCCs, and early-stage melanomas have a more favorable prognosis, whereas later-stage melanomas will require additional support, including psychosocial support, not only for the patient but for family members.

Postoperative instructions for patients who have had a wide local excision include providing written instructions for any dressing changes, instruction on signs and symptoms of infection, lymphedema precautions, and a phone number if the patient or family member has questions about the postoperative care. The nursing care plan should include education on preventing further skin lesions by avoiding sun exposure or tanning beds. Consistent application of sunscreen, even on cloudy days, along with the use of protective clothing such as a wide-brimmed hat, indicates that the patient understands self-care methods. Identification of suspicious lesions such as a mole that has changed in color or texture indicates a need for further evaluation.

It is imperative that instruction be provided to patients and family members for the possibility of recurrence, especially for those with a history of prolonged ultraviolet light exposure or early-stage melanomas. Educational materials are available through local community organizations and national organizations such as the American Cancer Society. Internet searches can unearth a wealth of information about the histology, treatment, and prognosis of the disease. Psychosocial considerations include the potential for serious body disfigurement from surgery or lymphedema from node dissections. It is important to assess patients' self-image as they cope with the cancer diagnosis and body disfigurement. They may benefit from participation in a support group or private counseling.

References

Dickson, P.V., & Gershenwald, J.E. (2011). Staging and prognosis of cutaneous melanoma. *Surgical Oncology Clinics of North America, 20,* 1–17. doi:10.1016/j.soc.2010.09.007

Dunn, R.M., Ignotz, R., Mole, T., Cockwill, J., & Smith, J.M. (2011). Assessment of gauze-based negative pressure wound therapy in the split-thickness skin graft clinical pathway—An observational study. *ePlasty, 11,* 116–126. Retrieved from http://www.ncbi.nlm.nih.gov/pmc/articles/PMC3060048

McGuire, L.K., Disa, J.J., Lee, E.H., Busam, K.J., & Nehal, K.S. (2012). Melanoma of the lentigo malignant subtype: Diagnostic challenges and current treatment paradigms. *Plastic and Reconstructive Surgery, 129,* 288e–299e. doi:10.1097/PRS.0b013e31823aeb72

National Cancer Institute. (2011, August 11). Sentinel lymph node biopsy. Retrieved from http://www.cancer.gov/cancertopics/factsheet/detection/sentinel-node-biopsy

Neto, J.P.D., Oliveira, F., Bertolli, E., Molina, A.S., Nishinari, K., Facure, L., & Fregnani, J.H. (2012). Isolated limb perfusion with hyperthermia and chemotherapy: Predictive factors for regional toxicity. *Clinics, 67,* 237–241. doi:10.6061/clinics/2012(03)06

Netscher, D.T., Leong, M., Orengo, I., Yang, D., Berg, C., & Krishnan, B. (2011). Cutaneous malignancies: Melanoma and nonmelanoma types. *Plastic and Reconstructive Surgery, 127,* 37e–56e. doi:10.1097/PRS.0b013e318206352b

Tufaro, A.P., Chuang, J.C., Prasad, N., Chuang, A., Chuang, T.C., & Fischer, A.C. (2011). Molecular markers in cutaneous squamous cell carcinoma. *International Journal of Surgical Oncology, 2011,* Article ID 231475. doi:10.1155/2011/231475

Viola, K.V., Jhaveri, M.B., Soulos, P.R., Turner, R.B., Tolpinrud, W.L., Doshi, D., & Gross, C.P. (2012). Mohs micrographic surgery and surgical excision for nonmelanoma skin cancer treatment in the Medicare population. *Archives of Dermatology, 148,* 473–477. doi:10.1001/archdermatol.2011.2456

Woods, C.C., Bacon, L.N., Ballard, B.R., & Beech, D.J. (2012). Subungual melanoma: Diagnosis and management. *Tennessee Medicine, 105,* 35–37, 42.

CHAPTER 15

Surgical Care of Brain Tumors

Susan D. Bell, MS, CNRN, CNP

Introduction

Surgery on the brain for tumor removal has been evolving for more than a century, and advances in the field have changed the approach and treatment significantly. Enhancements in neuroimaging allow improved anatomic and functional localization of tumors, while progress in surgical techniques and use of intraoperative adjuvant therapies make surgery safer and enable maximal tumor removal. A knowledgeable multidisciplinary team can enhance the patient experience with surgery and improve outcomes. The World Health Organization has classifications for more than 120 brain tumors, which are based on the predominant cell or tissue of origin and graded on the presence or absence of standard pathologic features (Osborn, Salzman, Thurnher, Rees, & Castillo, 2012). The most common types of primary malignant brain tumors are tumors of the neuroepithelial tissue such as astrocytomas (33.7%) and meningeal tumors such as meningiomas (35.5%) (Osborn et al., 2012).

Clinical Presentation

Most patients with primary brain tumors present with generalized complaints or a focal neurologic problem. Generalized symptoms such as fatigue, malaise, and unsteadiness are usually the result of increased intracranial pressure from tumor mass effect. More often, patients present with memory loss; cognitive changes; motor, language, or visual deficits; seizures; personality changes; nausea or vomiting; papilledema; or other focal neurologic signs relative to the location of the lesion (Chang et al., 2005). Although headaches are common in patients with brain tumors, headaches are rarely the sole presenting symptom and occur in only about 2% of cases

(Schankin et al., 2007). Nevertheless, patients who present with atypical headaches should be evaluated to rule out a tumor.

A brain magnetic resonance imaging (MRI) with gadolinium is the preferred diagnostic test for primary brain malignancies. After confirmation of a brain tumor, the patient is usually referred to a neurosurgeon to discuss treatment options. Anticonvulsants may be administered at presentation, especially if a seizure was the presenting symptom (Klimek & Dammers, 2010; Smith, 2010). Steroids (e.g., dexamethasone 4 mg three to four times a day) are also often administered at diagnosis, especially if the brain MRI demonstrates significant brain edema and the patient exhibits associated neurologic symptoms. Steroids should be taken with food; prophylactic medications often are administered to prevent gastrointestinal ulcers.

Surgical Management

The National Comprehensive Cancer Network (NCCN, 2013) guidelines for central nervous system cancers recommend maximal tumor removal when appropriate, with minimal surgical morbidity to provide an accurate diagnosis. The surgical plan is based upon pertinent patient and tumor factors such as patient age, medical history, neurologic examination, and performance status. Tumor type, location and number of lesions, grade, and vascular characteristics are also considered. Systemic imaging with computed tomography (CT) scans of the abdomen, chest, and pelvis may be indicated to identify any other malignant lesions and to verify the primary versus metastatic source of the lesion. Further neuroimaging such as single photon emission CT, positron-emission tomography scan, or functional MRI may be indicated to further differentiate and characterize any lesions. A cerebral angiogram may be warranted to identify the blood supply to the tumor.

Type of Surgery

The surgeon should discuss the objectives and plan for surgery with the patient and family: biopsy versus resection, awake versus asleep, length of the procedure, location of the incision, intraoperative adjuvant chemotherapy or radiation therapy, drains or catheters, and risks and benefits of surgery. Expectations of the surgeon with regard to improvement in symptoms and anticipated long-term sequelae should be discussed. The need for additional treatment after surgery (e.g., radiation therapy, chemotherapy) may be discussed, although specific interventions are dependent upon pathologic confirmation. Time for the patient and family to express their fears and concerns should be provided with appropriate psychological support. The timing of surgery (e.g., urgent versus elective) is based on tumor characteristics and patient symptoms, although most surgeries are planned, elective procedures. Any preoperative clinical trials should be offered, as applicable.

Preoperative Evaluation

Preoperative evaluation includes patient- and disease-specific blood work, anticonvulsant drug levels if appropriate, urinalysis, chest x-ray, and electrocardiogram. A history, physical, and comprehensive neurologic exam are obtained. Tolerance to previous surgery, family history of difficulties with anesthesia, and inquiries about medications should be discussed. Anticoagulants such as warfarin, clopidogrel, or aspirin should be stopped for an appropriate time frame, if possible. The use of herbal supplements should also be explored because of the potential for hematologic effects.

A methicillin-resistant *Staphylococcus aureus* (MRSA) nasal swab culture is obtained with the implementation of appropriate preoperative antibiotics. Those patients identified to have MRSA colonization or a prior history of MRSA infection are at higher risk for postoperative complications (Akins et al., 2010). To minimize the overall risk of infection, patients must shower and wash their hair with an antiseptic soap the night before surgery.

Intraoperative Management

After induction of general anesthesia, an arterial line, a urinary catheter, and sequential pneumatic compression devices are placed with a central venous catheter or large-bore IV lines. Preoperative images from the brain MRI or head CT are used to (a) plan the location and size of the craniotomy, (b) determine the relationship of the tumor to nearby critical brain structures, (c) serve as a guidance system to deeper subcortical structures, and (d) assist with tumor resection. An image-guided, three-dimensional stereotactic navigation system is used with or without a stereotactic frame to enhance the intraoperative plan (see Figure 15-1).

General neurosurgical principles are used to position the patient and minimize injury, promote venous return, and reduce brain retraction (St-Arnaud & Paquin, 2008). The patient is placed in one of four positions: supine, lateral, prone, or sitting. The patient's head is placed in the holding device to prevent movement during the surgery and secured with two to three metal screws into the skull (see Figure 15-2). Most often, the incision is made directly over the tumor yet behind the hairline for cosmetic reasons. The hair is shaved in a strip along the planned incision and subsequently scrubbed with an antiseptic surgical scrub. Immediately before the incision is made, IV steroids and an antibiotic are given; typically, IV mannitol (0.5 g/kg of body weight) and furosemide are also administered (St-Arnaud & Paquin, 2008).

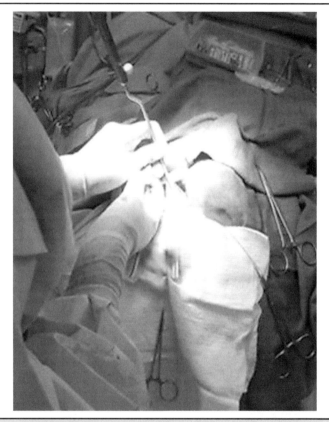

Figure 15-1. Use of Navigation System in Craniotomy

Note. Photo courtesy of Susan D. Bell, MS, CNRN, CNP, The Ohio State University. Used with permission.

The skin incision is created and carried down to the bone with cauterization of small vessels. The scalp flap is turned back and carefully rolled around gauze to prevent sharp kinks; the exposed flap is kept moist with antibiotic-soaked sponges during the procedure. One or more burr holes are created with a high-speed drill to penetrate the bone. A craniotome (specialized bone saw) is used to connect the burr holes and remove the bone flap (see Figure 15-3). The dura is carefully opened with avoidance of venous anatomy and reflected back with sutures. Once exposed, the abnormal tissue can usually be visualized and differentiated. Stereotactic and surface ultrasound can be used to localize the tumor if necessary. Tumors can either be debulked circumferentially or dissected in an outward direction. Tumor removal is completed with an ultrasonic aspirator, dissection, suction, and bipolar cautery. When tumors involve the speech or motor cortex,

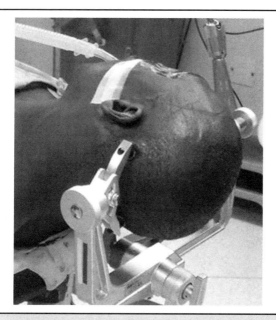

Figure 15-2. Patient Positioned in the Head-Holding Device

Note. Photo courtesy of Susan D. Bell, MS, CNRN, CNP, The Ohio State University. Used with permission.

the surgery may occur with only local anesthesia with cortical mapping and clinical monitoring (e.g., the awake craniotomy) (Chang et al., 2011; Sanai & Berger, 2010; Yordanova, Moritz-Gasser, & Duffau, 2011).

The goal of resection differs according to the tumor pathology. Meningiomas require complete removal of the tumor plus the dural attachment; intrinsic high-grade gliomas involve resection of the gross enhancing tumor; and resection of low-grade gliomas is based upon the abnormal signal on T2-weighted MRI images. Intraoperative techniques are used to maximize tumor resection and include intraoperative MRI and fluorescent dyes (e.g., 5-aminolevulinic acid) (Kubben et al., 2011; Kuhnt et al., 2011; Stummer et al., 2008). A meta-analysis of 1,111 patients with supratentorial malignant gliomas demonstrated an increase in overall survival in those patients treated with resection instead of biopsy (Tsitlakidis et al., 2010). Sanai, Polley, McDermott, Parsa, and Berger (2011) reported that newly diagnosed patients with glioblastoma who achieve a greater than 78% resection of malignant tissue have an increased median survival rate of 12.5 months.

After initial resection, a tissue sample is sent to the neuropathologist for a preliminary diagnosis to aid the surgeon in further surgical decision making. With the patient in the operating room, the surgeon and pathologist must answer the following questions (Castro et al., 2011).

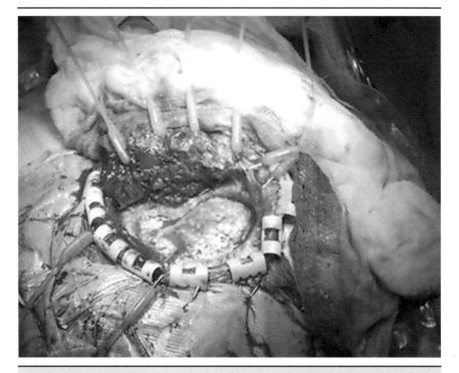

Figure 15-3. Exposed Brain Following Removal of Skull Bone

Note. Photo courtesy of Susan D. Bell, MS, CNRN, CNP, The Ohio State University. Used with permission.

- Was enough tissue excised to allow for a final pathologic diagnosis?
- Is the preliminary diagnosis likely to be more amenable to chemotherapy or radiation versus surgery?
- Can the preliminary diagnosis confirm the presence of tumor to proceed with placement of locoregional therapy, for example, chemotherapy wafers (polifeprosan 20 with carmustine implant), catheters for convection-enhanced therapy, or injection of viral/gene therapy?

After the surgeon has completed tumor resection and ensured hemostasis, the surgical cavity is irrigated with an antibiotic solution and packed with Surgicel®, an oxydized cellulose polymer used to induce blood clotting. The dura is closed in a watertight fashion, and the bone flap is replaced and secured with titanium plates and screws. The subcuticular structures are closed in separate layers with sutures; the skin is approximated and closed with sutures or staples. The patient is removed from the head-holding device, and a sterile dressing is applied.

Postoperative Care

After a craniotomy, patients typically spend one to two days in a neuro-intensive care unit for close observation, hourly vital signs, and neurologic measures. Optimal cardiovascular circulation and volume are maintained to provide for maximal brain perfusion; electrolytes, complete blood counts, and blood gas values are monitored several times per day. Airway patency and secretion management are critical, especially after endonasal approaches, as coughing can increase the patient's blood and intracranial pressures. Patients with preexisting hydrocephalus or third ventricular tumors may have a temporary postoperative ventriculostomy placed. A temporary lumbar drain may be placed after skull base surgeries to reduce the risk of cerebrospinal fluid (CSF) leakage (Bien, Bowdino, Moore, & Leibrock, 2007; Pepper, Lin, Sullivan, & Marentette, 2011).

A postoperative brain MRI is obtained within 24–48 hours to determine the extent of resection, postoperative surgical changes, and evidence of residual disease. Marked residual disease may be an indication for further surgery, perhaps even the next day.

In the initial postoperative period, the patient will be sleepy but should easily arouse and follow commands. It is beneficial to be familiar with the preoperative baseline neurologic examination in order to detect any postoperative deficits. The overall incidence of complications associated with brain tumor resection is 20%–35%, which includes neurologic, regional, and systemic events (Klein, Duffau, & Hamer, 2012). Neurologic deterioration should be reported immediately because increased brain swelling, hematoma formation, infarctions (e.g., venous, arterial), or pneumocephalus can occur rapidly after surgery. If complications are suspected, a head CT scan is performed; on occasion, surgical reexploration may be necessary. Patients can also neurologically decline secondary to seizures, hypoxia, or electrolyte abnormalities.

When the surgical procedure involves structures around the pituitary gland or hypothalamus, the patient should be monitored for the presence of diabetes insipidus, which can result in polyuria, polydipsia, and hypernatremia. The syndrome of inappropriate antidiuretic hormone can also occur, which causes water intoxication with associated hyponatremia, lethargy, and the possibility of seizures (Charalampaki, Ayyard, Kockro, & Perneczky, 2009).

The patient should be monitored for evidence of infection, although a low-grade fever or an elevated white blood cell count may be common the first 24–48 hours secondary to steroid administration and the surgery itself. The patient should be evaluated for CSF leakage and incision line drainage. Secondary to surgical site infection, meningitis is the next most common infection after a craniotomy (Barker, 2007). Antibiotic prophylaxis is effective in the prevention of surgical-site infections even in low-risk patients. Patients are maintained on prophylactic antibiotics for only 24 hours postoperatively because no evidence supports extending this time frame further (Barker, 2007).

Initiation of a steroid wean is dependent on the extent of resection, presence of postoperative swelling, length of time on preoperative steroids, and plan for postoperative treatment. The patient may complain of an increased headache or become more lethargic during the steroid wean. This is abnormal and should be called to the surgeon's attention. Anticonvulsant medications are continued for one week to three months after surgery. The prolonged use of anticonvulsants remains controversial (Klimek & Dammers, 2010; Komotar, Raper, Starke, Iorgulescu, & Gutin, 2011), although they may be continued indefinitely if the patient had a preoperative history of seizures or developed seizures in the postoperative period.

Pain and nausea should be evaluated after craniotomy. Thibault et al. (2007) reported that 76% of patients experienced moderate to severe pain for the first 48 hours after surgery. Frontal craniotomies were associated with less pain and required fewer opioids compared to posterior fossa procedures. Nausea can also occur frequently after craniotomy with documented incidence rates from 47% (Latz et al., 2011) to 56% (Thibault et al., 2007).

The surgical dressing is usually removed on postoperative day 2 and the incision left open to the air; ointments or creams are not recommended. A scarf or hat can be worn for cosmetic reasons. Most surgeons recommend maintaining a clean and dry incision until the sutures or staples are removed, which is about 7–10 days after surgery. Whether patients should shower and wash their hair is a controversial topic among surgeons. A prospective study randomized craniotomy patients at 72 hours after surgery to hair washing or no hair washing. No significant difference was reported in infection rates between the two groups (Ireland et al., 2007).

The patient's activity and diet are advanced as tolerated in preparation for discharge on postoperative day 3 or 4. The incidence of postoperative thromboembolytic complications after craniotomy for brain tumor ranges from 29% to 43% (Jenkins, Schiff, Mackman, & Key, 2010). The combined use of compression stockings, sequential pneumatic compression devices, and low-molecular-weight heparin is recommended (Knovich & Lesser, 2004), as well as early ambulation.

Conclusions

The science to support our understanding of brain tumor growth and development and therapy has exponentially increased. Improvements in outcomes are anticipated to be dramatic in the next decade. RNs and advanced practice nurses will continue to be integral members of the healthcare team for patients with brain tumors.

References

Akins, P.T., Belko, J., Banerjee, A., Guppy, K., Herbert, D., Slipchenko, T., ... Hawk, M. (2010). Perioperative management of neurosurgical patients with methicillin-resistant *Staphylococcus aureus. Journal of Neurosurgery, 112*, 54–61. doi:10.3171/2009.5.JNS081589

Barker, F.G. (2007). Efficacy of prophylactic antibiotics against meningitis after craniotomy: A meta-analysis. *Neurosurgery, 60*, 887–894. doi:10.1227/01.NEU.0000255425.31797.23

Bien, A.G., Bowdino, B., Moore, G., & Leibrock, L. (2007). Utilization of preoperative cerebrospinal fluid drain in skull base surgery. *Skull Base, 17*, 133–139. doi:10.1055/s-2007-970562

Castro, M.G., Candolfi, M., Kroeger, K., King, G.D., Curtin, J.F., Yagiz, K., ... Lowenstein, P.R. (2011). Gene therapy and targeted toxins for glioma. *Current Gene Therapy, 11*, 155–180. doi:10.2174/156652311795684722

Chang, E.F., Clark, A., Smith, J.S., Polley, M., Chang, S.M., Barbaro, N.M., ... Berger, M.S. (2011). Functional mapping-guided resection of low-grade gliomas in eloquent areas of the brain: Improvement of long-term survival. *Journal of Neurosurgery, 114*, 566–573. doi:10.3171/2010.6.JNS091246

Chang, S.M., Parney, I.F., Huang, W., Anderson, F.A., Asher, A.L., Bernstein, M., ... Laws, E.R. (2005). Patterns of care for adults with newly diagnosed malignant glioma. *JAMA, 293*, 557–564. doi:10.1001/jama.293.5.557

Charalampaki, P., Ayyard, A., Kockro, R.A., & Perneczky, A. (2009). Surgical complications after endoscopic transsphenoidal pituitary surgery. *Journal of Clinical Neuroscience, 16*, 786–789. doi:10.1016/j.jocn.2008.09.002

Ireland, S., Carlino, K., Gould, L., Frazier, F., Haycock, P., Ilton, S., ... Reddy, K. (2007). Shampoo after craniotomy: A pilot study. *Canadian Journal of Neuroscience Nursing, 29*, 14–19.

Jenkins, E.O., Schiff, D., Mackman, N., & Key, N.S. (2010). Venous thromboembolism in malignant gliomas. *Journal of Thrombolytic Haemostasis, 8*, 221–227. doi:10.1111/j.1538-7836.2009.03690.x

Klein, M., Duffau, H., & Hamer, P.C.D. (2012). Cognition and resective surgery for diffuse infiltrative glioma: An overview. *Journal of Neuro-Oncology, 108*, 309–318. doi:10.1007/s11060-012-0811-x

Klimek, M., & Dammers, R. (2010). Antiepileptic drug therapy in the perioperative course of neurosurgical patients. *Current Opinion in Anesthesiology, 23*, 564–567. doi:10.1097/ACO.0b013e32833e14f2

Knovich, M.A., & Lesser, G.J. (2004). The management of thromboembolic disease in patients with central nervous system malignancies. *Current Treatment Options in Oncology, 5*, 511–517.

Komotar, R.J., Raper, D.M., Starke, R.M., Iorgulescu, J.B., & Gutin, P.H. (2011). Prophylactic antiepileptic drug therapy in patients undergoing supratentorial meningioma resection: A systematic analysis of efficacy. *Journal of Neurosurgery, 115*, 483–490. doi:10.3171/2011.4.JNS101585

Kubben, P.L., ter Meulen, K.J., Schijns, O.E., ter Laak-Poort, M.P., van Overbeeke, J.J., & van Santbrink, H. (2011). Intraoperative MRI-guided resection of glioblastoma multiforme: A systematic review. *Lancet Oncology, 12*, 1062–1070. doi:10.1016/S1470-2045(11)70130-9

Kuhnt, D., Becker, A., Ganslandt, O., Bauer, M., Buchfelder, M., & Nimsky, C. (2011). Correlation of the extent of tumor volume resection and patient survival in surgery of glioblastoma multiforme with high-field intraoperative MRI guidance. *NeuroOncology, 13*, 1339–1348. doi:10.1093/neuonc/nor133

Latz, B., Mordhorst, C., Kerz, T., Schmidt, A., Schneider, A., Wisser, G., ... Engelhard, K. (2011). Postoperative nausea and vomiting in patients after craniotomy: Incidence and risk factors. *Journal of Neurosurgery, 114*, 491–496. doi:10.3171/2010.9.JNS10151

National Comprehensive Cancer Network. (2013). *NCCN Clinical Practice Guidelines in Oncology: Central nervous system cancers* [v.2.2013]. Retrieved from http://www.nccn.org/professionals/physician_gls/pdf/cns.pdf

Osborn, A.G., Salzman, K.L., Thurnher, M.M., Rees, J.H., & Castillo, M. (2012). The new World Health Organization classification of central nervous system tumors: What can the neuroradiologist really say? *American Journal of Neuroradiology, 33,* 795–802. doi:10.3174/ajnr.A2583

Pepper, J.P., Lin, E.M., Sullivan, S.E., & Marentette, L.J. (2011). Perioperative lumbar drain placement: An independent predictor of tension pneumocephalus and intracranial complications following anterior skull base surgery. *Laryngoscope, 121,* 68–73. doi:10.1002/lary.21409

Sanai, N., & Berger, M.S. (2010). Intraoperative stimulation techniques for functional pathway preservation and glioma resection. *Neurosurgical Focus, 28,* 1–9. doi:10.3171/2009.12.FOCUS09266

Sanai, N., Polley, M.Y., McDermott, M.W., Parsa, A.T., & Berger, M.S. (2011). An extent of resection threshold for newly diagnosed glioblastomas. *Journal of Neurosurgery, 15,* 3–8. doi:10.3171/2011.2.JNS10998

Schankin, C.J., Ferrari, U., Reinisch, V.M., Birnbaum, T., Goldbrunner, R., & Straube, A. (2007). Characteristics of brain tumor-associated headache. *Cephalalgia, 27,* 904–911. doi:10.1111/j.1468-2982.2007.01368.x

Smith, K.C. (2010). The management of seizures in brain tumor patients. *Journal of Neuroscience Nursing, 42,* 28–37.

St-Arnaud, D., & Paquin, M.J. (2008). Safe positioning for neurosurgical patients. *AORN Journal, 87,* 1156–1168. doi:10.1016/j.aorn.2008.03.004

Stummer, W., Reulen, H.J., Meinel, T., Pichlmeier, U., Schumacher, W., Tonn, J.C., … Pietsch, T. (2008). Extent of resection and survival in glioblastoma multiforme: Identification of and adjustment for bias. *Neurosurgery, 62,* 564–576. doi:10.1227/01.NEU.0000346230.80425.3A

Thibault, M., Girard, F., Moumdjian, R., Chouinard, P., Boudreault, D., & Ruel, M. (2007). Craniotomy site influences postoperative pain following neurosurgical procedures: A retrospective study. *Canadian Journal of Anaesthesia, 54,* 544–548. doi:10.1007/BF03022318

Tsitlakidis, A., Foroglou, N., Venetis, C.A., Patsalas, I., Hatzisotiriou, A., & Selviaridis, P. (2010). Biopsy versus resection in the management of malignant gliomas: A systematic review and meta-analysis. *Journal of Neurosurgery, 112,* 1020–1032. doi:10.3171/2009.7.JNS09758

Yordanova, Y.N., Moritz-Gasser, S., & Duffau, H. (2011). Awake surgery for WHO grade II gliomas within "noneloquent" areas in the left dominant hemisphere: Toward a "supratotal" resection. *Journal of Neurosurgery, 115,* 232–239. doi:10.3171/2011.3.JNS101333

CHAPTER 16

Surgical Care of Bone Cancers

Kristin Moore, RN, BSN

Introduction

Primary bone cancer, or sarcoma, is a rare cancer that starts in the bone. Primary soft tissue sarcomas are distinctly different from bone sarcomas, are treated with different regimens, and have different trajectories and outcomes. The term *bone cancer* is commonly confused with metastatic disease. Unlike sarcoma, metastatic bone disease represents a stage IV cancer, and treatment is based on mostly palliative measures. The most frequent sites of bone metastasis are long and flat bones with high levels of red blood cell production, such as the femur, humerus, pelvis, skull, ribs, and spine (American Academy of Orthopedic Surgeons [AAOS], 2012; Bickels, Dadia, & Lidar, 2009). This chapter will discuss sarcoma as a primary bone cancer and metastatic bone disease.

Primary Bone Cancer: Sarcoma

Incidence

The three main types of bone sarcoma are osteosarcoma, chondrosarcoma, and Ewing sarcoma. Each of these represents an extremely rare form of primary bone cancer. Osteosarcoma and Ewing sarcoma typically occur in the pediatric and adolescent age groups, and chondrosarcoma is typically seen in adults. The American Cancer Society (ACS, 2013) estimated 3,010 people were diagnosed in 2013 with a primary bone cancer; 40% were expected to have chondrosarcoma, 28% osteosarcoma, and 8% Ewing sarcoma.

Diagnosis

After a complete history and physical examination, multiple imaging studies are used to evaluate primary bone cancer. Plain radiographs with anteroposterior and lateral images are typically the first type of imaging studies obtained. Lesions smaller than 5 cm in diameter may not be visible on plain x-ray (Biermann, Holt, Lewis, Schwartz, & Yaszemski, 2009). Therefore, any suspicious lesion not apparent on plain films should be further imaged with a computed tomography (CT) scan or magnetic resonance imaging (MRI). MRI provides a three-dimensional image of the tumor and is usually the advanced imaging of choice for evaluation. The specific histologic type of bone cancer will be determined through biopsy of the lesion. Once the primary tumor site is confirmed, additional images may be warranted to determine the extent and degree of bony destruction as well as for complete staging. The multimodality treatment plan, with some combination of surgery, radiation, and chemotherapy, will be developed. MRI is used in planning the surgical excision, as well as following response to radiation or chemotherapy (Biermann et al., 2009).

Osteosarcoma

Osteosarcoma is the most common bone cancer in children and young adults 12–25 years old, with teenagers being the most commonly affected age group (ACS, 2012; National Comprehensive Cancer Network [NCCN], 2013). This corresponds to the time of rapid skeletal growth. Tumors most often occur in the distal or proximal end of the femur, tibia, or humerus. Osteosarcoma can also occur in older adults, typically those older than 60 years, although this is rare (ACS, 2013). Often, patients present with pain and swelling at the site of the tumor. As the pain and pressure progress, the patient may favor the limb, and a limp may be evident. Treatment includes neoadjuvant chemotherapy and surgery, followed by adjuvant chemotherapy. Limb salvage surgery is optimal, but depending on the location, size of tumor, and amount of bone destruction, amputation may be warranted (NCCN, 2013; Puri, Gulia, Jambhekar, & Laskar, 2012).

Chondrosarcoma

Chondrosarcoma is the second most common bone sarcoma and is primarily seen in those age 40 and older. This type of cancer develops from aberrant cartilage cells within the bone and is most common in the distal femur, proximal tibia, humerus, and pelvis. Chondrosarcoma is not chemotherapy or radiation sensitive; therefore, surgery with limb salvage or amputation is the treatment of choice.

Ewing Sarcoma

Approximately 500 cases of Ewing sarcoma are diagnosed each year (ACS, 2013). It is most common in patients 10–20 years old. Ewing sarcoma can occur anywhere in the body but is typically observed in the long bones of the arms and legs or in bones of the pelvis, chest, skull, or trunk. Ewing sarcoma arises from primitive mesenchymal stem cells (Subbiah & Kurzrock, 2012). Presenting symptoms include pain and swelling at the site of the tumor. Pathologic fractures can occur from seemingly minimal force at or near the site of the tumor because of tumor invasion. Ewing sarcoma is treated with both neoadjuvant and adjuvant chemotherapy followed by surgical resection. At the time of surgery, limb salvage is optimal for the patient, but amputation may be necessary (ACS, 2013; NCCN, 2013). In cases that are not in surgically resectable locations or if surgical margins are positive after resection, radiation may be used.

Metastatic Bone Disease

Incidence

Approximately 1.4 million new cancer cases are diagnosed each year in the United States; half of those are likely to metastasize to bone (ACS, 2013; Biermann et al., 2009). Half of the nearly 600,000 people who will die from cancer will have developed metastatic disease to the bone (ACS, 2013). Cancer metastasizes most commonly to the liver and lung, followed by the bone. Breast, prostate, thyroid, lung, and renal cell cancers represent more than 80% of all skeletal metastases. Patients who present with a solitary or limited metastasis versus multiple metastatic lesions may have an increased survival rate (Bickels et al., 2009; Biermann et al., 2009), although if one bony lesion responds to treatment, typically most or all lesions will respond.

Diagnosis

A complete physical assessment and medical history are essential prior to performing any radiographic testing. Assessment of any tender or painful areas and palpation for possible mass effects are indicated to detect abnormalities. Careful pain assessment is crucial to obtain an accurate diagnosis of possible metastatic disease. Only 20% of patients with skeletal metastasis will have significant symptoms. Many patients may be unaware they have metastatic bone disease because symptoms are often confused with exercise-induced or arthritic pain. Therefore, careful follow-up and imaging are warranted in patients with a clinical suspicion of bony metastatic disease.

Patients with symptomatic skeletal metastasis (see Figure 16-1) commonly present with constant pain that is not relieved by rest. Pain is typically worse at night and does not respond to usual interventions such as change of po-

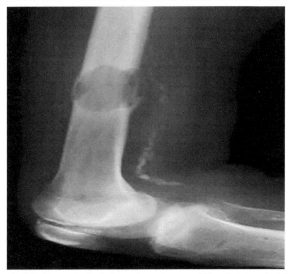

Lateral radiograph showing metastatic breast carcinoma of the distal part of the femoral di-aphysis. The lateral radiograph shows clear cortical destruction with tumor extension into the surrounding soft tissues.

Figure 16-1. Metastatic Bone Lesion

Note. From "Surgical Management of Metastatic Bone Disease," by J. Bickels, S. Dadia, and Z. Lidar, 2009, *Journal of Bone and Joint Surgery, 91,* p. 1506. doi:10.2106/JBJS.H.00175. Copyright 2009 by The Journal of Bone and Joint Surgery, Inc. All rights reserved. Reprinted with the permission of *The Journal of Bone and Joint Surgery,* www.jbjs.org.

sition or low doses of common pain relievers (ACS, 2013). Metastatic bone pain is often caused by the microscopic buckling of the bone secondary to weight bearing (Swanson, Pritchard, & Sim, 2000). These destructive chang-es may lead to pathologic bone fractures with replacement of normal bone with tumor or necrotic debris.

Diagnostic testing begins with x-rays to determine the type of bone changes caused by the lesion. Plain films can provide information about the lesion such as aggressive features, destruction of the cortex, perioste-al reactions, and fractures (Biermann et al., 2009). Osteolytic lesions oc-cur when the tumor is destroying the bone. This is commonly seen in solid tumors such as lung, thyroid, renal, and colon cancer. Osteoblastic lesions occur when the tumor is creating new bone to repair destruction, which is demonstrated in prostate, bladder, and stomach cancers. Metastatic breast cancer can present as osteolytic or osteoblastic lesions (AAOS, 2012). If metastatic disease is suspected, a CT scan or MRI can help determine the extent of disease and other possible complications, such as spinal metas-tasis with cord compression. Whole body bone scans may likewise be used to screen for metastatic disease. Positron-emission tomography is a newer technology that provides images of the entire body and evaluates increased metabolic activity (common in tumor deposits) and scans for additional lesions, although it may not fully demonstrate bony lesions. Physicians with significant expertise in bone tumor management can often differentiate between the lesions that can be safely managed through observation from those that are suspicious and need to be biopsied to confirm a diagnosis. Biopsies are often necessary for final diagnoses and can be obtained by fine needle aspiration or core needle, percutaneously under CT guidance, or as an open procedure (Bickels et al., 2009). Cancers such as renal cell, multiple myeloma, melanoma, and thyroid cancers may demonstrate false-negative results on nuclear medicine imaging studies, and these modalities may not appropriately identify metastatic lesions.

Preparation for Surgery

Multiple factors that are considered for surgical intervention in metastatic lesions, including location of tumor, size, specific bone involved, upper extremity versus lower extremity, presence of lytic or blastic lesions, and presence of pathologic fracture. Other considerations include the patient's general health condition, comorbid diseases, level of pain, and adequate adjacent bone for fixation. Lytic lesions have a higher rate of fracture than blastic lesions; therefore, fracture prevention with surgical fixation for lytic lesions has a much better outcome than fixation after a fracture occurs (Bickels et al., 2009). Generally, surgical intervention in the setting of metastatic disease is palliative, not curative, in nature. Expected surgery outcomes and changes in quality of life must be thoroughly discussed.

Preoperative Teaching

Standard preoperative testing and precautions are conducted prior to surgery. Avoidance of tobacco products is vital as smoking will delay healing because of constricted blood vessels and oxygen deprivation. Realistic expectations should be set for postoperative activity, incision-related pain level, and overall pain threshold secondary to metastatic bone disease. Chlorhexidine gluconate (CHG) soap is recommended for skin cleansing on the evening before and the morning of the surgery. This antimicrobial soap helps decrease skin infections and wound complications. Patients are prepped in the operating room with CHG and alcohol. Prophylactic IV antibiotics are administered at the start of surgery and immediately thereafter (Anderson et al., 2008).

Surgical Considerations

Lesions in the bone that are not radiation sensitive, such as metastatic renal cell carcinoma, are often surgically removed by curettage with placement of bone cement in the deficit, which allows for immediate weight bearing. Removal of tumors reduces the risk of hardware failure but increases the risk of infection and intraoperative blood loss.

Lesions that may respond to radiation therapy, such as metastatic breast cancer, are not removed but are stabilized with hardware. Subsequent radiation to the whole bone should be initiated two weeks postoperatively after appropriate wound healing. Metastatic renal cell carcinoma is a vascular tumor and is often embolized prior to surgical manipulation of the local tumor bed. Main vessels to the tumor are occluded by either coils or gel (see Figure 16-2) within 24 hours of surgery in order to diminish intraoperative blood loss and limit the need for perioperative transfusion (Bickels et al., 2009).

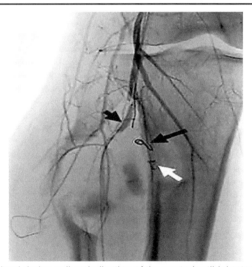

An angiogram obtained during coil embolization of the posterior tibial artery demonstrates successful coil placement of a proximal macrocoil (black arrow) and a distal microcoil (white arrow). A balloon can also be appreciated (short black arrow) in the anterior tibial artery to avoid thrombus and reflux of the coil.

Figure 16-2. Embolization of Main Tumor Vessels With Coils or Gel

Surgical Management

Intramedullary Nailing

The majority of weight-bearing bones, such as the femur and tibia, will require surgery with an intramedullary nail and screws if the patient develops pain from the lesion. This protects not only the weakened area of the lesion but the entire length of the bone, as well. Surgery takes one to two hours, and most patients will stay overnight for pain control. When a fracture is being repaired, partial weight bearing for six weeks post-op is indicated to allow for healing. When no fracture is present, weight bearing is allowed as tolerated.

Intramedullary Nailing of Non–Weight-Bearing Bones

Pain caused by fractures in non–weight-bearing bones can be treated by an intramedullary nail or plate and screws. Approximately 90% of patients experience a reduction in pain, if not complete pain relief, with some sort of fixation (Frassica & Frassica, 2003). Minimal activity restrictions are required after surgery unless a major muscle group (e.g., rotator cuff) is affected. Intramedullary nailing of the humerus, for example, involves surgery that takes one to two hours with an overnight stay to ensure pain control. Active range of motion of the shoulder is limited for six weeks to allow for the rotator cuff to heal; however, for plate and screws, activity restrictions are minimal (see Figure 16-3).

Hemiarthroplasty

A hemiarthroplasty is a partial joint replacement, which may be performed when a fracture or tumor disrupts smooth joint articulation, causing pain. It is often used in shoulder or hip fractures or tumors when a total joint replacement is either not necessary or not a good choice for the patient. When metastatic bone disease affects the femur and femur head and neck, a long-stem hemiarthroplasty prosthesis can be used. This surgery takes slightly longer, up to two hours, and has a hospital stay of two to three days. If a lesion develops distal from the stem, a plate and screws may be used (Biermann et al., 2009).

Girdlestone Procedure

Another type of surgery used for a femur head and neck lesion is called a Girdlestone procedure. This procedure is performed for pain control when a lengthy procedure cannot be tolerated. The fractured ball of the femur is

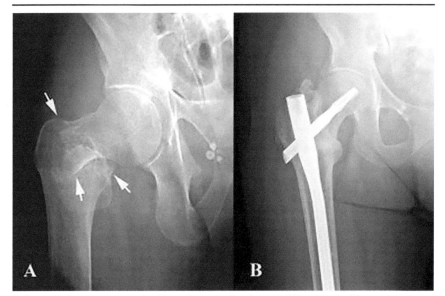

A: Preoperative anteroposterior hip radiograph showing a right basicervical femoral neck fracture after the patient experienced a low-energy fall (arrows). B: Postoperative radiograph made at 21 months following closed reduction and internal fixation with an intramedullary nail.

Figure 16-3. Intramedullary Nail Pinning to Reinforce Bone Strength

Note. From "Bilateral Pathologic Hip Fractures Associated With Antiretroviral Therapy: A Case Report," by B.J. Rebolledo, A. Unnauntana, and J.M. Lane, 2011, *Journal of Bone and Joint Surgery, 93,* p. e78(2). doi:10.2106/JBJS.J.00885. Copyright 2011 by The Journal of Bone and Joint Surgery, Inc. All rights reserved. Reprinted with the permission of *The Journal of Bone and Joint Surgery,* www.jbjs.org.

removed, setting the greater trochanter to rest on the pelvis. Although typically pain free, this shortens the leg about three inches, and a shoe lift is needed to balance the gait.

Replacement by Prosthesis

When significant cortical destruction has occurred in any bone, reconstruction using an oncologic prosthesis to replace the damaged bone is appropriate. This may also be an option if previous fixation has failed because of tumor progression or delayed healing due to radiation therapy. In situations where a fracture has occurred during radiation therapy, an oncologic prosthesis is used because the likelihood of the fracture healing is extremely low. This requires a major surgery. The destroyed bone must be completely removed and a metal joint and bone must be inserted (see Figure 16-4). A longer recovery and stricter activity restrictions are required during healing—three to six months or longer depending on the surgery required and location of the lesion. The surgeon must cut through the muscle and remove it from the bone. When the implant is in place, the muscle is sewn back to the hardware with strong suture. The patient must maintain a certain position to allow for healing of the muscle and surrounding tissues. The potential for dislocation during this healing period is extremely high. Hospital stays range from three to five days and may require an extended stay at a rehabilitation facility depending on the patient's physical ability. Physical therapy to restore function is required, yet long-term activity deficits can occur.

Pelvic Surgery

The majority of pelvic lesions are treated nonsurgically with radiation therapy. Prognosis and curative possibilities should be taken into consideration for this type of surgery, as rehabilitation for most pelvic surgeries can range from 3–12 months. Many of the muscles attached to the pelvis must be removed to locate the tumor. Once the tumor is removed, cement is often used to stabilize the area and to allow for immediate weight bearing. Hospital

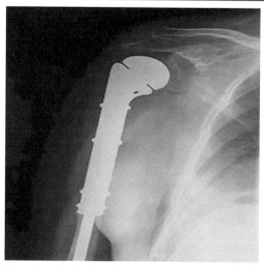

Anteroposterior plain radiograph showing the cemented proximal humeral endoprosthesis.

Figure 16-4. Shoulder-Forearm Replacement With Prosthesis

stays range from 3–14 days depending on the location, size, and extent of the surgery. More simple surgeries to perform curettage of the tumor, cement the deficit, and place stabilizing screws or pins allow the patient to ambulate as tolerated (see Figure 16-5).

Spinal Surgery

Many spinal lesions will respond to nonoperative treatment such as chemotherapy or radiation therapy. In situations where there is a displacement of the cord with neurologic deficits, emergency surgery is indicated. Other surgery indications include spinal instability, progressive neurologic deficit, intractable pain, or unresponsiveness to nonoperative treatment. Surgery allows for immediate stability for ambulation (Bickels et al., 2009). Multiple types of spinal surgery exist, but the goal remains the same: removal of the

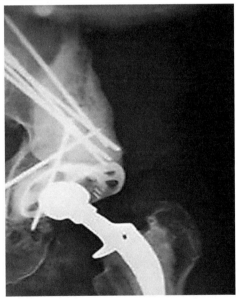

Anteroposterior radiograph of the left side of the pelvis, made after reconstruction with Steinmann pins and an antiprotrusio device as part of a total hip arthroplasty performed with cement.

Figure 16-5. Cement to Fill Postsurgical Deficit With Stabilizing Screws

Note. From "Instructional Course Lectures, The American Academy of Orthopedic Surgeons—Operative Treatment for Metastatic Disease of the Pelvis and the Proximal End of the Femur," by S.A. Rodeo, 2000, *Journal of Bone and Joint Surgery, 82,* p. 124. Copyright 2000 by The Journal of Bone and Joint Surgery, Inc. All rights reserved. Reprinted with the permission of *The Journal of Bone and Joint Surgery,* www. jbjs.org.

tumor, fixation of the bone, restoration of normal architecture and alignment, and maintenance of stability. Spinal surgeries include

- Vertebrectomy—removal of a portion of the vertebrae
- Vertebroplasty—injection of synthetic bone cement
- Kyphoplasty—inflation of a balloon to restore height followed by injection of the bone cement (see Figure 16-6)
- Laminectomy—removal of portion of the lamina.

Amputation

Amputation is rarely used for metastatic lesions. An amputation is indicated in situations where the bone and surrounding tissue are destroyed beyond repair, the tumor is surrounding vital structures such as the vessels or nerve, or the patient is experiencing intractable pain. Complete wound healing is critical before a prosthesis can be used; otherwise, the pressure of weight bearing could lead to wound dehiscence. When the wound is healed (typically in six weeks to three months), the patient can be fitted with a prosthesis and can begin physical therapy. Physical therapy is an important com-

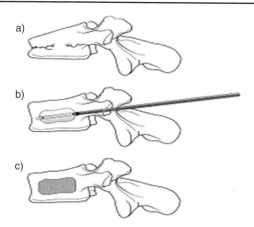

Restoration of vertebral height during kyphoplasty. (a) Vertebral space with compression: A fractured vertebra displaying loss of height. (b) Inflation and injection of space with cement: An inflated bone balloon displaces vertebral trabeculae and elevates the superior end plate, allowing some restoration of the height of the vertebral body. (c) Restored vertebral space: Removal of the balloon is followed by injection of methylmethacrylate into the void space.

Figure 16-6. Kyphoplasty

ponent of the overall outcome of any of these types of surgeries. Proper mechanics and gait training are imperative for maximum efficiency.

Nursing Management

Activity restrictions are dependent upon the location of the lesion, the mechanical integrity of the remaining bone, and the surgical construct. One advantage of having a prosthetic replacement versus internal fixation is the potential for immediate weight bearing and restoration of preoperative activity levels. Cementing a stem and intramedullary nails not associated with a fracture can allow immediate weight bearing. When placing an intramedullary nail through a pathologic fracture, it is best to partial weight bear for six weeks to allow for fracture healing. Allowing patients to bear weight sooner increases their quality of life, especially for those with a limited life expectancy.

Some postoperative issues affecting rehabilitation status are bone integrity, physical and overall medical status, and wound healing problems. Depending on the patient's overall physical and medical status, the healing time will vary. Those in need of adjuvant treatment, such as chemotherapy or radiation, and those who are immunocompromised will heal more slowly and will also have a depleted energy level. If at all possible, it is recommended that chemotherapy and radiation therapy be held until the surgical wound is completely healed. Any wound left unhealed during chemotherapy or radiation will not heal until the therapy is completed, if at all.

Standard postoperative wound care is to ensure that the incision stays clean and dry until the staples or sutures are removed at the two-week postoperative appointment. After that, the patient may shower but should not immerse the wound for another week after the staples or sutures are removed. Use of ointments and creams is discouraged until the wound is completely healed (Lagerquist et al., 2012). It is extremely important to keep the wound clean and dry because the ramifications of infected hardware will likely result in removal of the hardware and long-term IV antibiotics. Any postoperative wound complication will delay systemic treatment. Postoperative pin site care is just as important. Pin sites should be cleansed no more than once a week and inspected at each dressing change for signs of infection (W-Dahl & Toksvig-Larsen, 2003). A nonshedding swab soaked in alcohol-based solution should be used to clean not only the pin site but also the wound (W-Dahl & Toksvig-Larsen, 2004). Strict aseptic technique is used during the cleansing and dressing procedure while the patient is in the hospital. A clean technique should be taught for use at home (Santy, Vincent, & Duffield, 2009). The surgical incision as well as pin sites should be monitored for signs and symptoms of infection, which include pain, redness, or purulent drainage from the wound or pin sites (Santy et al., 2009).

Conclusions

The goals of surgical intervention in any bone malignancy are primarily to relieve pain, achieve local tumor control, and restore function that may allow for immediate use and provide mechanical stability. This also enhances the patient's quality of life and will allow for more independence; even nonambulatory patients are more likely to be able to transfer on their own. Importantly, it will provide both physical and psychological benefit to both the patient and family. Nonoperative management and appropriate use of contemporary, surgical, and reconstructive techniques can relieve pain and restore function, including ambulation.

Management of primary and metastatic bone cancers involves a multidisciplinary approach including the surgeon, medical physicians, nurses, and ancillary staff. Total patient well-being depends on the collaborative efforts of all involved. Patient care does not end after surgery but continues with ongoing cancer surveillance and survivorship guidance.

References

American Academy of Orthopedic Surgeons. (2012). Metastatic bone disease. Retrieved from http://orthoinfo.aaos.org/topic.cfm?topic=A00093

American Cancer Society. (2012). Bone metastasis. Retrieved from http://www.cancer.org/treatment/understandingyourdiagnosis/bonemetastasis/index

American Cancer Society. (2013). What are the key statistics about bone cancer? Retrieved from http://www.cancer.org/cancer/bonecancer/detailedguide/bone-cancer-key-statistics

Anderson, D., Kaye, K.S., Classen, D., Arias, K.M., Podgorny, K., Burstin, H., ... Yokoe, D.S. (2008). Strategies to prevent surgical site infections in acute care hospitals. *Infection Control and Hospital Epidemiology, 29*(Suppl. 1), S51–S61. doi:10.1086/591064

Bickels, J., Dadia, S., & Lidar, Z. (2009). Surgical management of metastatic bone disease. *Journal of Bone and Joint Surgery, 91*, 1503–1516. doi:10.2106/JBJS.H.00175

Biermann, J.S., Holt, G.E., Lewis, V.O., Schwartz, H.S., & Yaszemski, M.J. (2009). Metastatic bone disease: Diagnosis, evaluation, and treatment. *Journal of Bone and Joint Surgery, 91*, 1518–1530.

Frassica, F.J., & Frassica, D.A. (2003). Metastatic bone disease of the humerus. *Journal of the American Academy of Orthopedic Surgeons, 11*, 282–288.

Lagerquist, D., Dabrowski, M., Dock, C., Fox, A., Daymond, M., Sandau, K.E., & Halm, M. (2012). Care of external fixator pin sites. *American Journal of Critical Care, 21*, 288–292. doi:10.4037/ajcc2012600

National Comprehensive Cancer Network. (2013). *NCCN Clinical Practice Guidelines in Oncology: Bone cancer* [v.2.2013]. Retrieved from http://www.nccn.org/professionals/physician_gls/pdf/bone.pdf

Puri, A., Gulia, A., Jambhekar, N., & Laskar, S. (2012). The outcome of the treatment of diaphyseal primary bone sarcoma by resection, irradiation, and re-implantation of the host bone: Extracorporeal irradiation as an option for reconstruction in diaphyseal bone sarcomas. *Journal of Bone and Joint Surgery (British Volume), 94*, 982–988. doi:10.1302/0301-620X.94B7.28916

Santy, J., Vincent, M., & Duffield, B. (2009). The principles of caring for patients with Ilizarov external fixation. *Nursing Standard, 23*(26), 50–55.

Subbiah, V., & Kurzrock, R. (2012). Ewing's sarcoma: Overcoming the therapeutic plateau. *Discovery Medicine, 13*, 405–415.

Swanson, K.C., Pritchard, D.J., & Sim, F.H. (2000). Surgical treatment of metastatic disease of the femur. *Journal of the American Academy of Orthopedic Surgeons, 8*, 56–65.

W-Dahl, A., & Toksvig-Larsen, S. (2003). No difference between daily and weekly pin site care: A randomized study of 50 patients with external fixation. *Acta Orthopaedica Scandinavica, 74*, 704–708.

W-Dahl, A., & Toksvig-Larsen, S. (2004). Pin site care in external fixation sodium chloride or chlorhexidine solution as a cleansing agent. *Archives of Orthopedic and Trauma Surgery, 124*, 555–558.

CHAPTER 17

Surgical Care of Neuroendocrine and Other Endocrine Cancers

JoAnn Coleman, DNP, ACNP, AOCN®, GCN

Introduction

Neuroendocrine tumors (NETs) are a diverse group of primarily well-differentiated tumors that originate in neuroendocrine cells. These tumors can develop in multiple organs, particularly in the gastrointestinal (GI) tract (stomach, appendix, duodenum, and small intestine), the bronchopulmonary system (lung and thymus), the pancreas, and the colon and rectum. Most NETs secrete hormones that may be associated with a variety of clinical syndromes (Carrasquillo & Chen, 2010). NETs can be classified by site of origin, histology, grade, extent of disease, and functionality. Surgical resection is the treatment of choice for the vast majority of NETs, although surgery may not be feasible because of extensive or metastatic disease. Anatomic and functional imaging modalities are used to identify areas of NETs to stage the disease prior to surgery and to provide markers for subsequent surveillance (Carrasquillo & Chen, 2010). Although NETs are generally more indolent than adenocarcinomas, most NETs are classified as malignant and can show aggressive tumor behavior with metastases present at diagnosis (Modlin et al., 2008).

The incidence of gastroenteropancreatic NETs has increased over the past three decades (see Table 17-1). Initially considered rare tumors, gastroenteropancreatic NETs comprise 2% of all malignancies and are the second most common GI malignancy besides colorectal cancer (Schimmack, Svedja, Lawrence, Kidd, & Modlin, 2011). The increase in incidence and prevalence most likely reflects improvements in disease aware-

185

Table 17-1. Incidence of Neuroendocrine Tumors

Anatomic Site	Incidence
Bronchopulmonary system	25.3%
• Grade 1—Typical lung carcinoid	1%
• Grade 2—Atypical lung carcinoid	2%
• Grade 3—Large and small cell carcinomas	Rare
Gastrointestinal tract	67.5%
• Small intestine	41.8%
• Rectum	27.4%
• Stomach	8.7%
Pancreas (represents 10% of all pancreatic malignancies)	1%
• Gastrinomas	6%
• Insulinomas	4%
• Glucagonomas	2%
• VIPomas	1%

Note. Based on information from The NET Alliance, n.d., a Novartis Oncology Initiative.

ness and diagnostic techniques. NETs usually occur sporadically, but they can also be associated with various hereditary syndromes, such as *MEN-1* and *MEN-2* (multiple endocrine neoplasia types 1 and 2) genes, von Hippel-Lindau disease, and *NF1* (neurofibromatosis type 1) gene (Zhang & Nose, 2011).

Anatomy and Physiology

Neuroendocrine Tumors

NETs comprise the vast majority of neuroendocrine and endocrine tumors. An extensive review of pancreatic NETs, small bowel carcinoid tumor and carcinoid syndrome, bronchopulmonary and thymic NETs, and pheochromocytomas and paragangliomas is provided in Table 17-2.

Nonfunctional Neuroendocrine Tumors

Nonfunctional NETs histologically resemble other pancreatic NETs but do not secrete hormones that result in a detectable clinical syndrome. Most of the tumors do secrete chromogranin A, which can be detected in the serum and thus can be used to confirm the diagnosis (Lawrence et al., 2011). Most patients present with abdominal pain or

Table 17-2. Overview of Neuroendocrine Tumors

Neuroendocrine Tumor	Clinical Presentation	Hormone	Diagnostics	Preoperative Considerations	Surgery
Insulinoma • Most common in pancreatic neuroendocrine tumor • Affects women in 5th or 6th decade of life	Whipple's triad: low blood glucose level, symptoms of hypoglycemia at the time of the low blood glucose level, symptom relief with treatment of hypoglycemia Other hypoglycemic symptoms: headache, blurred vision, confusion, dizziness, lethargy, amnesia, diaphoresis, anxiety, tremor, palpitations, nausea, low serum glucose (< 40 mg/dl)	Insulin	Biochemical • Fasting serum insulin levels • Tolbutamide provocative test • Glucagon-stimulation test • IV calcium infusion test Imaging • CT • Transabdominal ultrasound • MRI • EUS • Arteriography with portal venous sampling • Intraoperative ultrasound	Localization of tumor (determines if laparoscopic resection possible) Control of hypoglycemia Diazoxide to control hypoglycemia (acts on beta cells to temporarily decrease insulin production)	Laparoscopic or open exploration Formal pancreatic resection Enucleation
Glucagonoma	4Ds—diabetes, dermatitis, DVT, depression May see cheilitis, anemia, weight loss, cachexia, hypoaminoacidemia, neuropsychiatric symptoms, elevated glucose levels, necrolytic migratory erythema	Glucagon PTH Gastrin Serotonin VIP Melanocyte-stimulating hormone	Biochemical • Serum glucagon level > 500 pg/ml Imaging • CT • MRI • SRS	Aggressive nutritional support due to catabolic state Rash treatment with zinc Heparin prophylaxis is for high occurrence of DVT Skin biopsy	Laparoscopic or open exploration Formal pancreatic resection

(Continued on next page)

Table 17-2. Overview of Neuroendocrine Tumors (Continued)

Neuroendocrine Tumor	Clinical Presentation	Hormone	Diagnostics	Preoperative Considerations	Surgery
VIPoma	WDHA syndrome—watery (secretory) diarrhea, hypokalemia, achlorhydria Hyperglycemia, hypercalcemia Abdominal pain, flushing, muscle weakness, weight loss	VIP	Biochemical • Serum VIP Imaging • CT or MRI • SRS	Correction of dehydration and metabolic abnormalities Aggressive nutritional support Initiation of octreotide	Laparoscopic or open exploration Formal pancreatic resection
Somatostatinoma	Diabetes, cholelithiasis, steatorrhea, anemia, weight loss	Somatostatin	Biochemical • Serum somatostatin Imaging • CT or MRI • SRS	Initiation of octreotide Correction of nutritional deficiencies	Laparoscopic or open exploration Formal pancreatic resection

(Continued on next page)

Table 17-2. Overview of Neuroendocrine Tumors (Continued)

Neuroendocrine Tumor	Clinical Presentation	Hormone	Diagnostics	Preoperative Considerations	Surgery
Gastrinoma	Idiopathic peptic ulcer disease, diarrheal conditions Combination of abdominal pain, diarrhea, heartburn, nausea, vomiting, fecal blood loss, weight loss Zollinger-Ellison syndrome with recurrent peptic ulcer disease Severe, resistant to treatment Prominent gastric rugal folds seen on endoscopy	Gastrin ACTH	Biochemical • Fasting serum gastrin • Secretin stimulation test • Gastrin stimulation test • Selective arterial secretin or calcium stimulation with sampling from hepatic veins Imaging • Ultrasound • CT • MRI • Angiography • SRS • EUS	Initiation or continuation of proton pump inhibitor Correction of nutritional deficiencies	Exploration of the gastrinoma triangle with possible pancreatic resection

(Continued on next page)

Table 17-2. Overview of Neuroendocrine Tumors (Continued)

Neuroendocrine Tumor	Clinical Presentation	Hormone	Diagnostics	Preoperative Considerations	Surgery
Small bowel carcinoid • Small, slow growing • Primarily found in the ileum • Male predominance in 6th decade of life • Also occurs in younger patients ages 40–60 years old	Hypercalcemia, Cushing syndrome, acromegaly, hypoglycemia, hypertension, gynecomastia, menstrual irregularity, abdominal pain, cramping, abdominal distention, nausea, vomiting, diarrhea, weight loss Small bowel obstruction Flushing, secretory diarrhea, palpitations, right-sided heart valve disease, bronchospasm	Serotonin Histamine Dopamine VIP 5-HTP Prostaglandins 5-HIAA	Biochemical • Chromogranin A • Associated labs with secreted hormones Imaging • CT • MRI • SRS • PET • Colonoscopy, small bowel enteroclysis • Capsule endoscopy • Cardiology evaluation for detection of cardiac abnormalities (right-sided heart problems)	Fluid and electrolyte repletion Correction of nutritional deficiencies Octreotide prophylaxis (pre-, intra-, and postoperatively) Corticosteroids Antihistamines Albuterol Astute anesthesia care to prevent carcinoid crisis (hypotension, flushing, tachycardia, bradycardia, bronchospasm, complete vasomotor collapse)	Right hemicolectomy most common

(Continued on next page)

Table 17-2. Overview of Neuroendocrine Tumors (Continued)

Neuroendocrine Tumor	Clinical Presentation	Hormone	Diagnostics	Preoperative Considerations	Surgery
Bronchopulmonary • Typical carcinoid • Atypical carcinoid • SCLC • Large cell neuroendocrine carcinoma	SCLC—hypercalcemia, Cushing syndrome, hyponatremia, SIADH Other symptoms: hemoptysis, cough, recurrent obstructive pulmonary infection, fever, chest discomfort, wheezing	Rare hypersecretory issues Chromogranin A Synaptophysin Neuron-specific enolase	Biochemical • ACTH • Growth hormone–releasing hormone • Insulin growth hormone 1 • ADH • Chromogranin A • Urine cortisol • 5-HIAA • Histamine metabolite Imaging • Chest x-ray • CT of chest, abdomen, pelvis • PET • SRS • Bronchoscopy	Assessment for paraneoplastic syndrome in SCLC such as SIADH and Cushing syndrome Biopsy (75% bronchial airway associated; 25% lung periphery)	Endobronchial excision of intraluminal typical carcinoid Anatomic resection—pneumonectomy or lobectomy Lung-sparing procedures, wedge resection, segmentectomy, and sleeve resection Thorascopic resection of peripheral lesions

(Continued on next page)

Table 17-2. Overview of Neuroendocrine Tumors (Continued)

Neuroendocrine Tumor	Clinical Presentation	Hormone	Diagnostics	Preoperative Considerations	Surgery
Thymus • Rare, sporadic tumors • Most are locally advanced with invasion into vital structures • Male predominance when associated with MEN-1	Incidental finding secondary to symptoms of paraneoplastic syndromes (in half of thymic tumors) Symptoms related to displacement or compression of adjacent thoracic structures Seen with Cushing syndrome and MEN-1	N-CAM Somatostatin ACTH	Biochemical • CD-56 • Neuron-specific enolase • Chromogranin A • Somatostatin • Synaptophysin Imaging • CT • MRI of head, neck, chest • SRS • PET/CT	—	Median sternotomy

(Continued on next page)

Table 17-2. Overview of Neuroendocrine Tumors (Continued)

Neuroendocrine Tumor	Clinical Presentation	Hormone	Diagnostics	Preoperative Considerations	Surgery
Pheochromocytoma • Secretes epinephrine • Rare, slow-growing tumor • 90% arise from chromaffin cells of adrenal medulla • Equal in men and women 40–60 years old • 25% due to genetic mutation	New-onset hypertension; often episodic, persistent, refractory to standard pharmacologic agents Triad of headache, palpitations, diaphoresis Other symptoms: anxiety, chest and abdominal pain, blurred vision, nausea and vomiting, tremor, pallor, flushing, tachycardia, postural hypotension, constipation, polyuria, polydipsia, hyperglycemia, hypercalcemia	Catecholamines	Biochemical • Plasma-free metanephrine test • Serum catecholamine • 24-hour urine catecholamines • Chromogranin A Imaging • CT with adrenal protocol • MRI • CT of neck and chest if no evidence of mass in abdomen • I-MIBG • PET	Alpha-blockade with phenoxybenzamine before surgery with last dose morning of surgery Beta-blockade as indicated Limitation in salt and fluid intake Anesthesia vigilance, especially during manipulation of tumor because of potential catecholamine surge Ligation of adrenal vein can cause abrupt hypotension.	Transabdominal laparoscopic adrenalectomy Open exploration Posterior retroperitoneal laparoscopic approach Bilateral adrenalectomy (cortical sparing)

(Continued on next page)

Table 17-2. Overview of Neuroendocrine Tumors (Continued)

Neuroendocrine Tumor	Clinical Presentation	Hormone	Diagnostics	Preoperative Considerations	Surgery
Paraganglioma • Equal occurrence in men and women 40–60 years old • Mostly located in abdomen • Head and neck tumors, likely carotid body tumors • Associated with von Hippel-Lindau, *MEN-2, SDH, NF1*	Hypertension	Normetanephrine	Biochemical • Plasma-free metanephrine test • Serum catecholamine • 24-hour urine catecholamines • Chromogranin A Imaging • CT • MRI	Same as for pheochromocytoma	Same as for pheochromocytoma

ACTH—adrenocorticotropic hormone; ADH—antidiuretic hormone; CD-56—cluster of differentiation 56; CT—computed tomography; DVT—deep vein thrombosis; EUS—endoscopic ultrasound; 5-HIAA—hydroxyindoleacetic; 5-HTP—hydroxytryptophan acid; I-MIBG—iodine-131 metaiodobenzylguanidine; MEN—multiple endocrine neoplasia; MRI—magnetic resonance imaging; N-CAM—neural cell adhesion molecule; NF1—neurofibromatosis type 1; PET—positron-emission tomography; PTH—parathyroid hormone; SCLC—small cell lung cancer; SDH—succinate dehydrogenase; SIADH—syndrome of inappropriate antidiuretic hormone; SRS—somatostatin-receptor scintigraphy; VIP—vasoactive intestinal peptide; VIPoma—vasoactive intestinal peptide

Note. Based on information from Boudreaux, 2011; Chen et al., 2010; Halperin & Kulke, 2012; Kalemkerian et al., 2011; Kooby & Chu, 2010; Mancuso et al., 2011; Ruffini et al., 2011; Saju et al., 2011.

other vague symptoms that prompts diagnostic studies (Falconi et al., 2012).

Neuroendocrine Tumor–Related Metastasis

Reddy and Clary (2010) reported that 50% of all patients with NETs have either regional or distant metastases at diagnosis. These patients have a poor prognosis with median survival of 33 months. The most frequent cause of death from NETs is liver failure because of hepatic replacement by tumor (Reddy & Clary, 2010). The goals of treatment include symptom management, biochemical control, tumor control, and improvement in quality of life.

Clinical Presentation

Patients with NETs may have silent indolent disease for years and typically become symptomatic with the occurrence of metastasis to the liver. Bone NETs can be a challenge to diagnose and often are discovered incidentally during routine screening, surgery, or abdominal imaging (see Table 17-2). NETs that arise in the GI tract can produce vague, nonspecific symptoms such as diarrhea, abdominal pain, flushing, and hypoglycemia that are easily mistaken for other conditions, such as irritable bowel syndrome and inflammatory bowel disease (Milan & Yeo, 2012). Patients may symptomatically suffer for years before NETs are correctly diagnosed. The estimated time to diagnosis for gastroenteropancreatic NETs is five to seven years (Modlin et al., 2008).

When symptoms raise the suspicion of NETs, serum or urine hormone tests are necessary to confirm diagnosis (see Table 17-2). Biomarker results, in the absence of pathologic diagnosis, should be confirmed with imaging and endoscopic techniques. Ideally, a tissue biopsy should be performed to provide confirmation of the malignancy (Bushnell & Baum, 2011; Vinik et al., 2010).

Surgical Management

Initial treatment of NETs is aimed at complete surgical resection of the primary tumors and associated nodal disease. In the absence of metastatic disease, exploratory surgery is performed with the goal of curative resection (see Table 17-2). The aim is to maintain a disease- and symptom-free state for as long as possible.

Metastatic Disease

In the presence of metastatic disease, often traditional surgery is not performed. Operative therapy is rarely curative, although it may be appropriate in select patients to achieve palliation through surgical debulking of the tumor. Surgery may be the only option for patients who experience life-threatening symptoms from hormonal hypersecretion for which other approaches have failed (National Comprehensive Cancer Network, 2013). Hepatic cytoreductive surgery can provide long-lasting benefit in some cases. Surgical options include formal hepatic lobe resections, nonanatomic mastectomies, or minimally invasive techniques such as radiofrequency ablation, cryoablation, microwave ablation, or laser-induced interstitial therapy (Strosberg, Cheema, & Kvols, 2011). In select cases, liver transplant may be considered if extrahepatic disease has been surgically controlled or eliminated (Tagkalos et al., 2011). Regional arterial therapies can be delivered in a segmental, lobar, or whole liver distribution. These include bland embolization, chemoembolization, radioactive microsphere embolization, and percutaneous hepatic perfusion (Strosberg et al., 2011).

Systemic Treatment

Excessive hormone secretions as evidenced by symptoms of severe flushing or persistent diarrhea need to be treated prior to any interventional treatment or surgical resection of functional NETs, as manipulation of the tumor can cause marked increases in hormone secretions. Careful intraoperative and anesthesia management are important to prevent and manage complications that may arise from these hormone surges (Boudreaux, 2011).

Postoperative Care

Postoperative nursing care of the patient who has undergone surgery for a NET is the same as for any patient having surgery for a solid organ tumor. The caveat to this care is that the nurse must be aware of the type of NET for which the patient had surgery and the particular functioning hormone or hormones associated with that tumor. Prompt identification and proactive interventions to control hypersecretion of hormones can significantly improve patient outcomes.

Discharge Planning

The best discharge planning program starts before surgery or related treatments and includes a multidisciplinary team approach with education of the patient and family. The postoperative NET patient needs routine education for activity, diet, care of surgical wounds, and any related tubes or drains. The patient may need to be instructed in subcutaneous administration of medications such as octreotide to control hypersecretory hormones. Referrals to resources such as the North American Neuroendocrine Tumor Society (www.nanets.net) or the Caring for Carcinoid Foundation (www .caringforcarcinoid.org) may benefit the patient and family. A complete family history is useful to identify potential genetic linkages and the need for genetic counseling.

Conclusions

Opportunities to conduct nursing research studies about these fascinating and challenging tumors are limitless and would enable the healthcare team to improve detection and diagnosis, surgical and nonsurgical interventions, and symptom management. A unique opportunity exists for collaborative nursing research among institutions with NET specialty clinics.

References

Boudreaux, J.P. (2011). Surgery for gastroenteropancreatic neuroendocrine tumors (GEPNETS). *Endocrinology and Metabolism Clinics of North America, 40,* 163–171. doi:10.1016/j.ecl.2010.12.004

Bushnell, D.L., & Baum, R.P. (2011). Standard imaging techniques for neuroendocrine tumors. *Endocrinology and Metabolism Clinics of North America, 40,* 153–162. doi:10.1016/j.ecl.2010.12.002

Carrasquillo, J.A., & Chen, C.C. (2010). Molecular imaging of neuroendocrine tumors. *Seminars in Oncology, 37,* 662–679. doi:10.1053/j.seminoncol.2010.10.015

Chen, H., Sippel, R.S., O'Dorisio, M.S., Vinik, A.I., Lloyd, R.V., & Pacak, K. (2010). The North American Neuroendocrine Tumor Society consensus guidelines for the diagnosis and management of neuroendocrine tumors: Pheochromocytoma, paraganglioma, and medullary thyroid cancer. *Pancreas, 39,* 775–783. doi:10.1097/MPA.0b013e3181ebb4f0

Falconi, M., Bartsch, D.K., Eriksson, B., Kloppel, G., Lopes, J.M., O'Connor, J., ... O'Toole, D. (2012). ENETS consensus guidelines for the management of patients with digestive neuroendocrine neoplasms of the digestive system: Well-differentiated pancreatic non-functioning tumors. *Neuroendocrinology, 95,* 120–134. doi:10.1159/000335587

Halperin, D.M., & Kulke, M.H. (2012). Management of pancreatic neuroendocrine tumors. *Gastroenterology Clinics of North America, 41,* 119–131. doi:10.1016/j.gtc.2011.12.003

Kalemkerian, G.P., Akerley, W., Bogner, P., Borghaei, H., Chow, L., Downey, R.J., ... Williams, C.C. (2011). NCCN clinical practice guidelines in oncology for small cell lung cancer. *Journal of the National Comprehensive Cancer Network, 9,* 1086–1113.

Kooby, D.A., & Chu, C.K. (2010). Laparoscopic management of pancreatic malignancies. *Surgical Clinics of North America, 90,* 427–446. doi:10.1016/j.suc.2009.12.011

Lawrence, B., Gustafsson, B.I., Kidd, M., Pavel, M., Svejda, B., & Modlin, I.M. (2011). The clinical relevance of chromogranin A as a biomarker for gastroenteropancreatic neuroendocrine tumors. *Endocrinology and Metabolism Clinics of North America, 40*, 111–134. doi:10.1016/j.ecl.2010.12.001

Mancuso, K., Kaye, A.D., Boudreaux, J.P., Fox, C.J., Lang, P., Kalarickal, P.L., ... Primeaux, P.J. (2011). Carcinoid syndrome and perioperative anesthetic considerations. *Journal of Clinical Anesthesia, 23*, 329–341. doi:10.1016/j.jclinane.2010.12.009

Milan, S.A., & Yeo, C.J. (2012). Neuroendocrine tumors of the pancreas. *Current Opinion in Oncology, 24*, 46–55. doi:10.1097/CCO.0b013e32834c554d

Modlin, I.M., Oberg, K., Chung, D.C., Jensen, R.T., de Herder, W.W., Thakker, R.V., ... Sundin, A. (2008). Gastroenteropancreatic neuroendocrine tumours. *Lancet Oncology, 9*, 61–72. doi:10.1016/S1470-2045(07)70410-2

National Comprehensive Cancer Network. (2013). *NCCN Clinical Practice Guidelines in Oncology: Neuroendocrine tumors* [v.2.2013]. Retrieved from http://www.nccn.org/professionals/physician_gls/pdf/neuroendocrine.pdf

The NET Alliance, a Novartis Oncology Initiative. (n.d.). High prevalence, increased incidence: Prevalence of NETs. Retrieved from http://www.neuroendocrinetumor.com/health-care-professional/prevalence-of-nets.jsp

Reddy, S.K., & Clary, B.M. (2010). Neuroendocrine liver metastases. *Surgical Clinics of North America, 90*, 853–861. doi:10.1016/j.suc.2010.04.016

Ruffini, E., Oliaro, A., Novero, D., Campisi, P., & Filosso, P.L. (2011). Neuroendocrine tumors of the thymus. *Thoracic Surgical Clinics, 21*, 12–23. doi:10.1016/j.thorsurg.2010.08.013

Saju, J., Wang, Y.Z., Boudreaux, J.P., Anthony, L.B., Campeau, R., Raines, D., ... Woltering, E.A. (2011). Neuroendocrine tumors: Current recommendations for diagnosis and surgical management. *Endocrinology and Metabolism Clinics of North America, 40*, 205–231. doi:10.1016/j.ecl.2010.08.004

Schimmack, S., Svedja, B., Lawrence, B., Kidd, M., & Modlin, I.R. (2011). The diversity and commonalities of gastroenteropancreatic neuroendocrine tumors. *Langenbeck's Archives of Surgery, 396*, 273–298. doi:10.1007/s00423-011-0739-1

Strosberg, J.R., Cheema, A., & Kvols, L. (2011). A review of systemic and liver-directed therapies for metastatic neuroendocrine tumors of the gastroenteropancreatic tract. *Cancer Control, 18*, 127–137.

Tagkalos, M.Z., Molmenti, P.A., Kobori, L., Fouzas, I., Beckebaum, S., & Sotiropoulos, G.C. (2011). Liver transplantation for hepatic metastases of neuroendocrine pancreatic tumors: A survival-based analysis. *Transplantation, 91*, 575–582. doi:10.1097/TP.0b013e3182081312

Vinik, A.I., Woltering, E.A., Warner, R.R.P., Caplin, M., O'Dorisio, T.M., Wiseman, G.A., ... Go, V.L.W. (2010). NANETS consensus guidelines for the diagnosis of neuroendocrine tumor. *Pancreas, 39*, 713–734. doi:10.1097/MPA.0b013e3181ebaffd

Zhang, Y., & Nose, V. (2011). Endocrine tumors as part of inherited tumor syndromes. *Advances in Anatomic Pathology, 18*, 206–218. doi:10.1097/PAP.0b013e3182169916

CHAPTER 18

Robotic Minimally Invasive Surgery

Donna Owen, RN, MS, CFNP, CPNP

Introduction

The use of robotic surgery has revolutionized hundreds of operations (Yu, Hevelone, Lipsitz, Kowalczyk, & Hu, 2012) and the pre-, peri-, and postsurgical care of patients (Francis & Winfield, 2006). The numbers of procedures that can be robotically performed have exponentially increased over the past two decades (Yu et al., 2012). Robotics is not a new concept, as it has been demonstrated in various forms over the past hundreds of years in such areas as literature, mathematics, entertainment, research, industry, and medicine. The first industrial robot, called Unimate®, was used at the General Motors automobile factory in New Jersey (Francis & Winfield, 2006). In 1985, a neurosurgical procedure called the Programmable Universal Manipulation Arm 560, or PUMA, was developed to orient a needle for brain biopsy under computed tomography guidance; it was later discontinued for safety reasons (Francis & Winfield, 2006).

The next robotic system was the PROBOT, developed by the Imperial College of England to assist in the transurethral resection of the prostate. In 1992, ROBODOC was developed by International Business Machines to aid in orthopedic surgery. In this same era, the National Aeronautics Space Administration began research in the area of robotic telepresence surgery through the Stanford Research Institute (Narula & Melvin, 2007). The modern use of robotics began in the military with a vision of a program that would allow for a remote surgery program and battlefield triage that was funded by the Defense Advanced Research Projects Agency (Yates, Vaessen, & Roupert, 2011). The fundamental aspect of the program was that surgery could be performed on a wounded person with a robotic base set up at a site near a war zone. The surgeon would work at a console and direct the robotic arms yet remain safe from warfare.

da Vinci® Surgical System

The prototype for the da Vinci® Surgical System was acquired from the military by Intuitive Surgical, Inc., who developed the commercial robotic system that is widely used in surgical suites today (Yates et al., 2011). This robotic system (see Figure 18-1) is a multi-armed, freestanding machine that is docked around the patient. As in laparoscopic surgery, the patient's abdomen is insufflated to provide intra-abdominal space. Trocars are strategically placed into the abdomen to allow access of the arms of the robot to the surgical area. The instrumentation is attached to the arms by the surgeon's assistants. The surgeon sits at a console separate from the robot and manipulates the arms of the robot to perform the surgery.

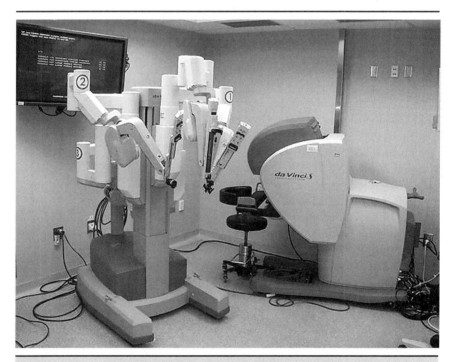

Figure 18-1. The da Vinci® Surgical System

Note. Photo courtesy of Edward Nickerson, The Ohio State University. Used with permission.

Use of Robotic Surgery

Robotic surgery can be incorporated into multiple surgical disciplines as a means to perform less invasive surgery on benign or malignant conditions. Current surgical uses include (a) urologic with radical prostatectomy, nephrectomy, partial nephrectomy, cystectomy, pyeloplasty, adrenalectomy, pelvic lymphadenectomy, and ureteroileal anastomosis strictures (Dangle & Abaza, 2012), (b) gynecologic with uterine myomectomy, fallopian tuberanastomosis, and hysterectomy for benign and malignant tumors (Liu et al., 2012), as well as ovarian tumor resection and pelvic and aortic lymphadenectomy (Holloway & Ahmad, 2012), (c) cardiovascular with mitral valve repair, internal mammary artery harvest, coronary artery bypass grafting, and epicardial lead placement (Francis & Winfield, 2006), (d) gastrointestinal with colorectal surgery (Leong & Kim, 2011), cholecystectomy, gastric bypass, Nissen fundoplication, Heller myotomy, splenectomy, and cyst and tumor excisions (Francis & Winfield, 2006), as well as pylorus-preserving pancreaticoduodenectomy (Zureikat, Nguyen, Bartlett, Zeh, & Moser, 2011), and (e) head and neck with skull-based surgery, oropharynx and tongue-based resection (Dallan et al., 2011), thyroidectomy, and facelift thyroidectomy (Terris & Singer, 2012).

Advantages of Robotic Surgery

The key concepts of robotic surgery include (a) improved visualization through optics that magnify and enhance the surgical field, (b) finer dissection techniques, (c) less invasion into the surgical fields, and (d) minimal blood loss (Yates et al., 2011). Robot-assisted surgery provides improved resolution for the surgeon with three-dimensional visual magnification of the surgical field and tumor margins. The scaling ability, seven degrees of movement, and ergonomics enable finer instrumentation with finer dissection and decreased blood loss. The robot is programmed to filter out human tremor or sudden movement that can be disruptive to the surgical procedure (Leong & Kim, 2011). These features allow for delicate dissection of organs and adjacent structures in the surgical field, enabling removal of the mass and potentially leaving the remainder of the organ intact (Yu et al., 2012). As robotic technology continues to improve, visualization will be increased, and robot haptic feedback will improve and allow unparalleled sensation for the surgeon that nearly eliminates tissue contact and injury (Simorov, Otte, Kopietz, & Oleynikov, 2012). By comparison, with an open incision approach, this fine dissection would not be possible and would necessitate complete removal of the organ.

With robotic surgery, patients typically experience rapid healing of port incisions, improved cosmetic outcomes, and an accelerated return to meaningful activities (Yu et al., 2012). These advantages are due to smaller entry sites with the absence of a large, painful incision. The need for postoperative narcotics with related side effects is decreased. The risk of infection is markedly decreased because of small entry incisions and potentially less internal organ manipulation (Yu et al., 2012). A clear surgical glue-like adhesive is used on the skin that seals the port sites and eases wound care; no external staples or sutures are used. Generally, the port sites can be gently washed with soap and water until healed. Blood loss is minimized because of the small port holes, which ultimately improves the patient's energy level. Some procedures allow for patient discharge on the day of surgery; otherwise, a short hospitalization may be necessary yet is far shorter than with an open procedure (Yu et al., 2012). Typically, the patient rapidly returns to normal activity level.

Disadvantages of Robotic Surgery

Cost

The overall advantages versus disadvantages of robot-assisted surgery are not clearly illustrated. Cost remains an issue with the purchase of the robot itself because not all facilities can justify the financial strain based on their surgery case quota versus the number and expertise of surgeons. The price of the da Vinci Surgical System at this writing is nearly $2.6 million, which includes the robot and the console (Health Quality Ontario, 2010). This does not include the cost of the instrumentation, another added cost per case as instrumentation is specific for the procedure being performed. Most instruments can be reused after sterilization but will need to be replaced after a certain number of sterilizations determined by manufacturer guidelines. The robot is able to detect if the instrument has exceeded its usage. The size of the robot is another negative factor, as the system consists of a console and the robot. Some operating rooms are not large enough to accommodate the size of the system. The da Vinci Surgical System has its own special equipment that is not interchangeable with other systems.

Surgical Proficiency

Port placement needs to be precise to aid in the proper implementation of the robotic instrumentation. If the port placement is not accurate, the robotic arms can collide or block the degree of rotation of another arm, thus interfering with the surgeon's ability to perform the operation. Patient positioning is critical for proper docking of the robotic system. If the patient's position changes, the system may need to be undocked, the position of the patient adjusted, and the system docked again. This can cost valuable time in the operating room and require the patient to remain under anesthesia for an extended time.

Other potential issues include (a) troubleshooting if the instrumentation fails, (b) addressing inadequate insufflation pressure in the abdomen, (c) correcting fogging of the scope, and (d) correcting lighting issues. The operating room nurse must be educated and in sync with all aspects of the system to aid in resolution of issues quickly and efficiently in order to prevent harm to the patient or the system.

The lack of trained surgeons is a disadvantage that exists in robotic surgery. Fellowships for robotic training are not easily found, and the number of applicants outnumbers the slots available. Some residencies incorporate time on the robot, but this time is shared with other residents, which can make it difficult to gain enough hours for proficiency. Virtual reality simulators are commercially available and have a role in the future of robotic training, but the cost is prohibitive for many facilities. There are basic skill sets with performance analysis and metrics software, but many do not contain procedural components necessary to advance the skill of the surgeon (Lallas, Davis, & Members of the Society of Urologic Robotic Surgeons, 2012).

Conclusions

Robotic surgery has replaced the open procedure in multiple urologic, gynecologic, cardiac, gastrointestinal, and head-and-neck operations. Although the immediate postoperative period may be markedly improved, the patient needs to be aware that internally the same surgery was completed. Postoperative pain can often be managed with non-narcotic medications, which enables the patient's gastrointestinal system to rapidly return to normal. Useful non-narcotic medications include ketorolac, acetaminophen, and simethicone. Recommended restrictions during the recovery period are still important and necessary for proper recovery.

References

Dallan, I., Seccia, V., Muscatello, L., Lenzi, R., Castelnuovo, P., Bignami, M., ... Vicini, C. (2011). Transoral endoscopic anatomy of the parapharyngeal space: A step-by-step logical approach with surgical considerations. *Head and Neck, 33,* 557–561. doi:10.1002/hed.21488

Dangle, P., & Abaza, R. (2012). Robot-assisted repair of ureteroileal anastomosis strictures: Initial cases and literature review. *Journal of Endourology, 26,* 372–376. doi:10.1089/end.2011.0423

Francis, P., & Winfield, H.N. (2006). Medical robotics: The impact on perioperative nursing practice. *Urologic Nursing, 26,* 99–108.

Health Quality Ontario. (2010). Robotic-assisted minimally invasive surgery for gynecologic and urologic oncology: An evidence-based analysis. *Ontario Health Technology Assessment Series, 10*(27), 1–118. Retrieved from http://www.ncbi.nlm.nih.gov/pmc/articles/PMC3382308

Holloway, R.W., & Ahmad, S. (2012). Robotic-assisted surgery in the management of endometrial cancer. *Journal of Obstetrics and Gynaecology Research, 38,* 1–8. doi:10.1111/j.1447-0756.2011.01744.x

Lallas, C.D., Davis, J.W., & Members of the Society of Urologic Robotic Surgeons. (2012). Robotic surgery training with commercially available simulation systems in 2011: A current review and practice pattern survey from the Society of Urologic Robotic Surgeons. *Journal of Endourology, 26,* 283–293. doi:10.1089/end.2011.0371

Leong, Q.M., & Kim, S.H. (2011). Robot-assisted rectal surgery for malignancy: A review of current literature. *Annals of Academic Medicine in Singapore, 40,* 460–466.

Liu, H., Lu, D., Wang, L., Shi, G., Song, H., & Clarke, J. (2012). Robotic surgery for benign gynaecological disease. *Cochrane Database of Systematic Reviews, 2.* doi:10.1002/14651858.CD008978.pub2

Narula, V.K., & Melvin, W.S. (2007). Robotic surgical systems. In V.R. Patel (Ed.), *Robotic urologic surgery* (pp. 5–14). London, England: Springer-Verlag.

Simorov, A., Otte, R.S., Kopietz, C.M., & Oleynikov, D. (2012). Review of surgical robotics user interface: What is the best way to control robotic surgery? *Surgical Endoscopy, 26,* 2117–2125. doi:10.1007/s00464-012-2182-y

Terris, D.J., & Singer, M.C. (2012). Robotic facelift thyroidectomy: Facilitating remote access surgery. *Head and Neck, 34,* 746–747. doi:10.1002/hed.22978

Yates, D.R., Vaessen, C., & Roupert, M. (2011). From Leonardo to da Vinci: The history of robot-assisted surgery in urology. *BJU International, 108,* 1708–1713. doi:10.1111/j.1464-410X2011.10576.x

Yu, H.Y., Hevelone, N.D., Lipsitz, S.R., Kowalczyk, K.J., & Hu, J.C. (2012). Use, costs and comparative effectiveness of robotic assisted, laparoscopic and open urological surgery. *Journal of Urology, 187,* 1392–1398. doi:10.1016/j.juro.2011.11.089

Zureikat, A.H., Nguyen, K.T., Bartlett, D.L., Zeh, H.J., & Moser, A.J. (2011). Robotic-assisted major pancreatic resection and reconstruction. *Archives of Surgery, 146,* 256–261. doi:10.1001/archsurg.2010.246

CHAPTER 19

Interventional Radiology: Diagnosis and Treatment

Gail M. Egan, MS, ANP

Introduction

Interventional radiology offers diagnostic and treatment options to patients prior to diagnosis, during treatment, and in the palliative phases of care. Before diagnosis, interventional radiology teams perform image-guided biopsies (e.g., ultrasound [US], computed tomography [CT], magnetic resonance imaging [MRI]) to establish a tissue diagnosis. Therapeutic options for cancer treatment include targeted transarterial embolization (e.g., insertion of particles with or without antineoplastic agents), thermal ablation (e.g., cryoablation, radiofrequency), and placement of medical devices. In the palliative phase of treatment, interventional radiology clinicians provide symptom relief with pain management interventions (e.g., kyphoplasty, vertebroplasty). Each of these interventions is performed in a minimally invasive manner using various imaging modalities to guide the clinician.

Interventional Radiology in the Diagnosis of Cancer

Biopsy

Image-guided biopsies (see Table 19-1) are one of the most frequently performed procedures in interventional radiology. Using coaxial needles guided with the assistance of CT, US, or fluoroscopic imaging, biopsies obtain a small core of tissue that is used to establish a diagnosis and provide disease information. The modality chosen to guide the needle depends on the size and location of the target lesion, its proximity to other structures, and the patient's overall body habitus. These biopsies are highly accurate, as

Table 19-1. Roles of Interventional Radiology in Cancer Treatment

Radiology Intervention	Description	Advantages
Biopsy		
Image-guided biopsy	Using coaxial needles with assistance of computed tomography (CT), ultrasound, or fluoroscopic guidance, a small core of tissue is taken for pathologic exam.	Provides accurate and real-time biopsy of nonpalpable lesion; noninvasive and minimizes trauma to area
Vascular Access		
Central vascular devices	Placed via fluoroscopy—real-time placement that enables the interventional radiology (IR) physician to accurately place catheter tip Enables complicated placement in the event of superior vena cava syndrome or other blockage of vasculature Under fluoroscopy, can examine central occlusions within or outside the catheter	Eliminates surgical time and space, is less expensive, IR physicians are more readily available than surgeons for central line placement, allows accurate tip positioning
Locoregional Therapies		
Transarterial chemoembolization	Used to treat primary and metastatic hepatic malignancies Enables delivery of chemotherapy via transhepatic arterial infusion	Noninvasive approach to locoregional therapy for chemotherapy infusion followed by embolization of vessels in liver
Radioembolization	Provides a local radiotherapeutic effect on primary or metastatic liver disease using yttrium-90	Exerts effect on liver without damage to surrounding organs. Involvement of IR enables visualization of adjacent vessels to ensure effective delivery and/or embolization.

(Continued on next page)

Table 19-1. Roles of Interventional Radiology in Cancer Treatment (Continued)

Radiology Intervention	Description	Advantages
Cryoablation	Uses in situ freezing to devitalize target tissue; the probe is placed percutaneously via fluoroscopy.	Provides of real-time and cross-sectional imaging to guide the probe accurately
Radiofrequency ablation	Achieves thermal ablation by heating the target tissue with electrical current	Enables localized therapy without systemic side effects
Microwave ablation	Uses high-frequency electromagnetic radiation; heat causes cellular death.	Faster than other methods with less procedural discomfort
Percutaneous ethanol injection	Via catheter, ethanol is injected directly into primary liver tumor, which causes cell death.	Real-time injection; noninvasive, nonsurgical procedure
Irreversible electroporation	Achieves nonthermal ablation; uses electrical fields to permeate cell membrane	Real-time placement of probes with CT guidance; spares neighboring structures and vessels
High-intensity focused ultrasound	Treats tumors of breast and liver via acoustic energy	Noninvasive, nonsurgical, but time-consuming and may require repeat treatments
Drain apparatus	Provides for percutaneous placement of drain to negative suction system: ascites, pleural effusions	Enables ongoing drainage when the patient is beyond treatment for the cancer
Pleurodesis	Enables placement of sclerosing agents into pleural space; creates irritation and barrier to fluid accumulation	Noninvasive, nonsurgical; prevents placement of chest tube
Percutaneous biliary drainage	Allows for percutaneous placement of biliary drain or internal stent	Noninvasive, nonsurgical approach to circumvent accumulating bile in palliative situation

(Continued on next page)

Table 19-1. Roles of Interventional Radiology in Cancer Treatment *(Continued)*		
Radiology Intervention	Description	Advantages
Celiac plexus block	The celiac plexus is injected with alcohol in an attempt to innervate nerve endings that are causing intractable pain.	Noninvasive, nonsurgical mechanism to relieve severe pain without systemic side effects of pain medication
Vertebroplasty	Involves placement of needle into fractured vertebral body through pedicle and injection of polymethyl methacrylate	Offers broad pain relief without surgery
Kyphoplasty/vertebroplasty (see Figure 16-6)	Provides relief of bone pain and simultaneous bone stabilization	Noninvasive surgery without long incisions to heal; bone repair without surgery

the needle is guided into the target using real-time imaging with confirmation of needle tip placement captured on the imaging screen. Targeted sites may include almost any organ or structure in the body. Image-guided biopsies are performed with a percutaneous approach. Local anesthetic is used to numb the skin overlying the target site; a small nick in the skin is used to facilitate insertion of the coaxial biopsy needle. Conscious sedation is often used in conjunction with local anesthetic, which is dependent on the target site and degree of difficulty of the biopsy. Most biopsies are performed on an outpatient basis, with a short recovery from sedation before release. Contraindications to percutaneous biopsy include uncorrectable coagulopathy and absence of a safe pathway to access the target lesion (Shankar, van Sonnenberg, Silverman, & Tuncali, 2002).

Imaging

US is used to guide the biopsy of superficial lesions that cannot be palpated, whereas deeper organ lesions require additional radiographic modalities. US is a real-time imaging modality, meaning that the operator can visualize needle placement as it happens, which allows for immediate adjustments in depth and trajectory. CT is an imaging guidance modality that provides excellent spatial resolution of lesions and neighboring structures. It is particularly useful for the biopsy of deep-seated lesions or those that present a technical challenge in location (e.g., retroperitoneal lymph nodes). Fluoroscopy is primarily used for biopsy of radiopaque lesions, such as lesions of vertebral bodies, the femur, or other bony structures. Fluoroscopy is used less often than CT or US to guide biopsy needles.

Potential complications of image-guided biopsies vary with the target site and overall condition of the patient. Potential complications of lung biopsies include pneumothorax, hemothorax, and hemoptysis. Pneumothorax is often asymptomatic and may require no intervention. Larger or expanding pneumothoraxes may require decompression with placement of a small-bore drainage catheter. Potential complications of intra-abdominal organ biopsy include bleeding and nontarget organ puncture. Upon completion of the biopsy, the patient is scanned again to assess for bleeding. Signs and symptoms of bleeding following the procedure would include hypotension and increasing pain. Repeat imaging is indicated if bleeding is suspected.

Interventional Radiology in Cancer Management

Vascular Access

A central vascular access device (VAD) or central line is most often used when reliable venous access for chemotherapy is required. Central VADs offer the patient reliable access for drug infusion coupled with access for venous sampling and contrast administration for imaging purposes. For optimal device function, the catheter tip should reside in the distal third of the superior vena cava (SVC) or atriocaval junction. Catheter tip position is verified with either a single-view chest x-ray (when the device is placed at the bedside) or with fluoroscopy for devices placed in interventional radiology or the operating room. Fluoroscopy has the additional advantage of allowing the clinician to adjust the tip position during the procedure and correct any malposition or directional problems. Accuracy of catheter tip placement is associated with optimal device performance for both infusion and sampling. In addition, poorly placed catheter tips are associated with an increased risk of catheter dysfunction, venous thrombosis, and stenosis (Gallieni, Pittiruti, & Biffi, 2008). New systems that verify catheter tip placement with electrocardiogram waveform feedback have been implemented in various clinical settings. These systems rely on feedback obtained from either a guide wire or a column of saline acting as endovascular electrodes, which detect changes in the height of the P wave or R wave as the catheter approaches the target tip location (Gallieni et al., 2008).

US-guided placement of central VADs has been shown to decrease technical failure, reduce the risk of puncture-related complications, and reduce procedure time. In a study comparing US-guided punctures with the traditional landmark approach to placing central VADs, Froelich et al. (2009) reported on 212 critically ill pediatric patients. They noted that US guidance reduced inadvertent arterial punctures, the number of punctures required to attain access, and procedure time.

Novel Access Sites

In patients with SVC stenosis or occlusion, catheter tip placement in the SVC is impossible. Several alternative access sites may be utilized in these patients. The azygos vein, a small vein that comes off the SVC, enlarges in the setting of SVC stenosis. A catheter tip may be placed here using fluoroscopic guidance. The azygos may not enlarge enough, however, to support the flow rates required for apheresis or hemodialysis. The common femoral vein is another alternate access site for central line placement. Central VADs may also be placed using a more direct approach into the inferior vena cava, using either a translumbar or transhepatic approach. The catheter is subsequently threaded into the inferior vena cava. To reduce the risk of infection, long-term central lines should be tunneled remotely from the puncture site when the common femoral vein is used.

Central Line Complications

One of the most common central VAD–related complications is persistent withdrawal occlusion (PWO). PWO is defined as the inability to aspirate at least 3 ml of free-flowing blood despite the ability to infuse fluids. Because an adequate blood return is one measure of accurate catheter tip placement and safety, PWO is a problem that needs to be addressed promptly. Central line occlusion occurs in up to 66% of adults with long-term catheters (Baskin et al., 2009). Device occlusion may occur for several reasons, including mechanical obstruction, tip malposition, drug precipitate, and thrombosis within or outside the catheter. Treatment is based on the etiology of the occlusion. Mechanical obstruction may be caused by catheter or IV tubing clamps, occluded injection caps, kinks in the catheter itself, or sutures that are too tight. Drug precipitates can be treated with solvents such as ethyl alcohol.

Thrombotic occlusions are common in patients with cancer and are more likely to occur in patients with a history of deep vein thrombosis, with subclavian vein placement, and with improper catheter tip position (Saber et al., 2011). Thrombotic catheter occlusions can be treated with an instillation of alteplase 2 mg in 2 ml sterile water for injection (or 110% of the catheter volume for larger devices) with a dwell time of 30–120 minutes. Higher-dose alteplase infusions may be more effective in the setting of recurrent PWO or an extensive fibrin sheath (Baskin et al., 2009). In cases where initial treatment fails or whenever the patient has discomfort with device use, imaging should be pursued with a single-view chest x-ray to determine whether the central VAD is intact or distorted. In cases where occlusion is not resolved and the chest x-ray is within normal limits, a catheter dye study can yield more information. A small amount of contrast, typically 5–10 ml, is injected into the catheter under fluoroscopy, with images saved in a video format. Treatment is initiated based on the patient's overall status and ability to tolerate the intervention, which may include disruption of the fibrin sheath with venoplasty or higher doses of alteplase infusion. Only in severe cases is device removal indicated (Baskin et al., 2009).

Central VAD–related infection is the second most common complication. Reported rates of central VAD–related infection range from 0.6%–27% depending on catheter location, catheter type, and immune status of the patient (Walser, 2012). Catheter-related bloodstream infections are diagnosed after the exclusion of other infectious causes. Device salvage may be attempted based on the cultured organism and the overall vascular access status of the patient. Fungal infections are difficult to treat with the device in place and most often require central line removal and subsequent replacement after the patient has been treated. Patients with recurrent infection and septic complications (e.g., endocarditis) often require device removal (Walser, 2012).

Interventional Radiology in Cancer Treatment

Locoregional Therapies

Locoregional therapy includes transarterial chemoembolization (TACE), thermal ablation (e.g., radiofrequency ablation [RFA], cryoablation), and radioembolization. These therapies are performed to treat primary and metastatic hepatic malignancies and renal cell carcinomas (Grasso et al., 2012; Gunven, 2008). They can also be used in other sites, such as lung masses and bone lesions. The goals of therapy are to halt or slow tumor growth and reduce tumor burden. Although initially developed as a treatment option in patients who are not candidates for surgery, these therapies are now used in conjunction with standard therapies as well as to treat small lesions in lieu of surgical resection (Grasso et al., 2012; Gunven, 2008). Locoregional therapies have become increasingly useful in the management of both primary and metastatic disease (Grasso et al., 2012; Gunven, 2008).

The patient's overall liver function, degree of cirrhosis, and performance status serve as predictors of the patient's ability to tolerate therapies. CT or MRI imaging is performed to evaluate the extent of liver disease. Cross-sectional imaging also identifies neighboring structures and assists clinicians to plan the trajectory of probe placement (Grasso et al., 2012; Gunven, 2008). These imaging studies are also used as baseline examinations for future comparison of post-treatment imaging, performed at three- to six-month intervals. Pretreatment laboratory analyses include a complete blood count with platelet level, coagulation studies (e.g., prothrombin time, partial thromboplastin time), and full chemistry profile with liver function panel (Gunven, 2008).

Transarterial Chemoembolization

The liver's anatomy and its rich vascular supply enable the liver to be a common site of metastatic disease (Riaz, Lewandowski, Kulik, & Salem, 2009). Liver tumors are primarily supplied via the arterial route; the portal vein supplies blood to the hepatic parenchyma. Thus, embolic agents and antineoplastic agents can be delivered via a transhepatic arterial infusion with preservation of overall liver function (Gunven, 2008).

TACE is a complex process that involves direct delivery of antineoplastic agents to the tumor site via its arterial supply. It is typically reserved for patients who are not candidates for surgical resection or ablative therapies (e.g., because of tumor size or location) or when systemic therapy has failed. Relative contraindications to TACE include replacement of more than 50% of the liver with tumor, hepatic encephalopathy, total bilirubin greater than 2 mg/dl, portal vein or biliary obstruction, and extensive extrahepatic disease with a limited life expectancy (Grasso et al., 2012; Lammer et al., 2010).

A small catheter is threaded under fluoroscopy from the common femoral artery to the blood supply of the targeted tumor, typically a primary or metastatic hepatic mass (see Figure 19-1). IV contrast is used to facilitate visualization as the operator guides the catheter to the artery supplying the tumor. A solution of embolic agents that is mixed with an antineoplastic agent is then injected until stasis is achieved, which robs the tumor of its blood supply and prolongs exposure of the tumor to the antineoplastic agent. The mixture may also include biocompatible nonresorbable hydrogel beads that bind with the antineoplastic agent and slowly disperse the drug over time. A liquid, radiopaque oil embolic agent, such as Ethiodol®, may be used; this agent adheres to the cell wall of the tumor and is actively transported into the cell to cause lysis (Lammer et al., 2010). The radiopaque nature of the substance stays within the tumor, which enhances post-treatment imaging and serves as a target for other probe-based ablative techniques. Overall, the reduction in arterial supply causes hypoxia and cell death. Adjacent, normal liver is spared as the portal vein remains patent (Lammer et al., 2010).

Many patients can experience a phenomenon known as postembolization syndrome (see Figure 19-2) and experience several days of low-grade fever, malaise, anorexia, nausea, and abdominal discomfort. These symptoms are related to tumor hypoxia and cell death with transportation of cell waste products. Postembolization syndrome is more common in patients with large-volume disease. These symptoms are generally self-limited, lasting for 24–72 hours, and managed with supportive therapy including hydration, antiemetics, acetaminophen, and opioid analgesics. Complications of TACE

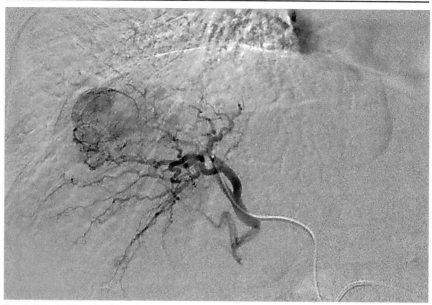

Dye is injected into the hepatic artery to identify the blood supply to the tumor.

Figure 19-1. Image Prior to Chemoembolization

Note. Photo courtesy of Gail Wych Davidson, MS, NP-C, OCN®, The Ohio State University. Used with permission.

include tumor lysis syndrome, liver failure, abscess formation, and gastric or duodenal mucosal erosion. Ischemic injury to neighboring organs may also occur with concomitant cholecystitis, pancreatitis (Guimaraes & Uflacker, 2011; Gunven, 2008), and bile duct necrosis.

Radioembolization

Radioembolization uses yttrium-90 (^{90}Y) to exert a local radiotherapeutic effect on primary or metastatic liver tumors with limited concurrent injury to surrounding normal tissue. ^{90}Y is a pure beta emitter, which makes it ideal for intra-arterial injection. It deteriorates to zirconium-90 and has a tissue penetration depth of 2.5 mm. ^{90}Y is loaded onto glass or resin microspheres, which are delivered through a microcatheter placed into the tumor blood supply. The microspheres serve as point sources of radiation therapy that preferentially locate to tumor tissue via the arterial vasculature; thus, normal hepatic parenchyma is largely spared. The half-life of ^{90}Y is 64.2 hours; thus, 94% of the radiation is emitted within the first 11 days of treatment (Guimaraes & Uflacker, 2011; Riaz et al., 2009).

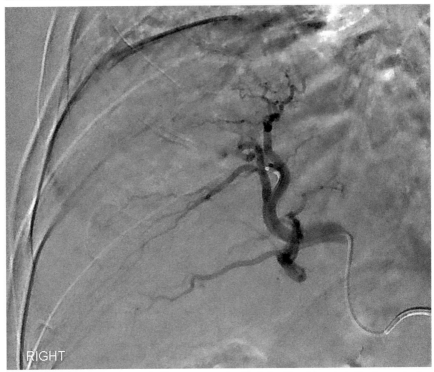

After chemotherapeutic and embolic agents are instilled, the blood supply to the tumor is diminished or ceased.

Figure 19-2. Image After Chemoembolization

Note. Photo courtesy of Gail Wych Davidson, MS, NP-C, OCN®, The Ohio State University. Used with permission.

Before a patient is treated with radioembolization, a hepatic angiogram is performed to define the hepatic arterial anatomy. The gastroduodenal artery and right gastric artery are also assessed, as reflux of ^{90}Y spheres can cause radiation enteritis. If these vessels are close to the intended arterial catheter placement for infusion, these vessels are embolized. Once the hepatic arterial supply to the tumor is identified, technetium-99m macroaggregated albumin (^{99m}Tc-labeled MAA) is injected as a predictor of how much ^{90}Y will pass through the liver to the lungs. The patient then undergoes a nuclear medicine perfusion scan, which assesses shunt to the lungs and tumor volume. If shunting to the lungs is extensive, the ^{90}Y dose may need to be reduced to avoid radiation pneumonitis. In patients with a shunt of more than 20%, the procedure is generally canceled to reduce the risk of pulmonary fibrosis (Riaz et al., 2009). The ^{90}Y dose is determined based on a ratio of tumor volume to normal hepatic volume and tumor vascularity. For example, a 4:1 ratio means that 80% of the ^{90}Y will be delivered to the tumor, with 20% going to normal liver (Guimaraes & Uflacker, 2011; Riaz et al., 2009). Once these calculations have been made, a specific dose of ^{90}Y is ordered for the patient, and infusion is scheduled one to two weeks following diagnostic angiogram. The ^{90}Y spheres are mixed with IV contrast and delivered via catheter placement in the hepatic artery. The patient's vasculature is visualized with fluoroscopy, with contrast opacification of the vasculature so that the catheter can be guided into position. The ^{90}Y spheres are delivered using a closed system to minimize the chance for room contamination (Guimaraes & Uflacker, 2011; Riaz et al., 2009).

Symptoms following treatment are minimal because radioembolization does not cause arterial occlusion. The most common side effects of ^{90}Y are fatigue, right upper quadrant or abdominal discomfort, decreased appetite, nausea, and diarrhea. Potential complications include gastritis, gastric or duodenal ulcer, radiation-induced hepatitis, and liver failure.

Cryoablation

Cryoablation uses in situ freezing to devitalize target tissue. The cryoablation probe is placed percutaneously into the target site. Cross-sectional imaging is used to guide the probe accurately to the center of the target lesion, with the ice ball extended 3–4 mm beyond the tumor to ensure complete ablation. The probe delivers liquid nitrogen or argon into an insulated probe, cooling the tumor to temperatures below $-20°C$. Cell death occurs from both direct damage due to intracellular ice formation and indirect damage to the cellular microvascular circulatory system. Cryoablation is useful for lesions less than 4 cm in size and in patients who are not surgical candidates. Multiple overlapping probes may be used when the tumor size is larger with ice balls of up to 8 cm. Renal cell carcinomas are particularly well suited to treatment with cryoablation because of their generally early diagnosis, slow-growing characteristics, and confinement to the kidney. Patients with a solitary kidney or bilateral renal tumors are also ideal candidates for cryoablation (Padma, Martinie, & Iannitti, 2009; Yang et al., 2012).

Radiofrequency Ablation

RFA is the most frequently used thermal ablation technique and is similar to cryoablation (see Figure 19-3). Instead of cooling the tumor, RFA heats the tumor using high-frequency (460–480 kHz) alternating electrical current. The current agitates the tissue and generates frictional heat that extends by conduction. The mass is heated to 60°C for four to six minutes and produces coagulative necrosis and irreversible cellular damage. An area at

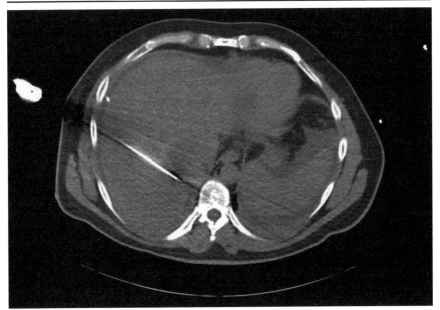

With computed tomography scan guidance, the ablation probe is positioned in the tumor. Heat (microwave or radiofrequency energy) or cold (cryo) is deployed through the probe to destroy the tumor.

Figure 19-3. Percutaneous Ablation

Note. Photo courtesy of Gail Wych Davidson, MS, NP-C, OCN®, The Ohio State University. Used with permission.

least 2 cm larger than the target lesion is ablated to achieve an adequate tumor-free margin. The largest RFA probe is 7 cm, meaning that the largest tumor that can be treated is 4–5 cm, unless overlapping ablations are performed. RFA can also be used to treat renal cell carcinoma. Local tumor therapy is particularly advantageous in patients with renal cell carcinoma who have a solitary kidney (Grasso et al., 2012). Heat-based thermal ablation techniques can cause vascular thrombosis. Therefore, bleeding is an unusual complication of RFA and thus RFA is useful in coagulopathic patients. More common complications include abscess formation and biliary injury (Grasso et al., 2012; Guimaraes & Uflacker, 2011).

Microwave Ablation

Microwave ablation uses high-frequency electromagnetic radiation that heats intracellular water molecules with a device that has a frequency of 900 MHz to 10 GHz. The heat generated causes coagulative necrosis and eventually cell death. Microwave technology is useful in achieving higher intratumoral temperatures, faster ablation times, and less procedural discomfort than RFA. The microwave probe generates higher temperatures than RFA; therefore, it is most useful for tumors located distantly from the gallbladder and biliary tree (Padma et al., 2009).

Advantages of local tumor ablation include limited morbidity and mortality, which makes these interventions viable options for patients who are poor surgical candidates. Interventions can also be performed sequentially or in multiple sessions, depending on the size, number, and location of lesions. The most common side effect is fatigue; however, other complications include thermal skin injury, abscess formation, adjacent organ damage, bleeding, and pain. Most interventions can be performed on an outpatient basis, which limits operational costs. The use of real-time imaging guidance allows the operator to clearly identify target lesions and place ablation probes accurately. Imaging also allows the clinician to assess the location of adjacent organs and take measures to reduce the risks of inadvertent ablation (Padma et al., 2009).

Percutaneous Ethanol Injection

Percutaneous ethanol injection (PEI) is one of the oldest strategies for treating hepatocellular cancer in a local fashion. It is most effective for treating small (less than 2 cm), easily accessible primary hepatic tumors. PEI involves the injection of ethanol directly into the tumor with a small needle guided by US or CT. Cell death results from coagulative necrosis and thrombosis of the tumor microcirculation. Multiple injections are often necessary to treat a small tumor because the ablation zone is unpredictable. This strategy has gained acceptance outside the United States, perhaps because of its limited cost. It has not demonstrated efficacy against metastatic tumors to the liver and leads to only about 70% necrosis in small hepatic lesions (Padma et al., 2009). In studies comparing PEI with RFA, RFA required fewer treatments and had about a 20% higher overall survival rate of three to four years (Guimaraes & Uflacker, 2011).

Irreversible Electroporation

Irreversible electroporation (IRE) is a nonthermal ablation technique that uses electrical fields to permeate the cell membrane. The membrane is permeabilized through the formation of nanoscale defects in the lipid bilayer, leading to cell death (Padma et al., 2009). Microsecond electrical pulses of 1,000–3,000 V are delivered to the target mass using percutaneous probes. The probes are placed in a similar fashion to other ablative probes, typically under real-time CT guidance. IRE may spare neighboring structures such as bile ducts and blood vessels in comparison to other ablation techniques, which makes it a compelling strategy for use in difficult-to-treat areas.

High-Intensity Focused Ultrasound

High-intensity focused ultrasound (HIFU) is a noninvasive method that has been used to treat malignancies of the breast and liver. The US beam generates heat as the acoustic energy is absorbed by the target tissue. This induces a coagulation necrosis as the tissue temperature reaches 60°C. Although HIFU is desirable because of its noninvasiveness, treatment times are long (four to six hours), and it may need to be repeated. In patients with unresectable hepatocellular carcinoma, the five-year survival rate following treatment with HIFU was 32% (Zhang et al., 2009). HIFU of the breast is not widely accepted in the United States as a treatment modality, given other available options.

Interventional Radiology in Palliative Care

Drain Apparatus

Malignant ascites is the accumulation of intraperitoneal fluid caused by an underlying cancer. A variety of cancers are associated with recurrent ascites, including ovarian, pancreatic, breast, and colon cancers. The exact etiology of malignant ascites is unknown but may be associated with obstructed lymphatic drainage, changes in vascular permeability, and sodium retention. Unlike the majority of patients with ascites whose conditions are caused by portal hypertension or cirrhosis, patients with malignant ascites rarely respond to medical therapy with protein replacement or diuretics (LeBlanc & Arnold, 2010). Instead, treatment is directed at the underlying cancer and palliative drainage.

Paracentesis can provide immediate relief of the symptoms associated with ascites, although it does not treat the underlying tumor. An US examination is performed to identify a safe target for drainage and to estimate fluid volume. Several drainage systems are available for paracentesis, such as the small pigtail drain and special drainage needles (e.g., Yueh needles). These systems provide efficient drainage when attached to a negative suction system. Small amounts of fluid may be easily withdrawn by hand if the underlying collection is small or if only a diagnostic aspiration is indicated. For patients with recurrent ascites, an indwelling peritoneal drain may be placed so that patients may drain in the convenience of their home. Tunneled catheter systems may also be placed that provide a stable and user-friendly option for home drainage (Tapping, Ling, & Razack, 2011). Potential complications of any type of paracentesis or drainage procedure include bleeding, hypotension, infection, and nontarget organ puncture.

Malignant pleural effusions are another common fluid-related complication of advanced cancer, with 150,000 new cases occurring in the United States annually (MacEachern & Tremblay, 2011). Malignant pleural effusions are associated most often with lung and breast cancers, with the patient exhibiting symptoms of dyspnea, fatigue, and cough. Treatment is targeted toward control of the underlying malignancy and relief of symptoms. Minimally invasive treatment involves thoracentesis and placement of a needle into the fluid-filled space between the visceral and parietal pleura. Fluid may be withdrawn by hand aspiration or by attachment to a suction device, which typically results in immediate symptom relief. Specimens may be sent to the laboratory for cytology and culture (MacEachern & Tremblay, 2011).

Repeated thoracentesis is not recommended for recurrent effusions. For inpatients, a multipurpose or pigtail drain may be placed and connected to underwater suction drainage. Small-bore catheters are as effective as larger-bore catheters in draining malignant pleural effusions (Fysh, Smith, & Lee, 2010) and are significantly more comfortable. Complications include catheter dislodgment, site bleeding, hemothorax, and pneumothorax. A tunneled catheter may be placed to facilitate repeated drainage, even in the home setting.

Other patients may be aided by pleurodesis, which is designed to obliterate the potential space in which fluid can accumulate. Performed through a pigtail catheter, sclerosing agents (e.g., talc, bleomycin, povidone iodine) are instilled into the pleural space and allowed to dwell for one to several days and then drained. The success of pleurodesis, as determined by lung re-expansion and obliteration of the pleural effusion, is estimated at 53%–60%, whereas spontaneous pleurodesis in patients with indwelling drainage catheters is estimated at 46% (Fysh et al., 2010; MacEachern & Tremblay, 2011). Complications from pleural drainage catheters include infection, catheter dislodgment, poor drainage, pneumothorax, fever, pain, and acute respiratory distress syndrome. Currently no consensus exists on whether patients with recurrent malignant pleural effusions are best served by repeated drainage versus pleurodesis, although both interventions may offer symptom relief and potential resolution of pleural effusions (Zahid, Routledge, Bille, & Scarci, 2011).

Patients with cholangiocarcinoma, primary or metastatic hepatic disease, or pancreatic cancers may benefit from decompression of obstructed biliary systems, which is evidenced by painless jaundice, anorexia, icterus, and elevated serum bilirubin. The purpose of percutaneous biliary drainage is to relieve pruritus, treat cholangitis, or decrease serum bilirubin to allow the administration of systemic antineoplastic agents that require hepatic metabolism or excretion. Contrast-enhanced CT imaging is obtained to evaluate for other hepatic disease and ascites, to assess anatomic land-marks, and to determine the level of biliary obstruction. Radiopaque land-marks are used to guide the initial needle puncture into the biliary tree under fluoroscopy. A guide wire is advanced through the biliary system, and a multiple-side-hole drainage catheter is advanced using a coaxial system (Tapping et al., 2011).

If the biliary system is totally obstructed, the drainage catheter is connected to a drainage bag. If the obstruction can be crossed with a guide wire, a biliary catheter can be advanced across the stenotic segment and into the small bowel. This is referred to as an *internal/external catheter* because it allows bile to drain into the external drainage bag as well as into the small bowel, although the primary goal is to achieve biliary drainage into the small bowel. The catheter serves as a stent because it provides structural support within the biliary tree. Subsequently, a patient may be a candidate for internal stent placement in the absence of active infection or bleeding in the biliary system. Patients with intraductal stones or tumor are typically not good candidates for internal stents, as long-term stent patency is unlikely. Percutaneous drainage catheters can remain in place for months or even years, with intermittent catheter exchange to ensure continued patency. Symptoms are rapidly relieved when biliary decompression is performed (Tapping et al., 2011).

Celiac Plexus Block

Abdominal pain is a common symptom in patients with pancreatic and upper gastrointestinal malignancies and is a challenge to control. Interventions in these cases are targeted to the celiac plexus, which is a complex network of nerves where the celiac trunk, superior mesenteric artery, and renal arteries branch from the abdominal aorta. The celiac plexus includes autonomic efferent nerves, which innervate the upper abdominal viscera, and afferent fibers, which innervate the abdominal viscera from the distal esophagus to the transverse colon (Erdek, Halpert, Fernández, & Cohen, 2010). Alcohol is the most commonly injected agent with fluoroscopy, US, or CT imaging to guide the needle to the celiac plexus with injection of 20–50 ml of the neurolytic agent. Symptom relief can be provided for months with reduction of systemic opioids. Potential complications include hypotension, paresthesia, and diarrhea (Markman & Philip, 2007).

Spine Interventions

At least 60% of patients with metastatic disease will experience involvement of bone (Biermann, Holt, Lewis, Schwartz, & Yaszemski, 2009). Bone metastasis is common in several cancers, including multiple myeloma (70%–95%), breast (65%–75%), and lung cancers (30%–40%) (vonMoos, Strasser, Gillessen, & Zaugg, 2008). These patients can experience pain, loss of structural integrity of bone, and potential fracture. Vertebral fractures are particularly common and are defined as reduction in height of the vertebral body of at least 20% from its initial dimensions. Initial evaluation of vertebral disease and compression fractures includes two-view radiographs. MRI is used to detect fracture age and to evaluate multilevel fractures (Rollinghoff et al., 2010). Conservative management strategies include bed rest, systemic opioid pain medications and nonsteroidal anti-inflammatory agents, and orthotics. These approaches carry with them the risks of immobilization, including deep vein thrombosis, pneumonia, skin breakdown, and accelerated bone resorption. Other potential treatments include external beam radiation therapy and systemic antineoplastic therapy. Vertebral augmentation techniques, such as kyphoplasty and vertebroplasty, offer minimally invasive alternatives for patients requiring pain control. They also provide simultaneous bone stabilization and may be used alone or in combination with standard therapy (Wu & Fourney, 2005).

Vertebroplasty involves placement of a needle into the fractured vertebral body through the vertebral pedicle with subsequent injection of polymethyl methacrylate (PMMA) into the compressed vertebral body. Kyphoplasty is a variant of vertebroplasty that consists of creation of a space within the vertebral body with insertion of a balloon (see Figure 16-6). The balloon is removed after inflation, and PMMA is injected into the newly created cavity. In either case, the PMMA stabilizes microfractures and reduces mechanical forces thought to contribute to pain control (Jha et al., 2010). PMMA may also contribute to pain control by destruction of pain receptors and nerve endings in the vertebral body. Patients with cancer were less likely to respond than patients with compression fractures of benign etiology such as osteoporosis. Patients who required treatment at multiple levels were also less likely to achieve pain control. Contraindications to vertebral augmentation include uncorrected coagulopathy, active infection, and bone cement allergy. The most common complications of vertebral augmentation include PMMA extravasation, balloon ruptures, bleeding, adjacent fractures, and neurologic compromise (Jha et al., 2009).

Conclusions

Procedures that involve interventional radiology occur across the entire cancer care continuum. Interventional radiology continues to evolve with greater involvement in patient care and innovative procedures to improve diagnostics and symptom management. Traditionally, interventional radiology focused on cancer diagnosis, interventions, and palliative care for inoperable cases. Today, interventional radiology is used in conjunction with all aspects of surgical and supportive cancer care to provide individualized personalized cancer care.

References

Baskin, J.L., Pui, C.H., Reiss, U., Wilimas, J.A., Metzger, M.L., Ribeiro, R.C., & Howard, S.C. (2009). Management of occlusion and thrombosis associated with long-term indwelling central venous catheters. *Lancet, 374,* 159–169. doi:10.1016/S0140-6736(09)60220-8

Biermann, J.S., Holt, G.E., Lewis, V.O., Schwartz, H.S., & Yaszemski, M.J. (2009). Metastatic bone disease: Diagnosis, evaluation, and treatment. *Journal of Bone and Joint Surgery, 91,* 1518–1530.

Erdek, M.A., Halpert, D.E., Fernández, M.G., & Cohen, S.P. (2010). Assessment of celiac plexus block and neurolysis outcomes and technique in the management of refractory visceral cancer pain. *Pain Medicine, 11,* 92–100. doi:10.1111/j.1526-4637.2009.00756.x

Froelich, C.D., Rigby, M.R., Rosenberg, E.S., Ruosha, L., Pei-Ling, J.R., Easley, K.A., & Stockwell, J.A. (2009). Ultrasound guided central venous catheter placement decreases complications and decreases placement attempts compared with the landmark technique in patients in a pediatric intensive care unit. *Critical Care Medicine, 37,* 1090–1096. doi:10.1097/CCM.0b013e31819b570e

Fysh, E.T.H., Smith, N.A., & Lee, Y.C.G. (2010). Optimal chest drain size: The rise of the small-bore pleural catheter. *Seminars in Respiratory and Critical Care Medicine, 31,* 760–768. doi:10.1055/s-0030-1269836

Gallieni, M., Pittiruti, M., & Biffi, R. (2008). Vascular access in oncology patients. *CA: A Cancer Journal for Clinicians, 58,* 323–346. doi:10.3322/CA.2008.0015

Grasso, R.F., Luppi, G., Faiella, E., Giurazza, F., Del Vescovo, R., Cazzato, R.L., & Zobel, B.B. (2012). Radiofrequency ablation of renal cell carcinoma in patients with a solitary kidney: A retrospective analysis of our experience. *La Radiologia Medica, 117,* 606–615. doi:10.1007/s11547-011-0758-6

Guimaraes, M., & Uflacker, R. (2011). Locoregional therapy for hepatocellular carcinoma. *Clinics in Liver Disease, 15,* 395–421. doi:10.1016/j.cld.2011.03.013

Gunven, P. (2008). Liver embolizations in oncology: A review: Part 1. Arterial (chemo) embolizations. *Medical Oncology, 15,* 1–11. doi:10.1007/s12032-007-0039-3

Jha, R.M., Hirsch, A.E., Yoo, A.J., Ozonoff, A., Growney, M., & Hirsch, J.A. (2010). Palliation of compression fractures in cancer patients by vertebral augmentation: A retrospective analysis. *Journal of Neurointerventional Surgery, 3,* 221–228. doi:10.1136/jnis.2010.002675

Lammer, J., Malagari, K., Vogl, T., Pilleul, F., Denys, A., Watkinson, A., ... Lencioni, R. (2010). Prospective randomized study of doxorubicin-eluting-bead embolization in the treatment of hepatocellular carcinoma: Results of the PRECISION V study. *Cardiovascular and Interventional Radiology, 33,* 41–52. doi:10.1007/s00270-009-9711-7

LeBlanc, K., & Arnold, R.M. (2010). Palliative treatment of malignant ascites. *Journal of Palliative Medicine, 13,* 1028–1029. doi:10.1089/jpm.2010.9799

MacEachern, P., & Tremblay, A. (2011). Pleural controversy: Pleurodesis versus indwelling pleural catheters for malignant effusions. *Respirology, 16,* 747–754. doi:10.1111/j.1440-1843.2011.01986.x

Markman, J.D., & Philip, A. (2007). Interventional approaches to pain management. *Anesthesiology Clinics, 25,* 883–898. doi:10.1016/j.anclin.2007.07.012

Padma, S., Martinie, J.B., & Iannitti, D.A. (2009). Liver tumor ablation: Percutaneous and open approaches. *Journal of Surgical Oncology, 100,* 619–634. doi:10.1002/jso.21364

Riaz, A., Lewandowski, R.J., Kulik, L., & Salem, R. (2009). Yttrium-90 radioembolization using TheraSphere in the management of primary and secondary liver tumors. *Quarterly Journal of Nuclear Medicine and Molecular Imaging, 53,* 311–316. Retrieved from http://www.minervamedica.it/en/journals/nuclear-med-molecular-imaging/article.php?cod=R39Y2009N03A0311

Rollinghoff, M., Zarghooni, K., Schluter-Brust, K., Sobottke, R., Schlegel, U., Eysel, P., & Delank, K.S. (2010). Indications and contraindications for vertebroplasty and kyphoplasty. *Archives of Orthopedic and Trauma Surgery, 130,* 765–774. doi:10.1007/s00402-010-1083-6

Saber, W., Moua, T., Williams, E.C., Verso, M., Agnelli, G., Coubain, S., … Lee, A.Y. (2011). Risk factors for catheter-related thrombosis (CRT) in cancer patients: A patient-level data (IPD) meta-analysis of clinical trials and prospective studies. *Journal of Thrombosis and Haemostasis, 9,* 312–319. doi:10.1111/j.1538-7836.2010.04126.x

Shankar, S., van Sonnenberg, E., Silverman, S.G., & Tuncali, K. (2002). Interventional radiology procedures in the liver: Biopsy, drainage, and ablation. *Hepatic Imaging and Intervention, 6,* 91–118.

Tapping, C.R., Ling, L., & Razack, A. (2011). PleurX drain use in the management of malignant ascites: Safety, complications, long term-patency and factors predictive of success. *British Journal of Radiology, 85,* 623–628. doi:10.1259/bjr/24538524

vonMoos, R., Strasser, F., Gillessen, S., & Zaugg, K. (2008). Metastatic bone pain: Treatment options with an emphasis on bisphosphonates. *Supportive Care in Cancer, 16,* 1105–1115. doi:10.1007/s00520-008-0487-0

Walser, E.M. (2012). Venous access ports: Indications, implantation technique, follow-up and complications. *Cardiovascular and Interventional Radiology, 35,* 751–764. doi:10.1007/s00270-011-0271-2

Wu, A.S., & Fourney, D.R. (2005). Supportive care aspects of vertebroplasty in patients with cancer. *Supportive Cancer Therapy, 2,* 98–104. doi:10.3816/SCT.2005.n.003

Yang, Y., Wang, C., Lu, Y., Bai, W., An, L., Qu, J., … Lv, J. (2012). Outcomes of ultrasound-guided percutaneous argon-helium cryoablation of hepatocellular carcinoma. *Journal of Hepatobiliary and Pancreatic Science, 19,* 674–684. doi:10.1007/s00534-011-0490-6

Zahid, I., Routledge, T., Bille, A., & Scarci, M. (2011). What is the best treatment for malignant pleural effusions? *Interactive Cardiovascular and Thoracic Surgery, 12,* 818–823. doi:10.1510/icvts.2010.254789

Zhang, L., Zhu, H., Jin, C., Zhou, K., Li, K., Su, H., … Wang, Z. (2009). High-intensity focused ultrasound (HIFU): Effective and safe therapy for hepatocellular carcinoma adjacent to major hepatic veins. *European Journal of Radiology, 19,* 437–444. doi:10.1007/s00330-008-1137-0

CHAPTER 20

Intraoperative Radiation Therapy

Louise Williams, BSN, RN, CNOR, and Sue A. Burke, BSN, RN, CNOR

Introduction

Radiation therapy (RT) is an important component in the multimodality treatment of cancer. RT primarily shrinks tumor mass and ultimately kills cancer cells. It may be the only treatment a patient receives or may be used in conjunction with surgery, chemotherapy, and biotherapy. Radiation treatments are performed in the outpatient setting when external beam RT (EBRT) is the selected mode. Some types of cancer respond to EBRT, such as cancers of the head and neck, breast, abdomen, pelvis, and thoracic regions and bone and soft tissue sarcomas.

RT may also be used at the time of surgical procedures; this is termed *intraoperative RT* (IORT). IORT differs from EBRT in that a single dose of radiation is delivered to a specific area with limited damage to the surrounding healthy tissue and structures. IORT may be used with or without chemotherapy and usually in combination with surgical resection of the tumor. Generally, only one area is treated, but it is possible to treat multiple sites, such as in the case of ovarian cancer when bilateral pelvic sidewalls are involved.

History of Intraoperative Radiation Therapy

The first IORT treatment was utilized in Japan in the early 1960s. IORT was first used in the United States in 1976 (Calvo, Meirino, & Orecchia, 2006). In the early days of IORT, hospitals transported anesthetized patients to the radiation oncology department, a difficult and potentially risky process. As progress was made in the application of IORT, some facilities constructed lead- or concrete-shielded operating rooms (ORs) and placed a dedicated linear accelerator for use in the OR only. This eliminated moving an anesthetized patient from one area to another and also ensured sterility of the patient and the operative field.

Use of Intraoperative Radiation Therapy

An advantage to IORT is the ability to visualize the tumor bed and direct the radiation beam to that area. This allows the surgeon and radiation oncologist to determine the exact area to be treated and the proposed margins after the surgical resection. In cases where the tumor resection is difficult and clear margins cannot be attained or when complete resection is not possible, IORT may be administered to treat and diminish tumor that may have remained after resection.

Margins of Tumor

Ideally, surgical resection with or without IORT will result in clear margins around the tumor with a predisposed rim of cancer-free tissue. Surgical margins are examined at the time of surgery, and subsequent IORT is aimed to eradicate malignant tissue up to 1 cm from the tumor margin (Sinha, 2008). Recurrent tumor most frequently occurs at or near the site of the original tumor, which supports the rationale to eradicate the positive tumor margins (Sinha, 2008). The provision of radiation in this setting enables higher individual radiation doses to be delivered with minimal exposure to normal and healthy tissues. Before IORT, the skin is retracted to move healthy tissue away from the field of radiation or healthy tissue is protected with the use of lead shields during the treatment. With IORT, further radiation treatment may not be required; therefore, the side effects experienced with EBRT can be eliminated.

Use in Breast Cancer

Recent advances in the treatment of breast cancer consider the use of IORT instead of six weeks of daily EBRT. This innovation is in part due to early detection and diagnosis of small breast tumors. Historically, women who underwent a lumpectomy were recommended to receive whole breast RT as part of their evidence-based treatment for breast cancer (Simone et al., 2012). Whole breast RT usually involves five to six weeks of daily (Monday through Friday) radiation treatments that require the patient to travel to the treatment center every day for the treatment period (Moore-Higgs, 2006).

Today, intraoperative partial breast radiation may be an option for some women who will require RT as part of their treatment plan. Several methods can potentially deliver partial breast IORT; these remain under study in clinical trials. Good or excellent cosmetic results were reported in 90% of women who received partial breast irradiation in clinical trials (Kimple et al., 2011; Moore-Higgs, 2006).

Physical Structure of Facility, Equipment, and Safety of Staff

Radiation treatments in the OR may be delivered by two different methods: IORT and high-dose-rate (HDR) radiation. The physical structure and safety of the staff must be intact prior to the delivery of these innovative approaches. Time, distance, and lead shields are the primary safety measures for the delivery of radiation. A dedicated surgical suite for IORT with concrete or lead shields is an expensive endeavor. In contrast, the development of the mobile linear accelerator with intact radiation shields increases the flexibility of OR space and eliminates the construction of a costly shielded room in order to deliver IORT (Abdel-Wahab, Rosenblatt, Holmberg, & Meghzifene, 2011).

However, the HDR-IORT mechanism still requires a room that is constructed with lead shields with the inclusion of lead-lined doors. A medical physicist and member of the radiation oncology team perform weekly quality safety checks. These precautions are paramount for the safety of the staff.

Equipment and Instruments

IORT uses a linear accelerator. In some facilities, it is stationary and the OR bed is moved to the accelerator, whereas other facilities have a mobile accelerator that is moved into place over the surgical field. A surgical clamp system such as an IORT Bookwalter bedpost clamp is attached to the rail on the side of the OR bed and an extension bar connects to the bedpost. This apparatus secures the Bookwalter mirror, applicator, and cone (see Figure 20-1). The applicators come in sizes that range from 3–10 cm, and the cones correspond to the sizes of the applicator and may be flat at the end or beveled at 15° or 30°. The beveled cones and rotation of the linear accelerator facilitate proper coverage (Biggs et al., 2011).

Sometimes rotating the OR bed or even repositioning the patient may be necessary to facilitate access to the desired area for treatment. A bolus or plastic disc may be inserted into the cone to increase the radiation dose to the surface tissue yet decrease the penetration depth of the beam of radiation (Biggs et al., 2011). These bolus inserts are available in sizes that correspond to the cones and are round for the flat cones and oval for the beveled cones. They come in two thicknesses, 5 mm and 10 mm. Lead shields are also available in various sizes and shapes. They are used to protect and shield normal tissues or structures that may be within the treatment area. The lead shields are wrapped in sterile plastic and may be covered with saline-soaked

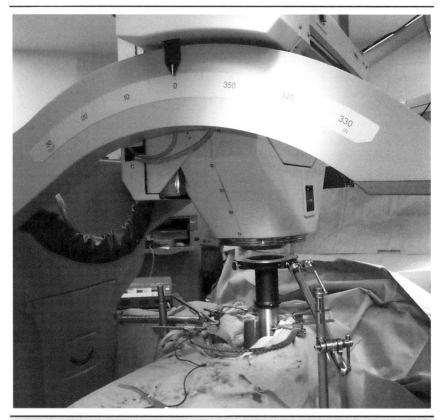

Figure 20-1. IORT Bookwalter Clamping Device Bedpost, Extension Bar, Applicator, Cone, and Mirror With Docked Linear Accelerator

Note. Photo courtesy of Sue A. Burke, BSN, RN, CNOR, The Ohio State University. Used with permission.

gauze to prevent the lead from coming in contact with patient tissue (Song, Delclos, Tomas, Crane, & Beddar, 2007).

Team Members

The provision of IORT requires a multidisciplinary approach that includes staff members from nursing, the surgery department, and the radiation oncology department. The surgical team may include the surgeon, fellows, residents, physician assistants, and medical students. The radiation oncology team includes the radiation oncologist, physicist, dosimetrist, and radiology oncology technologists. Preoperatively, the radiation oncologist evaluates the patient and collaborates with the surgeon as to whether the patient is a candidate for IORT. The perioperative nursing staff includes an RN circulator and scrub personnel, who could be either an RN or surgical technologist. Anesthesia providers and pathologists are also members of this team.

Preparation

The perioperative nursing staff has responsibilities that begin before the patient even enters the OR suite. The RN should turn on and verify the function of the monitors and video equipment in the anteroom. The OR setup includes verification of the patient's position during the procedure and procurement of the correct OR bed and necessary positioning devices. The specialized OR bed must enable the linear accelerator to access any part of the patient that requires radiation. In addition, the OR bed must allow access for C-arm images if anticipated for the operative procedure. The position of the patient and the location of the area to be treated will dictate the orientation of the OR bed. The RN and the surgical technician gather the sterile supplies and equipment needed for the case and any instruments needed by the radiation oncologist. The perioperative nursing staff is responsible for the safe care of the patient during the entire procedure. The RN helps position the patient on the OR bed, with full knowledge of the operative and radiation needs. The RN circulator notifies the radiation oncology team to allow them time to prepare the RT equipment and perform the required safety checks (Song et al., 2007).

During IORT or HDR-IORT treatments, all staff must leave the main OR room. A mobile lead shield may be placed in front of the door between the OR and the anteroom where the personnel will remain scrubbed during the treatment period. Equipment to monitor the patient is located in the anteroom so that crucial observations can occur. Continuous visualization of the surgical field, the treatment area, and the patient is achieved with monitors and cameras in the OR that can be rotated to various angles. The patient monitor allows the anesthesia care provider to observe the patient's vital signs, electrocardiogram, and any other parameters, such as an arterial line. Any changes in the patient's condition can be observed and the treatment may be immediately interrupted, if necessary. An emergency shut-off system is connected to the doors of the OR and will automatically shut off the radiation source if a door is inadvertently opened. This emergency shut-off may also be used if the patient's condition critically changes during the radiation treatment (Abdel-Wahab et al., 2011).

Precautions

The IORT procedure is performed with the patient under general anesthesia. The anesthesia care provider induces the patient, monitors hemodynamic status, and administers fluids and blood products as needed. The surgeon is the person responsible for the entire procedure; the surgeon and assistants make the incision and resect the tumor. When necessary, other specialty surgeons may be consulted to assist with the safe resection of the tumor. For example, if the tumor involves structures such as major blood vessels, ureter, or bladder, a vascular surgeon or urologist may be consulted. The tumor specimen may be sent after resection to the pathologist to ensure clear surgical margins. This information at the time of surgery may help to determine the area of IORT.

After completion of the tumor resection, the radiation oncologist and surgeon confirm the size of the tumor bed to be irradiated. The radiation oncologist selects the appropriate size applicator and cone based on the size of the treatment area and prescribes the dose of radiation based on the extent of the tumor, adjacent critical structures, patient anatomy, residual tumor, and history of previous RT (Beddar et al., 2001). The medical physicist and dosimetrist collaborate with the radiation oncologist to develop the computerized treatment plan to deliver the highest dose to the tumor bed, with inclusion of constraints such as tissue tolerance and possible long-term side effects. The radiation oncology technologist places the applicator and cone and is the last person to leave the room. He or she verifies that all other personnel have exited and all safety measures are intact.

At the end of the treatment, all staff reenter the room. After aseptically putting on gowns and gloves, the radiation oncologist removes the applicator and cone. The radiation oncologist may place gold seeds or hemoclips in the treatment area as markers at the resection margin. Gold seeds are more radiopaque and will not be confused with hemoclips used to obtain hemostasis during the surgical resection of the tumor. Gold seeds can be used as markers to plan EBRT that may be required to complete the patient's treatment (Nag, Koc, Schuller, Tippin, & Grecula, 2005).

High-Dose-Rate Intraoperative Radiation Therapy

The equipment and supplies required for HDR treatment are different than those needed for IORT. HDR treatment times are usually longer than IORT. The remote afterloader, a computer-controlled machine, delivers the HDR treatments. The remote afterloader may be kept in the radiation oncology department to be used for outpatient treatments and brought to the shielded OR when needed. The Harrison-Anderson-Mick (HAM) applicators are flexible silicone pads with imbedded catheters that provide access to body surfaces that cannot be accessed with the rigid applicators and cones used in IORT (Willett, Czito, & Tyler, 2007). The catheters are 10 mm apart but parallel to each other (Song et al., 2007).

The width of the HAM applicator depends on the size of the area to be treated and may range from 3–24 cm. Sterile, hollow transfer tubes connect from the catheters in the HAM applicator to the HDR afterloader in proper order and position (see Figures 20-2 and 20-3). A metal wire called a check cable is used to verify correct connections. The computer-controlled HDR afterloader contains a small radiation source attached to a thin cable or wire. After the transfer tubes are connected to the afterloader, the source is extended outside the afterloader, passing through the transfer tubes to the tumor site. As with IORT, all staff and equipment safety precautions must be observed. After treatment is completed, the radiation source is retracted into the HDR afterloader.

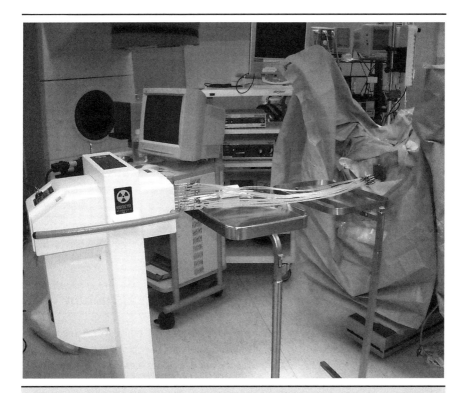

Figure 20-2. High-Dose-Rate Treatment Afterloader, Transfer Cables, Needles, and Template

Note. Photo courtesy of Sue A. Burke, BSN, RN, CNOR, The Ohio State University. Used with permission.

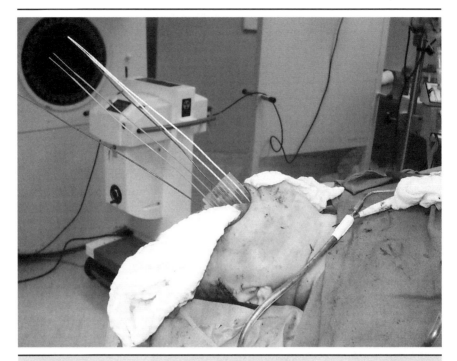

Figure 20-3. High-Dose-Rate With Silastic Block for Maxillary and Palate Treatment

Note. Photo courtesy of Sue A. Burke, BSN, RN, CNOR, The Ohio State University. Used with permission.

Brachytherapy

The word *brachytherapy* comes from the Greek word *brachy*, which means "short." In cancer treatment, this refers to the short distance from the radioactive source to the site of the tumor (Randall, 2008). Some brachytherapy implants, such as prostate seeds, are permanent, whereas others, such as the ring and tandem used to treat cervical cancer, are removable. Randall (2008) classified brachytherapy in three variables: (a) dose rate (high or low), (b) permanent or removable implant, and (c) location of the implant, such as interstitial or intracavitary. An interstitial implant is placed in or around the tumor without the benefit of using a body cavity. Prostate seeds are an example of an interstitial implant. Intracavitary implant refers to placing the radiation source into a body cavity such as the vagina, cervix, or uterus. These intracavitary implants are removed after completion of the treatment plan.

Prostate Brachytherapy

Prostate cancer treatment using the brachytherapy method with low-dose radioactive seeds is an outpatient procedure. With the patient under anesthesia, the radiation oncologist places implants with ultrasound guidance in a percutaneous transperineal approach with preloaded needles that contain the radioactive seeds. The radioactive seeds are placed according to predetermined coordinates. A computed tomography scan or magnetic resonance imaging may be performed after completion of the brachytherapy implants to verify seed location (Marcus, Jani, Godette, & Rossi, 2010).

The room, trash, suction canisters, and linens are scanned before they are removed from the room to ensure no radioactive seeds are left behind. If any seeds are found, they should not be picked up with the hand but should be retrieved using V-block forceps and placed in a lead-lined container. The radioactivity can last two to three months. The patient and family should be educated regarding precautions to observe at home.

Cervical and Vaginal Cancer Radiation

Removable, intracavitary brachytherapy implants may be used to treat cervical and vaginal cancers. In the past, low-dose-rate (LDR) RT was the accepted treatment modality for these types of cancer. Manufacturers have stopped making LDR equipment, which leaves HDR as one of the alternative treatments (Valentin, 2005). HDR treatments for cervical cancer may require several treatments performed on an outpatient basis. Radioactive material is inserted at each treatment for a few minutes and then removed. The applicators used for HDR RT may be the ring and tandem, the Fletcher-Suit-Delclos, or the Smit sleeve (see Figure 20-4). The applicator is inserted and

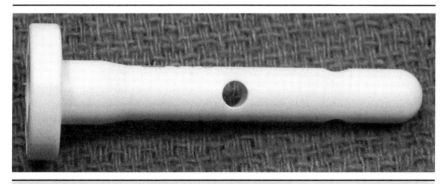

Figure 20-4. Smit Sleeve

Note. Photo courtesy of Sue A. Burke, BSN, RN, CNOR, The Ohio State University. Used with permission.

sutured in place with the patient in the OR and under anesthesia. One advantage of HDR treatment is that the patient does not have to stay still for long periods of time as the treatment is short, lasting 1–12 minutes (Valentin, 2005). Another advantage is that outpatient treatments allow the patient to be at home with family between treatments, preventing the feeling of isolation that may occur during the inpatient LDR treatment and also decreasing the risks associated with prolonged bed rest.

Another type of brachytherapy, eye plaque, is used to treat choroidal melanoma. Melanoma may develop in the vascular support layer of the eye, the uveal tract. The most common location is in the choroid, the posterior portion of the uveal tract located under the retina (Mishra, Quivey, Daftari, & Char, 2010). This low-dose brachytherapy utilizes the iodine-125 isotope. The placement of the eye plaque is done using local anesthesia. The eye is dilated to facilitate tumor location. Before the radioactive plaque is placed, a dummy plaque is placed and the position verified. The radiation oncologist may use ultrasound to ensure proper placement (see Figure 20-5). A lead patch is placed over the eye with the implant and no further shielding is required. The implant usually remains in place for four days. At the end of the treatment period, the patient returns to the hospital to have the implant removed. For many years, enucleation was the standard treatment for this disease. This treatment provides patients an opportunity for possible vision preservation.

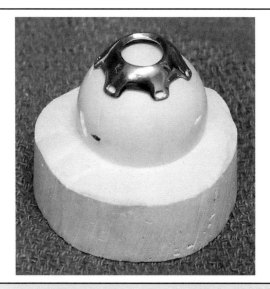

Figure 20-5. Eye Plaque Device on Ocular Mold for Choroidal Melanoma

Note. Photo courtesy of Sue A. Burke, BSN, RN, CNOR, The Ohio State University. Used with permission.

Conclusions

Technologic advances have made IORT a treatment option for more patients in more facilities. A collaborative and coordinated multidisciplinary team effort is necessary to provide these services. The mobile linear accelerator makes it possible to perform the IORT in the OR, eliminating the need to transfer the patient to the radiology department. HDR devices allow for more ambulatory treatment options, decreasing the need for expensive hospital stays. With greater access and the availability of clinical trials, these treatment modalities may result in improved patient satisfaction and outcomes.

References

Abdel-Wahab, M., Rosenblatt, E., Holmberg, O., & Meghzifene, A. (2011). Safety in radiation oncology: The role of international initiatives by the International Atomic Energy Agency. *Journal of the American College of Radiology, 8,* 789–794. doi:10.1016/j.jacr.2011.07.014

Beddar, A., Domanovic, M., Kubu, M., Ellis, R., Sibata, C., & Kinsella, T. (2001). Mobile linear accelerators for intraoperative radiation therapy. *AORN Journal, 74,* 700–705.

Biggs, P., Willet, C.G., Rutten, H., Ciocca, M., Gunderson, L.L., & Calvo, F.A. (2011). Intraoperative electron beam irradiation: Physics and techniques. In L.L. Gunderson, C.G. Willett, F.A. Calvo, & L.B. Harrison (Eds.), *Intraoperative irradiation: Techniques and results* (2nd ed., pp. 51–72). New York, NY: Humana Press.

Calvo, F.A., Meirino, R.M., & Orecchia, R. (2006). Intraoperative radiation therapy first part: Rationale and techniques. *Critical Reviews in Oncology/Hematology, 59,* 106–115. doi:10.1016/j.critrevonc.2005.11.004

Kimple, R.J., Klauber-DeMore, N., Kuzmiak, C.M., Pavic, D., Lian, J., Livasy, C.A., ... Ollila, D.W. (2011). Cosmetic outcomes for accelerated partial breast irradiation before surgical excision of early-stage breast cancer using single-dose intraoperative radiotherapy. *International Journal of Radiation Oncology, Biology, Physics, 79,* 400–407. doi:10.1016/j.ijrobp.2009.10.032

Marcus, D., Jani, A., Godette, K., & Rossi, P. (2010). A review of low-dose-rate prostate brachytherapy—Techniques and outcomes. *Journal of the National Medical Association, 102,* 500–510.

Mishra, K.K., Quivey, J.M., Daftari, I.K., & Char, D.H. (2010). Uveal melanoma. In R.T. Hoppe, T.L. Phillips, & M. Roach (Eds.), *Leibel and Phillips textbook of radiation oncology* (3rd ed., pp. 1400–1421). Philadelphia, PA: Elsevier Saunders.

Moore-Higgs, G. (2006). Radiation options for early stage breast cancer. *Seminars in Oncology Nursing, 22,* 233–241. doi:10.1016/j.soncn.2006.07.005

Nag, S., Koc, M., Schuller, D., Tippin, D., & Grecula, J. (2005). Intraoperative single fraction high-dose-rate brachytherapy for head and neck cancers. *Brachytherapy, 4,* 217–223. doi:10.1016/j.brachy.2005.06.002

Randall, M. (2008). Brachytherapy for gynecologic cancers. *Journal of Gynecologic Oncology Nursing, 18,* 5–10.

Simone, N.L., Dan, T., Shih, J., Smith, S.L., Sciuto, L., Lita, E., ... Camphausen, K. (2012). Twenty-five year results of the National Cancer Institute randomized breast conservation trial. *Breast Cancer Research and Treatment, 132,* 197–203. doi:10.1007/s10549-011-1867-6

Sinha, A. (2008). Intraoperative radiation therapy. *Radiation Therapist, 17*(1), 17–32.

Song, G., Delclos, M., Tomas, L., Crane, C., & Beddar, S. (2007). High-dose-rate remote after-loaders for intraoperative radiation therapy. *AORN Journal, 86,* 827–836.

Valentin, J. (2005). Prevention of high-dose-rate brachytherapy accidents. *Annals of the International Commission on Radiological Procedures, 35,* 1–51. doi:10.1016/j.icrp.2005.05.002

Willett, C., Czito, B., & Tyler, D. (2007). Intraoperative radiation therapy. *Journal of Clinical Oncology, 25,* 971–977. doi:10.1200/JCO.2006.10.0255

CHAPTER 21

Reconstructive Surgery

Deborah Anne Miller, RN, MSN, and Michael J. Miller, MD

Introduction

Microvascular surgery is a technique that allows replacement of impaired tissues with healthy tissue obtained from a distant location on the patient's body. Microvascular surgery allows surgical treatment of multiple solid tumor types previously considered inoperable because of unacceptable risks related to morbidity or mortality. Microvascular surgical procedures are technically complex, and success requires a multidisciplinary cancer care team. Reconstructive microvascular surgery has become an integral part of surgical oncology with a significant impact on oncology nursing. Focused care of patients undergoing these specialized procedures is necessary to optimize outcomes (Bhama, Davis, Bhrany, Lam, & Futran, 2013). This chapter will review the physiology of microvascular surgery as the basis for insightful nursing management.

Reconstructive Microvascular Surgery

Reconstructive microvascular surgery involves the transfer of tissues as surgical flaps with a preserved blood supply. Tissues of all types can be transferred including muscle, fat, bone, peripheral nerve, and viscera. Figures 21-1 through 21-7 demonstrate the use of surgical flaps.

Types of Surgical Flaps

The two basic types of surgical flaps are pedicled and free flaps. Pedicled flaps are transferred without interruption of the vasculature, which contains at least one vein and one artery. Examples of clinical conditions that may be reconstructed with a rotational or pedicled flap include partial breast or mastectomy deformities (see Figure 21-1) and nonhealing wounds from soft

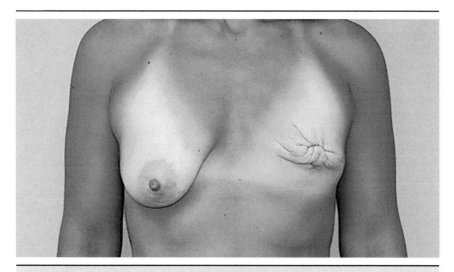

Figure 21-1. Absence of Breast Secondary to Mastectomy/Defect With Scar Tissue

Note. Photo courtesy of Michael J. Miller, MD, The Ohio State University Wexner Medical Center. Used with permission.

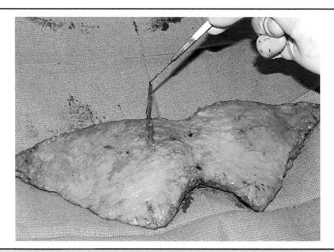

Figure 21-2. Deep Inferior Epigastric Perforator Free Flap With Vascular Pedicle Harvested From Lower Abdomen for Bilateral Breast Reconstruction

Note. Photo courtesy of Michael J. Miller, MD, The Ohio State University Wexner Medical Center. Used with permission.

tissue sarcoma (see Figure 21-4). The free flap is completely detached, or free, from the host at the time of tissue transfer. The vascular pedicle is cut and then reattached at the area of reconstruction. Reattachment of the pedicle requires connection of blood vessels (e.g., vein and artery) that are less than 5 mm in diameter. This procedure is performed under the operating microscope, hence the term *microvascular surgery* (Heffelfinger et al., 2013). Flap success is contingent upon the maintenance of patency at the microvascular anastomosis during the postoperative period. Clinical conditions that benefit from free flaps include breast reconstructions after total mastectomy (see Figures 21-2 and 21-3) and head and neck reconstructions (Lundberg et al., 2013).

The factors that affect blood flow at the microvascular anastomosis guide nursing management of these patients. The sutured blood vessels are at risk for blood clot formation secondary to the injured vascular endothelium and initiation of the clotting cascade from platelet adherence (Selber et al., 2013). Although platelets are essential to the healing process, excessive accumulation can occlude the pedicle vessels and ultimately lead to loss of the free flap. The critical factor that prevents excess accumulation of platelets is the force of blood across the anastomosis. Thus, an uninterrupted high flow of blood through the microvascular anastomosis is essential to sustained patency (Selber et al., 2013).

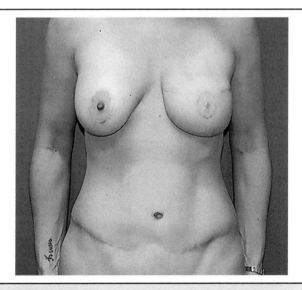

Figure 21-3. Successful Unilateral Deep Inferior Epigastric Perforator Flap Reconstruction Two Years After Surgery

Note. Photo courtesy of Michael J. Miller, MD, The Ohio State University Wexner Medical Center. Used with permission.

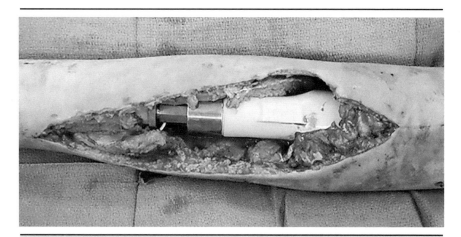

Figure 21-4. Revision of Nonhealing Wound Secondary to Resection of Sarcoma and Insertion of Artificial Prosthesis in Lower Extremity

Note. Photo courtesy of Michael J. Miller, MD, The Ohio State University Wexner Medical Center. Used with permission.

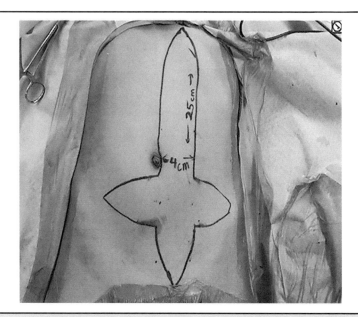

Figure 21-5. Intraoperative Flap Planning of Abdominal Tissue and Vessels for Revision of Lower Leg Wound

Note. Photo courtesy of Michael J. Miller, MD, The Ohio State University Wexner Medical Center. Used with permission.

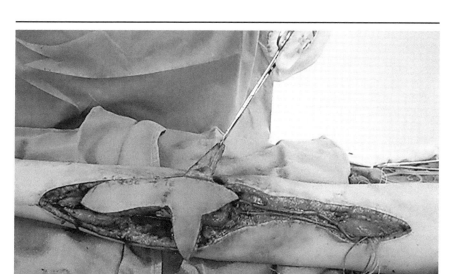

Figure 21-6. Preparation of Flap for Placement in Lower Extremity Defect

Note. Photo courtesy of Michael J. Miller, MD, The Ohio State University Wexner Medical Center. Used with permission.

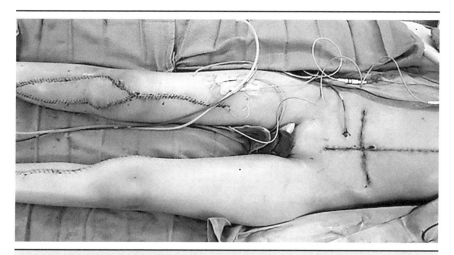

Figure 21-7. Appearance of Completed Revision With Flap: Closed Abdominal Wound as Visualized in Operating Room

Note. Photo courtesy of Michael J. Miller, MD, The Ohio State University Wexner Medical Center. Used with permission.

Factors that indirectly affect nursing care after reconstructive microsurgery include the length and complexity of the surgery, comorbid conditions, and psychosocial issues. These procedures are often combined with surgical resection of the tumor, which requires many hours to complete and involves operating simultaneously on two or more locations. Oncology reconstruction is often performed on older adults with surgical risk factors, such as diabetes mellitus, high blood pressure, cardiopulmonary dysfunction, or vascular disease (Abdel-Galil & Mitchell, 2009; Serletti, Higgins, Moran, & Orlando, 2000). Each coexisting disorder must be managed and coordinated in consult with other specialists as to not threaten the overall recovery of the patient and success of the free tissue transfer (McAnneny, Durden, Pearson, & Tiwari, 2012). The emotional and psychosocial effects of the cancer diagnosis with the potential deformities and impact on quality of life should be assessed as they relate to supportive care, coping, patient education, and discharge planning (Maciejewski et al., 2010; Temple-Oberle et al., 2013).

Nursing Management

Caring for patients after free flap surgery requires a well-functioning care team with sound knowledge, timely communication, and attention to detail (Bhama et al., 2013). In addition to the routine postoperative care for general safe recovery, further information is needed to guide nursing interventions toward promoting and ensuring maximum blood flow through the flap (Abdel-Galil & Mitchell, 2009).

Postanesthesia Care Unit Nursing

Gentle emergence from anesthesia is essential after reconstructive microvascular surgery. Agitation, coughing, shivering, extreme Valsalva maneuver, or excessive movement can cause hemorrhage, hematoma formation, or disruption of the microvascular anastomosis. Head and neck and extremity free flaps are particularly at risk for complications from these causes (Dobrut, Maciejewski, & Półtorak, 2013). Head and neck patients often have a history of alcohol and tobacco abuse and are prone to experience postoperative agitation and symptoms of withdrawal (Patel et al., 2010). Nurses may manage alcohol withdrawal according to institutional guidelines and clinical pathways, and no direct adverse effects would be expected unless doses of high levels of sedation cause systemic hypotension. Nicotine patches should not be used because they have a potential adverse effect on microvascular anastomotic patency (Nahabedian, Singh, Deune, Silverman, & Tufaro, 2004).

Patient Positioning

The patient must be positioned to avoid compression on the flap pedicle, especially if vein grafts have been harvested. In fact, the type of flap (free or pedicled), patient position, flap monitoring, and flap condition (Horng, Chen, Lee, & Horng, 2010) are additional features that often require a nurse-nurse visual report and has become best practice when caring for these complex patients.

Flaps placed on the head are often revascularized from the large vessels in the neck (e.g., external carotid artery, internal jugular vein). Head movement may cause stretching, folding, or compression of the vascular pedicle. The head should be maintained in neutral position without excessive cervical rotation or flexion. A pillow should not be used; sedated patients can have the head stabilized with sand bags placed on either side. Special care must be taken to prevent patients from lying directly on flaps placed on the cranium, torso, or extremities. When the flap pedicle is in the axilla, it is important to keep patients in a supine position with the arms slightly abducted when they are in bed (Abdel-Galil & Mitchell, 2009). Positioning is also of particular importance in cases involving the extremities. Extremity free flaps should be elevated to reduce soft tissue swelling and prevent elevated venous pressure. Wrap dressings often used in extremity surgeries are contraindicated because of possible flap pedicle compression. Negative-pressure wound therapy may be useful in large flap reconstruction of extensive head and neck surgeries and may decrease major wound complications (Schmedes, Banks, Malin, Srinivas, & Skoner, 2012). Ambulation is often delayed, beginning only with dangling the extremity approximately seven days after surgery.

Devices

Devices commonly used for postoperative care must be carefully placed to avoid compressing the flap pedicle or disrupting the flap. Oxygen masks and tubing, wire leads, arterial and venous lines, catheters, wound drains, and other attachments must not place pressure in the area of the flap or flap pedicle. Tracheotomy tubes should be sutured into place rather than secured with collars. In microsurgical breast reconstruction, brassieres may be used but must not compress the flap pedicle.

Temperature Control

Patients might experience hypothermia after long surgical procedures. Large open wounds may exist for hours with limited areas available for warming devices. Hypothermia can promote soft tissue bleeding, hematoma, and flap compromise (Abdel-Galil & Mitchell, 2009). Body and ambient room temperatures directly affect flap circulation. The skin is a thermoregulatory organ that responds to decreased temperature with vasoconstriction. Nursing interventions include monitoring of body temperature, maintaining a warm ambient room temperature in both the postanesthesia unit and surgical floor unit, and covering the patient with warm blankets. Direct heating of the transferred tissue using a radiant source is not usually necessary and may be harmful because the flap tissue lacks sensation (Abdel-Galil & Mitchell, 2009).

Pain Control

Immediate postoperative analgesia in microvascular surgery is similar to that with other major surgical procedures. As the patient enters the postoperative period, a surge in catecholamines and prothrombotic mediators (e.g., plasminogen-1 activator inhibitor, cortisol) occurs. This stress response may result in vasoconstriction detrimental to success of the flap because changes can occur to large, small, and microvessels. Adequate analgesia is therefore vital in an attempt to thwart this stress response (Abdelhamid, Davies, Adam, Vohra, & Bradbury, 2012).

Opioids are the most common option and work best when used in combination with other pain management techniques. This approach results in lower pain scores and reduced need for analgesics after surgery (Jin & Chung, 2001; Silvesti, Svartling, Pitkanen, & Rosenberg, 2000). These drugs and interventions do not affect flap perfusion unless hypotension or hematoma formation occurs. Epidural blocks facilitate pain control and decrease catecholamine concentrations in plasma associated with the surgical stress response.

Hemodynamic Support and Fluid Management

Good overall hemodynamic support, oxygenation, and maintenance of hydration are essential (Rahmanian-Schwarz, Rothenberger, Amr, Jaminet, & Schaller, 2012). The complexity and length of the procedure can create challenges in fluid management because fluid losses can be high. The aim is to maintain intravascular volume for optimal tissue perfusion, especially to the surgical flap. In a study of 23 patients with breast cancer who underwent deep inferior epigastric perforator flap breast reconstruction, drops in the skin oxygen supply, as well as in blood flow on postoperative day 3, were significant for flap failure (Rahmanian-Schwarz et al., 2012). Consequently, postoperative hypovolemia may be adverse for the free tissue transfer even if it appears to be systemically tolerated by the patient. Mild hypervolemia may challenge flap perfusion by increasing cardiac output, venous return, and reflex peripheral vasodilation, although it is a fine balance. Likewise, the volume of blood loss secondary to the complex surgery may negatively affect the flap. It is recommended to maintain a nondiluted hemoglobin level greater than 10 g/dl and hematocrit level greater than 30% in the postoperative period (Hill et al., 2012). In most cases, fluid and blood volume management are sufficient to maintain optimal blood pressure and cardiac output. Diuretics (e.g., furosemide) are avoided when possible because decreased intravascular volume can have an adverse effect on flap blood flow, with resultant platelet aggregation at the venous anastomosis and a compensatory increase in the levels of circulating catecholamine (Rahmanian-Schwarz et al., 2012). Vasoactive drugs, such as sodium nitroprusside and phenylephrine, must be used with caution because of potential adverse effects on flap perfusion. A study in head and neck reconstruction failed to document an adverse effect from intraoperative vasopressors on microvascular flap success, although these findings cannot be extrapolated to all reconstructive procedures (Monroe, Cannady, Ghanem, Swide, & Wax, 2011). Inotropes (e.g., digoxin, isoproterenol, dopamine) used in doses at which minimal vasopressor activity occurs are not detrimental to flap perfusion.

Anticoagulation

Routine anticoagulation with either antiplatelet drugs (e.g., aspirin, dextran) or anticoagulants (e.g., heparin) is not indicated in uncomplicated microvascular tissue transfer operations (Nahabedian, 2011). If complications occur such as postoperative pedicle thrombosis, the patient may be anticoagulated after emergency surgery that successfully reestablishes flow. The nurse should work with the surgeon to monitor the level of anticoagulation, adjust the dosages as ordered, and observe for signs of hematoma formation. In a comparative study of patients with microvascular free tissue transfer, aspirin as compared to low-molecular-weight heparin, a combination, or a heparin drip demonstrated no significant improvement ($p = 0.002$) in the prevention of complications and may be associated with increased adverse events (Lighthall, Cain, Ghanem, & Wax, 2013).

Wound Management

Patients who undergo microvascular surgery usually have at least two surgical sites: the tissue donor site and the recipient site where the actual reconstruction was performed (see Figures 21-5 through 21-7). Additional wounds may be on the extremities where vein grafts were harvested or an area adjacent to the primary defect that was explored to identify appropriate recipient vessels to revascularize the flap. Nursing management would include dressing changes; observation for erythema, fluid collection, and hematoma; and maintenance of skin graft donor site dressings, with detailed documentation and communication. Drain care is of particular importance, as subcutaneous or deep wound drains might be present at multiple sites. The location of each drain, as well as the amount and color of drainage, should be documented and reported to the surgical team, particularly if drainage amounts are unexpectedly low or high.

Monitoring Flap Tissue Perfusion

Frequent monitoring of flap tissue perfusion is vital to ensure flap survival (Nahabedian, 2011). Early detection of pedicle thrombosis was identified as the most important factor for successful salvage of flaps complicated by this condition; use of bedside high-resolution ultrasound may provide improved surveillance (Lamby et al., 2009). The importance of nursing in this role cannot be overstated, as critical thinking and timely communication provide the foundation for successful postoperative care.

Flap perfusion is assessed using a combination of clinical signs supplemented at times with devices able to measure different indicators related to tissue blood flow and oxygenation. Clinical signs are color, temperature, turgor, bleeding, and capillary refill time (Beier et al., 2013; Buntic, 2013).

Color

The color of the visible skin should be compared with that of well-perfused skin in the surrounding area. Venous congestion may be present if the color is notably darker than surrounding tissues. If it is pale, then arterial obstruction is possible. Exposed portions of muscle flaps should have a rich, red color. These color changes are visible in most patients except very dark-skinned people.

Temperature

The flap should be warm. However, even a poorly perfused flap can be warmed by heat transferred from surrounding tissues. Significant changes in temperature different than surrounding tissues might be an indication of decreased perfusion of the flap.

Turgor

Tissue turgor refers to the ability of tissues to be deformed by direct pressure and then return to normal shape. It is controlled primarily by the total amount of fluid inside of them. A flap with arterial occlusion can seem flaccid and deflated, whereas a flap with venous obstruction can feel tense and bulging.

Bleeding

Bleeding from the flap edges can be another sign of increased pressure inside the flap caused by venous obstruction. This is especially true if the bleeding appears to be a new onset in the postoperative period.

Capillary Refill Time

This is the most reliable clinical sign of adequate flap tissue perfusion. The capillary refill time is the time it takes for normal color to return to tissues after direct pressure is applied and then suddenly released. It is obtained in free tissue transfers by gentle digital pressure applied to the surface of the flap—enough to cause blanching. The pressure is released and the point of application observed for return of color. Normal capillary refill time is approximately 2 seconds. If the return is brisk (i.e., less than 2 seconds), venous congestion and outflow compromise may be present. If it is prolonged (i.e., more than 2 seconds), arterial occlusion might exist (Beier et al., 2013; Buntic, 2013).

The nurse should be able to interpret these signs to distinguish between arterial insufficiency and venous congestion. In arterial insufficiency, the tissue is flaccid, pale, and cool and has slow or absent capillary refill. In venous congestion, the tissue has a purple appearance and is engorged, extended, or taut and warm to touch (Buntic, 2013).

Muscle flaps covered with skin grafts have slightly different characteristics, yet the overall principles of flap monitoring still apply. Temperature and capillary refill are generally not helpful, yet the use of a surface Doppler is often indicated. Percutaneous Doppler ultrasound devices are the most commonly used aids (Buntic, 2013). The surgeon will often mark the site where a signal can be obtained and should clearly identify this for the nursing staff. The visible skin graft on muscle flaps will have a poor color in the immediate postoperative period because it is not yet revascularized from the muscle surface, a process that requires approximately five days. If the graft is meshed, the underlying muscle may be visible and should appear red. When muscle flaps become venous congested, they appear dark blue or black, and increased bleeding may occur from the margins or exposed surfaces and loss of the venous signal. Signs of arterial occlusion include a flap where the turgor is flaccid, color is pale, no bleeding occurs on pinprick, and the arterial sign is lost (Buntic, 2013).

Buried flaps, such as the fibular flap without a skin paddle, are the most difficult to monitor because of the lack of visible surface characteristics; however, advances in medical devices have expanded the options available. The most widely used device is the implantable ultrasound probe. This consists of a tiny (1 mm diameter) Doppler crystal that is implanted immediately adjacent to the flap pedicle at the time of surgery. It transmits a sound pulse at 20 MHz frequency and then receives the sound waves reflected from the formed elements circulating in the bloodstream through the pedicle (Buntic, 2013). With this or any other specialized device used for flap monitoring, it is important to communicate with the surgeon to understand how to properly interpret information the machine provides, as well as how to troubleshoot possible problems to avoid false-positive findings.

Preparations for Emergent Repeat Surgery

When signs appear that suggest a problem with flap perfusion related to loss of blood flow through the flap pedicle, the patient must be immediately returned to the operating room to reestablish flow. The successful salvage of a failing free flap is directly related to the amount of time required to restore perfusion to the flap. Therefore, the standard postoperative care of every patient who has had reconstructive microvascular surgery must include preparedness of the nursing, anesthesia, and operating room staff to accommodate emergency microvascular surgery.

Leech Therapy

The medicinal leech (*Hirudo medicinalis*) is a freshwater worm approximately 8–10 cm in length. The primary indication for leech therapy in surgical flaps is to treat venous congestion (Chepeha, Nussenbaum, Bradford, & Teknos, 2002). Leeches are indicated in microvascular surgery only after it is confirmed that venous congestion is not caused by reversible obstruction of the flap pedicle. Leeches are not a substitute for flap reexploration or for treatment of arterial insufficiency.

Leech therapy entails an initial attachment period lasting 20–45 minutes and a postattachment period, during which the site continues to bleed for hours (Yantis, O'Toole, & Ring, 2009). The postattachment phase provides the primary therapeutic benefit. Bleeding is promoted from the tiny wound caused by the leech because vasodilators and anticoagulants in the leech's saliva are injected (Yantis et al., 2009).

A physician order for leech therapy should contain the number of leeches for use, the specific location for attachment, and the frequency of the therapy. Prophylactic antibiotics are also indicated because of the risk of infection by a specific organism, *Aeromonas hydrophila,* known to be associated with leech bites. Nursing management includes assessment, patient education, attachment of the leeches per institutional policy, and frequent containment and monitoring of leech therapy.

Conclusions

Reconstructive microvascular surgery has become an important part of surgical oncology. Microvascular surgery cases are technically complicated, usually lengthy, and often performed in patients with significant comorbidities. Nursing management of these patients requires an appreciation of the unique factors that affect the outcome in this specialized type of surgery. The most important underlying principle of nursing care is to maintain maximum blood flow across the microvascular anastomosis to prevent excess platelet accumulation and flap pedicle thrombosis while maintaining an overall patient recovery. Attention to detail is necessary as patients emerge from anesthesia, particularly in their positioning, placement of medical devices, and management of pain. Sound knowledge and critical thinking skills guide practice as nurses provide assessment of infection risk with multiple wound sites, decreased mobility, hemodynamic support, and fluid management.

Postoperative monitoring of flap tissue perfusion is an essential function of oncology nursing. Timely communication with the microvascular team and facilitation of prompt return of the patient to the operating room at the first sign of flap compromise will give patients the best opportunity for successful outcomes. As with all oncology care, close cooperation among all members of the multidisciplinary team provides the foundation essential for patient well-being, treatment, and recovery.

References

Abdel-Galil, K., & Mitchell, D. (2009). Postoperative monitoring of microsurgical free tissue transfers for head and neck reconstruction: A systematic review of current techniques—part I. Non-invasive techniques. *British Journal of Oral and Maxillofacial Surgery, 47,* 351–355. doi:10.1016/j.bjoms.2008.11.013

Abdelhamid, M.F., Davies, R.S., Adam, D.J., Vohra, R.K., & Bradbury, A.W. (2012). Changes in thrombin generation, fibrinolysis, platelet and endothelial cell activity, and inflammation following endovascular abdominal aortic aneurysm repair. *Journal of Vascular Surgery, 55,* 41–46. doi:10.1016/j.jvs.2011.07.094

Beier, J.P., Horch, R.E., Arkudas, A., Dragu, A., Schmitz, M., & Kneser, U. (2013). Decision-making in DIEP and ms-TRAM flaps: The potential role for a combined laser Doppler spectrophotometry system. *Plastic, Reconstructive, and Aesthetic Surgery, 66,* 73–79. doi:10.1016/j.bjps.2012.08.040

Bhama, P.K., Davis, G.E., Bhrany, A.D., Lam, D.J., & Futran, N.D. (2013). The effects of intensive care unit staffing on patient outcomes following microvascular free flap reconstruction of the head and neck: A pilot study. *Otolaryngology—Head and Neck Surgery, 139,* 37–42. doi:10.1001/jamaoto.2013.1132

Buntic, R.F. (2013). Flap and replant monitoring. Retrieved from http://www.microsurgeon.org/monitoring

Chepeha, D.B., Nussenbaum, B., Bradford, C.R., & Teknos, T.N. (2002). Leech therapy for patients with surgically unsalvageable venous obstruction after revascularized free tissue transfer. *Archives of Otolaryngology—Head and Neck Surgery, 128,* 960–965.

Dobrut, M., Maciejewski, A., & Półtorak, S. (2013). An evaluation of the efficacy of microvascular breast reconstruction techniques. *Polish Journal of Surgery, 85,* 6–11. doi:10.2478/pjs-2013-0002

Heffelfinger, R., Murchison, A.P., Parkes, W., Krein, H., Curry, J., Evans, J.J., & Bilyk, J.R. (2013). Microvascular free flap reconstruction of orbitocraniofacial defects. *Orbit, 32,* 95–101. doi:10.3109/01676830.2103.76446

Hill, J.B., Patel, A., Del Corral, G.A., Sexton, K.W., Ehrenfeld, J.M., Guillamondegui, O.D., & Shack, R.B. (2012). Preoperative anemia predicts thrombosis and free flap failure in microvascular reconstruction. *Annals of Plastic Surgery, 69,* 364–367. doi:10.1097/SAP.0b013e31823ed606

Horng, S.Y., Chen, C.K., Lee, C.H., & Horng, S.L. (2010). Quantitative relationship between vascular kinking and twisting. *Annals of Vascular Surgery, 24,* 1154–1155. doi:10.1016/j.avsg.2010.07.023

Jin, F., & Chung, F. (2001). Multimodal analgesia for postoperative pain control. *Journal of Clinical Anesthesia, 13,* 524–539.

Lamby, P., Prantl, L., Schreml, S., Pfister, K., Mueller, M.P., Clevert, D.A., & Jung, E.M. (2009). Improvements in high resolution ultrasound for postoperative investigation of capillary microperfusion after free tissue transfer. *Clinical Hemorheology and Microcirculation, 43,* 35–49. doi:10.3233/CH-2009-1219

Lighthall, J.G., Cain, R., Ghanem, T.A., & Wax, M.K. (2013). Effect of postoperative aspirin on outcomes in microvascular free tissue transfer surgery. *Otolaryngology—Head and Neck Surgery, 148,* 40–46. doi:10.1177/0194599812463320

Lundberg, J., Thorarinsson, A., Karlsson, P., Ringberg, A., Frisell, J., Hatschek, T., ... Elander, A. (2013). When is the deep inferior epigastric artery flap indicated for breast reconstruction in patients not treated with radiotherapy? *Annals of Plastic Surgery.* Advance online publication. doi:10.1097/SAP.0b013e31826cafd0

Maciejewski, O., Smeets, R., Gerhards, F., Kolk, A., Kloss, F., Stein, J.M., ... Yekta, S.S. (2010). Gender specific quality of life in patients with oral squamous cell carcinomas. *Head and Face Medicine, 6,* 21. doi:10.1186/1746-160X-6-21

McAnneny, A., Durden, F., Pearson, G.D., & Tiwari, P. (2012). Intra-flap thrombosis secondary to acute sickle crisis: A case report. *Microsurgery, 32,* 585–587. doi:10.1002/micr.22024

Monroe, M.M., Cannady, S.B., Ghanem, T.A., Swide, C.E., & Wax, M.K. (2011). Safety of vasopressor use in head and neck microvascular reconstruction: A prospective observational study. *Otolaryngology—Head and Neck Surgery, 144,* 877–882. doi:10.1177/0194599811401313

Nahabedian, M.Y. (2011). Free tissue transfer flaps. Retrieved from http://edmedicine.medscape.com/article/1284841-overview

Nahabedian, M.Y., Singh, N., Deune, E.G., Silverman, R., & Tufaro, A. (2004). Recipient vessel analysis for microvascular reconstruction of the head and neck. *Annals of Plastic Surgery, 52,* 148–155. doi:10.1097/01.sap.0000095409.32437.d4

Patel, R.S., McCluskey, S.A., Goldstein, D.P., Minkovich, L., Irish, J.C., Brown, D.H., ... Gilbert, R.W. (2010). Clinicopathologic and therapeutic risk factors for perioperative complications and prolonged hospital stay in free flap reconstruction of the head and neck. *Head and Neck, 32,* 1345–1353. doi:10.1002/hed.21331

Rahmanian-Schwarz, A., Rothenberger, J., Amr, A., Jaminet, P., & Schaller, H.E. (2012). A postoperative analysis of perfusion dynamics in deep inferior epigastric perforator flap breast reconstruction: A noninvasive quantitative measurement of flap oxygen saturation and blood flow. *Annals of Plastic Surgery, 69,* 535–539. doi:10.1097/SAP.0b013e31821bd484

Schmedes, G.W., Banks, C.A., Malin, B.T., Srinivas, P.B., & Skoner, J.M. (2012). Massive flap donor sites and the role of negative pressure wound therapy. *Otolaryngology—Head and Neck Surgery, 147,* 1049–1053. doi:10.1177/0194599812459015

Selber, J.C., Garvey, P.B., Clemens, M.W., Chang, E.I., Zhang, H., & Hanasono, M.M. (2013). A prospective study of transit-time flow volume measurement for intraoperative evaluation and optimization of free flaps. *Plastic and Reconstructive Surgery, 131,* 270–280. doi:10.1097/PRS.0b013e3182789c91

Serletti, J.M., Higgins, J.P., Moran, S., & Orlando, G.S. (2000). Factors affecting outcome in free-tissue transfer in the elderly. *Plastic and Reconstructive Surgery, 106,* 66–70.

Silvesti, M., Svartling, N., Pitkanen, M., & Rosenberg, P.H. (2000). Comparison of intravenous patient-controlled analgesia with tramadol versus morphine after microvascular breast reconstruction. *European Journal of Anaesthesiology, 17,* 448–455.

Temple-Oberle, C.F., Ayeni, O., Cook, E.F., Bettger-Hahn, M., Mychailyshyn, N., & MacDermid, J. (2013). The breast reconstruction satisfaction questionnaire (BRECON-31): An affirmative analysis. *Journal of Surgical Oncology, 107,* 451–455. doi:10.1002/jso.23258

Yantis, M., O'Toole, K.N., & Ring, P. (2009). Leech therapy. *American Journal of Nursing, 109*(4), 36–42. doi:10.1097/01.NAJ.0000348601.01489.77

CHAPTER 22

Nutritional Care of the Surgical Patient

Terezie Tolar Mosby, EdD, MS, RD, IBCLC, LDN

Introduction

Patient nutritional status is important for the optimal outcome of an expected surgery. Often, patients with malignancies are already malnourished before a surgical procedure is scheduled. Malnutrition includes both overnutrition (obesity) and undernutrition. Both conditions increase the risk for postsurgical complications. In this chapter, the importance of adequate nutrition, screening, and assessment, as well as nutritional care across the operative continuum, will be reviewed.

Importance of Adequate Nutrition

Nearly 34% of adults in the United States are overweight, and more than 34% are obese (Flegal, Carroll, Kit, & Ogden, 2012). Obese patients have increased risks for atherosclerotic cardiovascular disease, heart failure, systemic hypertension and pulmonary hypertension related to sleep apnea and obesity hypoventilation, cardiac arrhythmias, deep vein thrombosis, pulmonary embolism, and poor exercise capacity. Therefore, obesity predisposes patients to perioperative and postoperative complications.

Conversely, undernutrition is a common problem in patients with cancer. Protein-calorie malnutrition poses significant issues in patients with cancer, most commonly in patients with upper gastrointestinal (GI) tumors and patients with lung cancer (Bovio, Fonte, & Baiardi, 2014). These include anorexia, nausea, vomiting, dysphagia for solid and liquid food sources, dry mouth, chewing disturbances, hypogeusia, dysgeusia, and hiccups (Bovio et al., 2014). In a study of 243 patients with thoracic cancer, 35% were malnourished with a reduced median survival rate of 155 days less than those with improved nutrition (19% vs. 41%; p < 0.01 for both values) (Percival et al., 2013). Undernutrition may result from an inadequate diet or from an inability to absorb or metabolize nutrients. Food intake may be insufficient to supply calories or protein or may be deficient in one or more essential vitamins or minerals. Protein-energy malnutrition is also known as protein-calorie malnutrition. It develops in children and adults whose consumption of protein and energy (measured in calories) is insufficient to satisfy the body's nutritional needs. Protein malnutrition has been found to alter the pharmacokinetics of chemotherapy drugs such as doxorubicin and epirubicin, with one study in rats showing prolonged exposure of the heart to the drugs; this course of action is of concern for protein-malnourished patients (El-Demerdash, Ali, El-Taher, & Hamada, 2012).

Undernutrition in Patients With Cancer

Various reasons exists for undernutrition in patients with cancer, including progression of neoplastic disease, inability to consume adequate calories, obstruction, or psychosocial issues (National Cancer Institute [NCI], 2011). Patients with cancer may experience side effects of treatment and symptoms related to disease that may further impair nutritional status, including anorexia, nausea and vomiting, diarrhea, constipation, stomatitis, mucositis, dysphagia, alteration of taste and smell, pain, depression, and anxiety (Bovio et al., 2013). In addition, surgery itself can predispose patients to a catabolic state because of the inability to have adequate oral intake prior to surgery, nothing-per-mouth status before and after surgery, and increased calorie and protein requirements after surgery. Often patients are in a catabolic state before surgery or become catabolic soon after.

Catabolisms are pathways of metabolism that involve the breakdown and oxidation of fuels and provision of metabolic energy (Icard & Lincet, 2013). People who are undernourished or suffering from cachexia may be in a catabolic state as they break down their body tissues without replacement. Malnutrition can contribute to the incidence and severity of treatment side effects that impair the immune system and therefore increase the risk for infections, impaired wound healing, decreased mobility, and negative effects on the kidneys, heart, and GI tract. Malnourished patients can require longer intubation, prolonged surgical recovery, increased length of hospital stay, and increased readmission rates (Icard & Lincet, 2013). These negative effects all lead to increased hospital costs.

The role of medical nutrition therapy is to prevent or reverse malnutrition of patients before and after surgery. Because each patient is unique with a different state of nutritional status, age, gender, and disease burden, an individualized approach to each patient's nutritional management is important.

Nutrition Screening and Assessment

Appropriate assessment of the nutritional status of a patient is necessary for medical nutritional therapy development. An individualized approach enables the clinician to screen and assess each patient with establishment of measurable outcomes.

Nutrition Screening

Nutrition screening serves as identification of an individual's nutritional, health, functional, and behavioral status and is the first step in a comprehensive nutritional assessment (McCallum, 2006). Nutrition screening should be performed within 24–72 hours after patient admission and should be repeated regularly to identify cancer-related malnutrition and cachexia and patients at risk for such conditions. Nutrition screening can be performed by any appropriately trained healthcare professional (Mosby, Barr, & Pencharz, 2009). Screening may include factors such as change in weight (recent weight loss or weight gain), food allergies, diet order, and the presence of symptoms such as nausea, emesis, diarrhea, constipation, and changes in appetite and oral intake. Screening should be simple, efficient, quick, reliable, and inexpensive. These concepts can be adapted in the outpatient setting by oncology professionals.

Nutrition Assessment

Unlike nutrition screening, nutrition assessment should be performed by a professional who is trained in nutrition assessment, such as a registered dietitian. Nutrition assessment consists of three parts: (a) data collection, (b) data evaluation, and (c) interpretation of findings. Data collection should include diagnosis, historical data, biochemical and anthropometric data, and a nutrition-focused physical examination. This accurate nutrition history and assessment is most important in older adults (Farrer et al., 2013). Oncologic diagnoses predispose patients to increased risk for malnutrition. Patients with aerodigestive cancers (e.g., esophageal, gastric, pancreatic, liver, gallbladder, bile duct, small and large intestine) can have severe weight loss because of changes in normal digestion and absorption (Thomas, 2006).

Historical data include medical history, diet history, oral intake history, and weight history. Questions about the psychological status of the patient should be asked with special attention to stress and depression. Lifestyle items such as tobacco and alcohol use are important as alcohol abuse is a major risk factor for head and neck cancers and can itself lead to malnutrition (NCI, 2011). Assessment of patient use of over-the-counter medications, vitamins, and dietary and herbal supplements is crucial because all herbal medications and some vitamins need to be discontinued two weeks before surgery, as the synergistic effect of herbs and medications may increase bleeding, activate immunosuppressive drugs, or have other negative side effects. Oral intake can be assessed using 24-hour dietary recall or food records.

Biochemical data include visceral protein (e.g., albumin, transferrin, prealbumin, retinol-binding protein), total lymphocyte count, hemoglobin, hematocrit, lipid profiles, and blood glucose level. Additional studies may be performed, such as nitrogen balance studies or delayed hypersensitivity tests. Creatinine height index can be obtained, which is a measurement of the 24-hour urinary excretion of creatinine, generally related to the patient's muscle mass and an indicator of malnutrition. Anthropometric data include weight, height, mid-arm muscle circumference, triceps skin fold, body mass index (BMI), and waist-to-hip ratio. The nutrition-focused physical examination should include overall musculature, adipose fat stores, and visual examination of tongue, gums, lips, and mucosal membranes, as well as hair, skin, nails, and eyes. Hand grip strength is an important prognostic factor (Chen, Ho-Chang, Huang, & Hung, 2011) and has been shown to predict mortality from all causes (Angst et al., 2010).

Calorie requirements can be calculated and compared with actual patient caloric intake. Another option is to estimate calorie needs with indirect calorimetry, a measurement of the amount of heat generated in an oxidation reaction by determination of the intake or consumption of oxygen, or measurement of the amount of carbon dioxide or nitrogen released. These data are subsequently translated into a heat equivalent. Indirect calorimetry is useful but reserved for the research setting because of the cost involved. Ideal body weight should be calculated and recorded with comparison to the patient's actual weight. Weight change can be calculated in one-week and one- and six-month intervals. BMI is calculated with height and weight measurements with classification of nutritional status.

Patient-specific laboratory values are compared with reference values to determine possible nutritional deficits. For example, the normal albumin level is 3.5–5 g/dl, and albumin has a half-life of approximately 20 days. Although many factors can influence albumin level, the preoperative level of albumin has been found to be an excellent predictor of surgical outcome (Lin et al., 2011). A reverse relationship has been found between serum albumin level and postoperative morbidity and mortality. The normal level of prealbumin is 16–40 mg/dl, and prealbumin has a short half-life of just two to three days. It is a favorable marker for acute nutritional status changes (Huang et al., 2012).

Nutrition Interventions

Preoperative Nutritional Aspects

All attempts should be made to optimize the nutritional status of patients before surgery. In part, time is a consideration, although preoperative modifications can occur; diet, dietary supplements, appetite stimulants, pharmaconutrients, or nutritional support can all be used. More aggressive approaches should be implemented for patients who are undernourished.

Obese Patients

Obese patients are those with a BMI greater than 30 kg/m²; morbidly obese patients are those with a BMI greater than 40 kg/m² (Centers for Disease Control and Prevention, 2011). Obesity increases the incidence and severity of comorbidities and influences tolerance of the prescribed regimen and overall patient outcomes. Obese patients may have protein-energy malnutrition, known as sarcopenic obesity. When there is an interval of at least a month before surgery, gradual weight loss should be recommended and accomplished by decreased oral calorie consumption, enteral nutrition (EN), or parenteral nutrition (PN). A high-protein, hypocaloric regimen is recommended to reduce the fat mass, improve insulin sensitivity, and preserve lean body mass. If EN is used, the formula should have a low ratio of nonprotein calories to nitrogen with a variety of added pharmaconutrient agents to modulate immune responses and reduce inflammation (McClave et al., 2011).

Undernourished Patients

Diet modifications can be incorporated for patients who are allowed to have oral intake and are able to consume at least 75% of their estimated calorie needs. Diet modification can consist of increased calories in the diet by adding more calorie-dense food or by modifying food consistency to allow the patient to consume more calories. Examples of calorie-dense foods are peanut butter, nuts, trail mix, cheese, high-calorie smoothies, and "extras," such as putting sour cream on baked potatoes, gravy on meats, butter on vegetables, mayonnaise on sandwiches, and cream cheese on fruits.

Supplements

Many dietary supplements are on the market, and they can be chosen based on the patient's preference and medical condition. Typically, dietary supplements with higher protein content are recommended, although modular products can be added to the patient's food to supply additional calories, protein, or fat. Fortified foods on the market are in forms of pudding, cereals, ice cream, and ice pops.

Appetite Stimulants

Many patients with cancer report poor appetite. Initiation of appetite stimulants such as progestational agents, glucocorticoids, cannabinoids, antihistamines, antidepressants/antipsychotics, anti-inflammatory agents, metabolic inhibitors, and anabolic agents can be considered if it is medically appropriate to increase the patient's oral intake (NCI, 2011). The most commonly used appetite stimulants are cyproheptadine, dronabinol, and megestrol acetate.

Nutritional Support

Nutritional support should be considered for adult patients who meet the following criteria (Centers for Disease Control and Prevention, 2011).
- BMI less than 18.5
- Unintentional weight loss greater than 10% over the past three to six months
- BMI less than 20 and unintentional weight loss greater than 10% over the past three to six months
- Minimal intake for more than five days or no intake for five days or longer
- Poor GI absorption, high nutrient losses, or increased nutritional needs

Nutritional support can be used as primary therapy or as a supplemental therapy to oral intake. Calories provided via nutritional support depend on usual oral intake and individual calorie requirements. The goal is to provide 25–30 Kcal/kg of actual body weight (or in obese patients, adjusted body weight) and 0.8–1.5 g/kg/day of protein (in intensive care unit, up to 2.5 g/kg/day).

Enteral Nutrition

Early initiation of EN (Seres, Valcarcel, & Guillaume, 2013) has been promoted as the preferred route of nutritional support because it is more physiologically congruent to food and less expensive than PN. Benefits of EN include improved maintenance of GI mucosal integrity and decreased bacterial translocation, infectious complications, multiorgan failure, and death. EN should be started preoperatively when the patient is severely malnourished. Evidence exists for preoperative EN relative to clinical outcomes of surgery, when surgery is elective, or when surgery can be delayed for 7–10 days (Seres et al., 2013).

Contraindications to EN include complete bowel obstruction, intractable vomiting, colonic fistula, shock, and GI bleeding. If the patient is found to have incompetence of the gastroesophageal junction, the patient's head should be elevated to prevent aspiration and development of aspiration pneumonia. For long-term enteral feedings (three months or longer), gastrostomy or jejunostomy should be performed (Seres et al., 2013).

Parenteral Nutrition

PN should be used if EN is contraindicated because of intestinal obstruction, diffuse peritonitis, intractable vomiting, paralytic ileus, severe GI bleeding, uncorrectable diarrhea, or intestinal ischemia (Motoori et al., 2012). Patients who are well nourished or mildly malnourished will not benefit from PN. It therefore should be initiated only in patients who are severely malnourished and undergoing elective major surgery (e.g., bowel resection) or those receiving intensive therapy associated with hematopoietic stem cell transplantation (Habschmidt, Bacon, Gregoire, & Rasmussen, 2012). PN may be administered through a central venous catheter, peripherally inserted central catheter, or midline catheter. A midline is a peripheral catheter suitable for delivery of PN for periods of less than 14 days (Shepherd, 2009). Long-term administration of PN is costly and may cause atrophy of intestinal mucosa and a host of other possible complications.

Immunonutrition

Immunonutrition is immunity-enhancing nutrition that helps to decrease the risk of postoperative infections (Osland, Hossain, Khan, & Memon, 2014). Immune-enhanced formula may contain glutamine (e.g., amino acid), arginine, RNA, omega-3 fatty acids, or a combination of any of these supplements. Preoperative administration of such supplemented enteral formulas can significantly reduce postoperative infections and decrease length of stay for patients undergoing cancer-related surgery (Osland et al., 2014). Oral glutamine may be initiated when solid foods are allowed; omega-3 fatty acids can start about three days after surgery to ensure lack of interference with normal blood clotting.

Other supplements such as vitamins (e.g., vitamin C) and minerals (e.g., zinc), herbs (e.g., turmeric), and probiotics can be used if medically indicated. Antioxidants appear to interact best if obtained from food sources. Turmeric is a potential antioxidant and has been used after surgery for its anti-inflammatory and antibiotic properties (Gautam, Gao, & Dulchavsky, 2007). Probiotics are used to improve the integrity of the gut mucosal barrier, the balance of the gut microbiota, and the rate of infection (Lundell, 2011). Probiotics can also be taken in the form of capsules or yogurt.

Perioperative and Postoperative Guidelines

Every institution and surgical and anesthesia team has guidelines regarding the length of preoperative and postoperative fasting. Fasting before surgery may induce hyperglycemia caused by transitory insulin resistance, a phenomenon of metabolic response to stress. Overnight fasting may also cause dehydration. New guidelines have significantly decreased the period of fasting before surgery (Roberts, 2013), although this evidence has not translated to the bedside. Current recommendations of the German Society of Anesthesiology and Intensive Care Medicine call for withholding solid food for six hours and clear liquids for two hours before surgery (Breuer et al., 2010). A clear liquid diet consists of foods with low residue content that are in liquid form to minimize the load of food that requires intestinal digestion, such as electrolyte replacement solutions, water, ginger ale, sweetened tea or coffee, fat-free broth, plain gelatin, and strained fruit juices. The diet is used preoperatively and postoperatively until bowel function returns. It is nutritionally inadequate and should not be used for more than two days as the sole source of nutrition.

Dietary recommendations immediately after surgery will depend on factors such as the type of surgery, tumor location, and nutritional status of the patient. There is a reported benefit of early postoperative alimentation. A short-term status of nothing by mouth followed by a clear liquid diet for the first 6–24 hours after surgery may be recommended with advancement to full-liquid diet, pureed diet, soft diet, and then full diet. Advancement of diet will depend on recovery from anesthesia, the type and extent of surgery, and individual tolerance of the prescribed diet.

Medical nutrition therapy consists of diet modification, dietary supplements, modular boosters, appetite stimulants, immunonutrition, and nutritional support and should be personalized to each patient. Surgery can lead to increased energy requirements; wound healing and recovery will increase the needs and requirements for macronutrients and micronutrients. During postoperative stress, short-term hypocaloric feedings with 1–2 g of protein per kilogram per day may reduce metabolic complications and support a reduction in negative nitrogen balance.

Surgery can cause mechanical or physiologic barriers to adequate nutrition. Surgical therapy for aerodigestive cancers can result in gastric paresis, alterations in digestion, malabsorption of nutrients, hyperglycemia, elevated lipid levels, hepatic encephalopathy, fluid and electrolyte imbalance, anastomotic and chyle leaks, dumping syndrome, and vitamin and mineral deficiencies. Individualized nutritional therapy can help relieve or reduce these problems.

Short gut syndrome can develop after extensive bowel resection and may lead to malnutrition. Short gut syndrome is a malabsorption disorder caused by the surgical removal of the small intestine or, rarely, the complete dysfunction of a large segment of bowel. It usually does not develop unless more than two-thirds of the small intestine has been removed. Dumping syndrome is a group of symptoms likely to develop if part or all of the stomach was surgically removed or bypassed. It is also called *rapid gastric emptying*. It occurs when undigested contents of the stomach are transported or "dumped" into the small intestine too rapidly. Symptoms include abdominal cramps, nausea, sweating, and low blood pressure. Foods high in sugar may promote dumping syndrome and should be avoided.

In general, dietary recommendations after surgery include small, frequent meals, easily chewed foods, protein-rich foods, and foods and drinks low in sugar. A well-balanced diet with the recommended amounts of essential nutrients and calories will promote good wound healing. Early ambulation is important and may increase advancement of nutrition therapy. Finally, proper nutrition and adequate rest may help prevent or treat fatigue (NCI, 2011). Constipation is a common side effect of surgery caused by anesthesia and pain-related medications. A high-fiber diet with increased water intake will help improve this complication and encourage bowel regularity.

Conclusions

Nutritional status is important for optimal outcomes of surgery, surgical recovery, and quality of life. All patients should be assessed for nutritional risk. Based on the assessment, an individualized plan for nutritional intervention should be developed and executed. Nurses with experience in surgical oncology should incorporate nutrition screening in routine patient care and consult with dietary professionals for complex nutrition assessments and interventions.

References

Angst, F., Drerup, S., Werle, S., Herren, D.B., Simmen, B.R., & Goldhahn, J. (2010). Prediction of grip and key pinch strength in 978 healthy subjects. *British Medical Journal of Musculoskeletal Disorders, 11*, 94. doi:10.1186/1471-2474-11-94

Bovio, G., Fonte, M.L., & Baiardi, P. (2014). Prevalence of upper gastrointestinal symptoms and their influence on nutritional state and performance status in patients with different primary tumors receiving palliative care. *American Journal of Hospital and Palliative Care, 31*, 20–26. doi:10.1177/1049909112474713

Breuer, J.P., Bosse, G., Prochnow, L., Seifert, S., Langelotz, C., Wassilew, G., ... Spies, C. (2010). Reduced preoperative fasting periods. Current status after a survey of patients and colleagues. *Anaesthesist, 59*, 607–613. doi:10.1007/s00101-010-1736-4

Centers for Disease Control and Prevention. (2011). Healthy weight—It's not a diet, it's a lifestyle! Retrieved from http://www.cdc.gov/healthyweight/index.html

Chen, C.H., Ho-Chang, Huang, Y.Z., & Hung, T.T. (2011). Hand-grip strength is a simple and effective outcome predictor in esophageal cancer following esophagectomy with reconstruction: A prospective study. *Journal of Cardiothoracic Surgery, 6,* 98. doi:10.1186/1749-8090-6-98

El-Demerdash, E., Ali, A.A., El-Taher, D.E., & Hamada, F.M. (2012). Effect of low-protein diet on anthracycline pharmacokinetics and cardiotoxicity. *Journal of Pharmacy and Pharmacology, 64,* 344–354. doi:10.1111/j.2042-7158.2011.01413

Farrer, K., Donaldson, E., Blackett, B., Lloyd, H., Forde, C., Melia, D., & Lal, S. (2013). Nutritional screening of elderly patients: A health improvement approach to practice. *Journal of Human Nutrition and Dietetics.* Advance online publication. doi:10.1111/jhn.12073

Flegal, K.M., Carroll, M.D., Kit, B.K., & Ogden, C.L. (2012). Prevalence of obesity and trends in the distribution of body mass index among US adults, 1999–2010. *JAMA, 307,* 491–497. doi:10.1001/jama.2012.39

Gautam, S.C., Gao, X., & Dulchavsky, S. (2007). Immunomodulation by curcumin. *Advances in Experimental Medicine and Biology, 595,* 321–341. doi:10.1007/978-0-387-46401-5_14

Habschmidt, M.G., Bacon, C.A., Gregoire, M.B., & Rasmussen, H.E. (2012). Medical nutrition therapy provided to adult hematopoietic stem cell transplantation patients. *Nutrition in Clinical Practice, 27,* 655–660. doi:10.1177/0884533612457179

Huang, L., Li, J., Yan, J.J., Liu, C.F., Wu, M.C., & Yan, Y.Q. (2012). Prealbumin is predictive for postoperative liver insufficiency in patients undergoing liver resection. *World Journal of Gastroenterology, 18,* 7021–7025. doi:10.3748/wjg.v18.i47.7021

Icard, P., & Lincet, H. (2013). The cancer tumor: A metabolic parasite? *Bulletin du Cancer, 100,* 427–433. doi:10.1684/bdc.2013.1742

Lin, Y., Samardzic, H., Adamson, R.H., Renkin, E.M., Clark, J.F., Reed, R.K., & Curry, F.R. (2011). Phosphodiesterase 4 inhibition attenuates atrial natriuretic peptide-induced vascular hyperpermeability and loss of plasma volume. *Journal of Physiology, 589,* 341–353. doi:10.1113/jphysiol.2010.199588

Lundell, L. (2011). Use of probiotics in abdominal surgery. *Digestive Diseases, 29,* 570–573. doi:10.1159/000332984

McCallum, P.D. (2006). Nutrition screening and assessment in oncology. In L. Elliott, L.L. Molseed, P.D. McCallum, & B. Grant (Eds.), *The clinical guide to oncology nutrition* (2nd ed., pp. 44–53). Chicago, IL: American Dietetic Association.

McClave, S.A., Kushner, R., Van Way, C.W., III, Cave, M., DeLegge, M., Dibaise, J., ... Ochoa, J. (2011). Nutrition therapy of the severely obese, critically ill patient: Summation of conclusions and recommendations. *Journal of Parenteral and Enteral Nutrition, 35*(Suppl. 5), 88S–96S. doi:10.1177/0148607111415111

Mosby, T.T., Barr, R.D., & Pencharz, P.B. (2009). Nutritional assessment of children with cancer. *Journal of Pediatric Oncology Nursing, 26,* 186–197. doi:10.1177/1043454209340326

Motoori, M., Yano, M., Yasuda, T., Miyata, H., Peng, Y.F., Yamasaki, M., ... Doki, Y. (2012). Relationship between immunological parameters and the severity of neutropenia and effect of enteral nutrition on immune status during neoadjuvant chemotherapy on patients with advanced esophageal cancer. *Oncology, 83,* 91–100. doi:10.1159/000339694

National Cancer Institute. (2011, November 30). Nutrition in cancer (PDQ®) [Health professional version]. Retrieved from http://www.cancer.gov/cancertopics/pdq/supportivecare/nutrition/HealthProfessional

Osland, E., Hossain, M.B., Khan, S., & Memon, M.A. (2014). Effect of timing of pharmaconutrition (immunonutrition) administration on outcomes of elective surgery for gastrointestinal malignancies: A systematic review and meta-analysis. *Journal of Parenteral and Enteral Nutrition, 38,* 53–69. doi:10.1177/0148607112474825

Percival, C., Hussain, Z., Zadora-Chrzastowska, S., White, G., Maddocks, M., & Wilcock, A. (2013). Providing nutritional support to patients with thoracic cancer: Findings of a

dedicated rehabilitation service. *Respiratory Medicine, 107,* 753–761. doi:10.1016/j.rmed
.2013.01.012

Roberts, S. (2013). Preoperative fasting: A clinical audit. *Journal of Perioperative Practice, 23,* 11–16.

Seres, D.S., Valcarcel, M., & Guillaume, A. (2013). Advantages of enteral nutrition over parenteral nutrition. *Therapeutic Advances in Gastroenterology, 6,* 157–167. doi:10.1177/1756283X12467564

Shepherd, A. (2009). Nutrition support 2: Exploring different methods of administration. *Nursing Times.* Retrieved from http://www.nursingtimes.net/nutrition-support-2-exploring-different-methods-of-administration/1987729.article

Thomas, S. (2006). Nutritional implications of surgical oncology. In L. Elliott, L.L. Molseed, P.D. McCallum, & B. Grant (Eds.), *The clinical guide to oncology nutrition* (2nd ed., pp. 94–109). Chicago, IL: American Dietetic Association.

CHAPTER 23

Surgical Wounds and Ostomy Care

Molly Pierce, RN, BSN, ET, CWOCN, and Kelli Bergstrom, RN, BSN, ET, CWOCN

Introduction

Surgery disrupts the protective skin barrier. Incisional wounds typically heal by primary intention where the wound edges are approximated and secured. Wound healing is a priority concern for nursing care in the postoperative period. The incision may be covered by an occlusive dressing, which can be removed 24–48 hours postoperatively and left open to air. The Centers for Disease Control and Prevention guidelines for prevention of surgical infections (Mangram et al., 1999) state that as the incision heals, it becomes impenetrable to bacteria by day 2–3. When the dressing is removed, the nurse should assess the incision site carefully, observing for the presence of epithelial resurfacing, wound closure, healing ridge, and change in the incision appearance. Because of the normal inflammatory response of healing, the area around the incision may be slightly red and swollen, but the skin should be of normal color and temperature. Clean technique is used when managing the incision and changing the dressing. The evidence is insufficient to support sterile technique over clean technique for bedside dressing changes in decreasing infection rates for incisions and wounds (Flores, 2008).

In some cases, wounds are intentionally left open to heal by secondary intention and allowed to heal by scar formation. Four phases are involved with this type of wound healing: (a) hemostasis, (b) inflammation, (c) proliferation, and (d) maturation. Healing is a complex process that overlaps and does not always occur in an orderly fashion. In some cases, surgical site healing can be delayed because of many different factors, such as infection, medical conditions (e.g., diabetes; vascular, renal, or pulmonary disease), obesity, certain medications (e.g., anti-inflammatories, steroids), chemotherapy, radiation, stress, age, and nutrition (e.g., inadequate intake of protein, calories, vitamins A and C, zinc, magnesium, copper, and iron). These factors can lead to *wound dehiscence*, a separation and disruption of previously joined wound edges or evisceration in which the wound edges separate to the extent that the intestines protrude through the wound. The wound then heals by tertiary intention (Doughty & Sparks-Defiese, 2012).

Skin and Wound Assessment

Accurate assessment of the wound is required for appropriate management. Frequency of wound assessment is based on institutional policies; however, the standard of care is to assess the wound with each dressing change or alteration in patient condition, with healing reassessment every one to two weeks. The anatomic location is important to note in order to determine what dressing or healing modality should be selected. The extent of tissue involvement guides the selection of interventions and determines the length of time the healing process may require (Farren & Martelly-Kebreau, 2011).

The amount and type of tissue in the wound base should be assessed to determine the presence of viable or nonviable tissue. Viable tissue is described using shades of red and pink, whereas nonviable tissue can be yellow slough or black eschar. Wounds are measured using metric units and should include length, width, and depth, as well as the presence and location of undermining and tunneling (Ousey & Cook, 2011). The edge of the wound should also be assessed for attachment to the wound bed, which provides information about epithelial advancement. The *periwound*, or the area around the wound, needs to be assessed and be a part of routine care. Assessment includes color, texture, skin temperature, and integrity. The presence and severity of pain should also be addressed because it can indicate infection or inappropriate wound management (Nix, 2012). Wound exudate is essential to wound healing because the right amount and mixture of growth factors will contribute to the wound healing process; however, excessive amounts of drainage can prevent healing and signify infection. Characteristics of the exudate should include amount, type, consistency, and odor. Although most wounds have an odor, extremely odorous wounds with purulent exudate can suggest infection (Ousey & Cook, 2011). Figure 23-1 is an example of an open wound; consider these characteristics for documentation.

Wound Infection

Bacteria are inevitable in any wound, as a wound not a sterile environment. Overload can occur with increased bacteria quantity, virulence, and

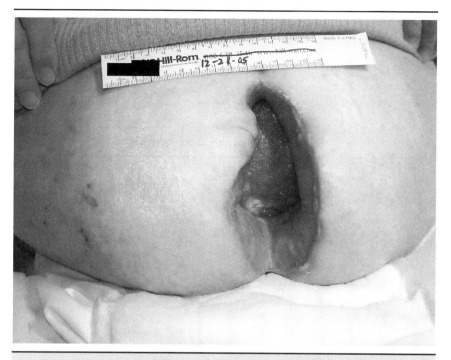

Figure 23-1. Large Abdominal Wound Healing by Secondary Intent

Note. Photo courtesy of Molly Pierce, RN, BSN, ET, CWOCN, The Ohio State University Wexner Medical Center. Used with permission.

decreased host defenses. Four states of infection development exist: contamination, colonization, critical colonization, and infection. Signs of infection can be subtle, especially for chronic wounds. These include a change in color and consistency, new or increased presence of slough, poor evidence of granulation tissue formation, erythema around the wound, increased pain, offensive odor, and an increase in wound size (Cook & Ousey, 2011). Steroids can often mask signs of infection, so a full clinical assessment is critical. A wound culture may be required if the wound has shown no healing for two weeks. Several culture methods are available. The most common and least invasive method is the swab technique, where a swab or applicator is moistened and rotated on the clean wound surface. The gold standard for wound culture is tissue biopsy, in which a piece of the wound tissue free of necrotic material is removed with a scalpel or punch biopsy. Wound healing cannot proceed if the source of infection is not addressed. Management includes local or topical treatments and systemic therapies. Debridement should be conducted to remove nonviable necrotic tissue, a breeding ground for bacteria, from the surface of the wound (Nix, 2012).

Wound Debridement

Debridement options include autolysis, chemical, mechanical, and sharp. Autolytic debridement involves intrinsic enzymes and macrophages to remove necrotic tissue. A semiocclusive or occlusive moisture-retentive dressing is placed on the wound to promote softening of the dead tissue (Benbow, 2011). Nonviable tissue can also be removed with the help of enzymes through a chemical process. Collagenase is a topically applied enzymatic agent that digests slough and dissolves collagen anchors. Diluted sodium hypochlorite solution (Dakin's solution) has a long history as a disinfectant and debriding agent; however, its use is controversial because of toxicity risks and lack of evidence to support its effectiveness. Fly larvae are another form of chemical debridement because the larvae secrete enzymes to break down necrotic tissue, which the larvae then ingest. This therapy is only considered when other forms of debridement are unsuccessful. Mechanical debridement uses conventional wet-to-dry gauze dressings in which saline-moistened gauze is applied to a heavily necrotic wound bed and allowed to dry. This method is controversial because dressing changes can be painful, it is nonselective where viable tissue is also removed, and it can lead to periwound maceration if the dressing is too moist (Ramundo, 2012). Sharp debridement includes conservative and surgical methods. Conservative sharp debridement involves the use of sterile surgical instruments to remove loosely adherent, nonviable tissue. This method can be combined with other forms of debridement but can be very uncomfortable for the patient with risk of blood loss. Surgical sharp debridement is typically reserved for wounds with a large amount of necrotic tissue or an infectious process that necessitates immediate removal of the tissue performed in the operating room by a surgeon (Benbow, 2011).

Wound Dressings

Dressing selection is based on the wound size, location, amount and type of drainage, and presence of necrotic tissue or infection. The purpose of all dressings is to maintain a closed, moist environment to promote healing. Many categories of wound dressings will help promote healing. No single product is right for every type of wound, and considerations need to be based on patient needs, frequency of dressing changes, cost, comfort, ease of use, and evidence-based practice guidelines.

Gauze is the most widely known dressing that absorbs exudate and supports wound debridement; however, some studies suggest that these dressings can lead to patient discomfort, prolonged inflammation, localized hypothermia, risk of infection, increased costs, and increased nursing time. Gauze should no longer be considered the standard of wound care (Ryan, 2008). A hydrogel dressing should be considered for wounds requiring moisture because it is designed to rehydrate the wound. Hydrocolloids, a polymer dressing that gels on contact with drainage, and composite dressings, which combine an absorbent layer with a semi- or nonadherent surface, are ideal for wounds with minimal exudate. When wounds have moderate to heavy exudate, appropriate choices include alginates and hydrofibers, fiber-spun dressings that gel and conform to the wound bed, along with a polyurethane foam, which absorbs fluid and wicks it away from the wound bed, and specialty absorptive dressings that are multilayered and provide a semi- or nonadherent layer with absorptive layers of fibers (Rolstad, Bryant, & Nix, 2012). See Figure 23-2 for an example of a wound requiring layered, nonadherent, absorptive dressings.

A contact layer is a single layer of perforated polymer sheet that is used directly on the wound bed to protect it from direct contact when used with other dressings. Antimicrobial dressings impregnated with silver or iodine come in a variety of dressing types and assist in the management of infected wounds by killing or inhibiting a broad spectrum of organisms. Another dressing option that is becoming more readily used for wound care is

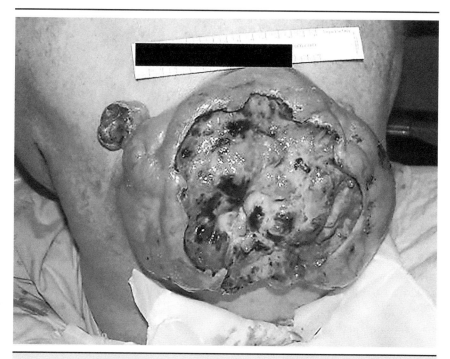

Figure 23-2. Wound Requiring Absorptive Wound Dressings

Note. Photo courtesy of Molly Pierce, RN, BSN, ET, CWOCN, The Ohio State University Wexner Medical Center. Used with permission.

the negative-pressure wound therapy system. This system uses controlled negative pressure to assist in wound healing by evacuating excess exudate, maintaining a closed, moist environment, stimulating granulation tissue formation, promoting blood flow to the wound bed, and decreasing bacterial burden (Myles, 2006). Figure 23-3 demonstrates a wound managed by negative-pressure therapy.

Pressure Ulcers

Surgical patients are at a high risk for developing pressure ulcers because of immobility during intra- and postoperative periods, as well as anesthesia administration, which causes decreased pressure sensations and hypoperfusion. Other factors include preexisting skin conditions, age, comorbid dis-

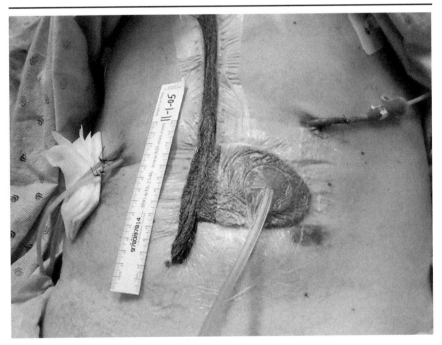

Product-specific dressing supplies must be used for negative-pressure wound therapy. The dressing is placed in the wound bed, and an occlusive transparent film covers the wound and adjacent skin. Suction tubing attached to the negative-pressure therapy machine is applied to the wound dressing, and negative pressure is initiated per prescribed settings.

Figure 23-3. Wound Managed With Negative-Pressure Therapy

Note. Photo courtesy of Kelli Bergstrom, RN, BSN, ET, CWOCN, The Ohio State University Wexner Medical Center. Used with permission.

eases, malnutrition, smoking, and anemia (Cherry & Moss, 2011). A *pressure ulcer* is an area of localized injury to the skin or subcutaneous tissue over a bony prominence that is caused by pressure alone or in combination with shear and friction. Pressure ulcers are classified according to the extent of tissue involvement and documented as stages I–IV, unstageable, and suspected deep tissue injury (Black et al., 2011).

Pressure ulcer prevention is essential to decrease not only the discomfort and cost to the patient but also the cost to the hospital and overall health-care system. A pressure ulcer prevention program should be in place at every institution. Risk assessment for pressure ulcers is done with a standardized rating tool, such as the Braden scale, upon patient admission and every 48 hours or with a change in the patient's condition. The Braden scale enables nurses to score patient skin on six variables (sensory perception, moisture, subscales of activity, mobility, nutrition, and friction and shear). Each subscale has a score of 1–4, with the exception of friction and shear, which is 1–3 (Copeland-Fields & Hoshiko, 1989; U.S. National Library of Medicine, 2013). Higher scores indicate healthy skin; a score of 12 or less is very concerning for the development of pressure sores (Copeland-Fields & Hoshiko, 1989). Pressure reduction techniques are essential for preventing and managing existing pressure ulcers. Frequent patient repositioning, at least every two hours while lying in a bed and every 15 minutes while sitting in a chair, is the standard of care, although no specific research evidence supports this frequency. Patients who are incontinent are susceptible to skin damage; therefore, frequent cleansing routines, scheduled toileting, use of incontinence products, and application of moisture barrier ointments are important. Support surfaces are the cornerstone in elimination of pressure because they maximize contact and distribute weight evenly over a large surface area. Contact surfaces include beds, chairs, and operating room tables (Pieper, 2012).

Radiation-Induced Skin Alterations

Radiation is a common treatment modality and a palliative intervention for several types of cancers. Skin-related side effects are common with radiation therapy. About 85%–95% of patients with cancer who receive radiation therapy will develop some degree of radiation skin damage (Dendaas, 2012; Feight, Baney, Bruce, & McQuestion, 2011). Despite the frequent occurrence of these side effects, evidence-based standards of care are limited, and variations in skin care recommendations for use in the prevention and treatment of radiation-induced skin changes are often based on expert opinion rather than research evidence (Dendaas, 2012).

Radiation-induced skin reactions can occur within one to four weeks after initial treatment and persist for two to four weeks following completion of treatment. These adverse effects can occur on areas of the body that are exposed to radiation, particularly where the outer skin is thin and smooth (Dendaas, 2012; Feight et al., 2011). The severity of skin reaction varies greatly among individuals, depending on preexisting health conditions, skin condition, race, lifestyle choices, age, nutritional status, type and total dose of radiation, and concurrent chemotherapy or immunosuppressant therapy (Dendaas, 2012; Feight et al., 2011). Skin reactions can range from no reaction to moist, painful ulcerations and even necrosis (see Figure 23-4). Patients can experience irritation, discomfort, pain, burning, or itching at the site. This affects activities of daily living and leads to a decrease in quality of life and possible treatment interruptions. The management of irradiated skin includes promoting skin integrity, providing comfort, maintaining cleanliness, reducing pain, protecting from trauma, preventing infection, and supporting wound healing (Dendaas, 2012; Feight et al., 2011).

Tubes and Drains

Surgical tubes and drains are used in a wide variety of surgeries and are common in the postoperative period. Several types of tubes and drains are

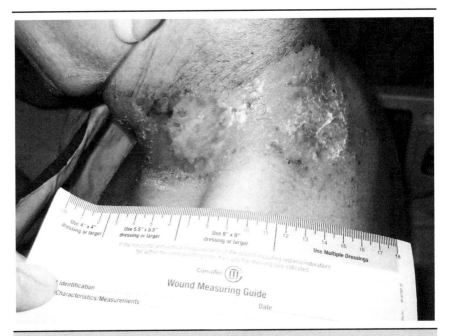

Figure 23-4. Radiation Burn in a Patient Receiving Radiation Therapy to the Neck

Note. Photo courtesy of Molly Pierce, RN, BSN, ET, CWOCN, The Ohio State University Wexner Medical Center. Used with permission.

employed, and management of these depends on their type, purpose, and location. It is important that the nurse know the purpose of the drain or tube. An example of this includes jejunostomy or gastrostomy tubes, which can be used for enteral feedings or decompression of the gastrointestinal system. Management includes ensuring that the tubes and drains are free of kinks, are adequately secured with an appropriate securement device, remain in the dependent position for drainage, and are emptied on a routine basis. The amount, color, and consistency of the drainage from these tubes and drains must be documented. In a recent study of patients with breast cancer with Jackson-Pratt drains, patients were randomized 1:1 to standard care with alcohol swabs around the site versus standard care plus chlorhexidine patch at the exit site; the drainage bulb was also irrigated with dilute sodium hypochlorite twice a day (Degnim et al., 2013). Significant differences (p = 0.004) were noted between the two arms: no infections were reported among the 58 participants in the chlorhexidine arm (Degnim et al., 2013).

The insertion site is assessed for signs of leakage or infection. A dressing, such as foam or gauze, can be used around the site to absorb drainage. If skin irritation occurs around the tube/drain site due to leakage, moisture barrier ointments can be applied to protect the skin from further breakdown. If leakage increases, a pouching system can be implemented to contain and quantify the drainage and a surgeon consulted for management.

Ostomies

Ostomy care begins with a diagnosis that could result in a physical alteration in elimination. Cancers that may require an ostomy include genitourinary (bladder, prostate, or urethral), gastrointestinal (colon, rectum, or gastrointestinal stromal tumor), gynecologic (ovarian, uterine, endometrial, or cervical), and musculoskeletal (sarcoma, chondroma, and liposarcoma). Treatment modalities that can lead to ostomies include radiation enteritis or fistula formation (Sliesoraitis & Tawfik, 2011). In cases where a cure is not an option, surgery may be done as a palliative measure to prevent large or small bowel obstruction.

Psychologically, patients can have a difficult time adjusting to an ostomy. Patients experience a change in body image as well as psychological distress regarding participating in daily activities; caring for the ostomy away from home; and managing odor, noise, or leakage issues (Pittman, 2011). Patients and their support team should be educated about the ostomy and have the opportunity to ask questions. Education begins preoperatively and continues throughout hospitalization. Meeting with a certified ostomy nurse before surgery also often leads to decreased anxiety. The American Urologic Association and the American Association of Colon and Rectal Surgeons endorse having a certified ostomy nurse mark a stoma location preoperatively because proper location of the stoma will help with management issues in the future and avoid unnecessary problems for the patient. The United Ostomy Associations of America (n.d.) has affiliates across the nation. Patients and families can attend support groups to obtain firsthand knowledge from other people who have ostomies.

Ostomy Assessment and Care

A *stoma* is a surgically created opening in the skin constructed to drain stool or urine. An *ostomy pouch* is worn over the stoma to collect the drainage. Small bowel stomas are called *ileostomies* and produce large amounts of liquid stool, whereas large bowel or colon stomas are called *colostomies* and produce semisolid or solid stool, possibly at predictable intervals. Urinary diversions, often made from small bowel, are called *ileal conduits* and produce urine with mucus. Stomas can be an end or loop of bowel and should have a moist, pink appearance similar to the mucous membranes of the mouth. Viability of the stoma is a concern if the stoma turns black, dark purple, or dusky and may necessitate reoperation. The stoma is swollen during the first four to six weeks postoperatively, and the stoma needs to be measured with every pouch change. Once the swelling resolves, a precut pouch of the correct size may be worn. Stomas typically shrink after construction; however, stomas may prolapse or enlarge if tumor burden has increased or a hernia has developed. Abdominal binders have been designed to address this issue if surgery to fix the stoma is not an option. If the patient's nutritional status is poor, a separation between the stoma and the skin edge (mucocutaneous junction separation) may occur, and filling this defect with stoma powder and cutting the pouch the size of the stoma will promote healing.

The peristomal skin (skin around the stoma) should be dry and intact. If the pouch has leaked, the skin may be red, raw, or bleeding. Ostomy drainage, particularly the digestive enzymes of an ileostomy, can spill onto the skin if the pouch fit is incorrect. Pouches are made to fit flat and convex surfaces. A convex appliance is used when the stoma is at or below skin level to reduce drainage onto the peristomal skin. An ostomy belt may be used to hold the appliance close to the abdomen so it does not fall off as easily. Cleansing the stoma and the peristomal skin does not require special soaps; regular lotion-free soap can be used. Figure 23-5 demonstrates stoma measurement for selecting the properly sized appliance.

Bladder and Bowel Diversion Options

Continent diversions are possible for both bladder and bowel diversions in select patient populations. Continent urinary diversions, such as a neo-

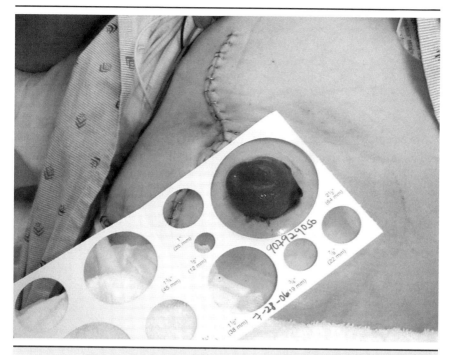

Figure 23-5. Measuring Stoma for Appliance Sizing

Note. Photo courtesy of Molly Pierce, RN, BSN, ET, CWOCN, The Ohio State University Wexner Medical Center. Used with permission.

bladder, are pouches that are able to be catheterized but require additional small bowel or ileum to construct a conduit. Preoperative counseling and education are focused on management of the diversion. The patient must understand that complete continence is not always possible. The interval for draining the pouch or neobladder varies from one to two hours initially and progresses to four to eight hours in a couple of months. Nighttime continence with a neobladder is markedly better one year after surgery. Patients with continent bowel diversions such as a J-pouch (colon removed, ileum connected to the anus) may have more frequent bowel movements. Patients with a Kock pouch (internal reservoir for stool constructed with ileum) require a catheter to drain the pouch periodically.

Incontinent diversions such as an ileal conduit for urine and ileostomy or colostomy for stool are performed for primary cancers and as a consequence of side effects from treatment. Urinary tract infections are more prevalent after a urinary diversion because both ureters are shortened during the procedure. Old urine standing in a pouch can colonize. Obtaining a urine specimen for a bacterial count is done with a catheter, although applying a clean pouch and collecting from it is acceptable. Some colostomies leave a rectal stump or blind pouch behind. This piece of colon may produce mucus and may benefit from half an enema once a month or a glycerin suppository to expel this mucus (Snyder, Richter, & Hill, 2010).

Ostomy Appliances

Several manufacturers produce ostomy appliances and pouches. One-piece pouches have a built-in adhesive that allows them to stick to the skin. Two-piece pouches have the adhesive as a cut-to-fit or precut disc. The pouch sticks or snaps onto the disc, depending on the design. All of the pouches (one- or two-piece) can be transparent or opaque. They should hold or adhere to the body for at least three days, although some are changed weekly. When selecting a design, dexterity and neuropathy should be considered. Learning how to empty the ostomy appliance and apply a new one will be the first steps toward independence for the patient (Snyder et al., 2010).

Patient Concerns

Patient concerns that emerge with an ostomy include bowel activity, odor, noise, clothing options, diet or food selection, medications, travel, and activities. Patients report that after having contrast for a computed tomography scan, they usually need to empty their pouch before they get home. Diatrizoic acid (Gastrografin®) has a laxative effect. Frequent stooling may increase the need to change pouches more often, using an excess number of supplies. Conversely, a decrease in ostomy activity can occur, which can lead to significant problems if not corrected. Suppositories generally do not promote evacuation of stool because there is no sphincter to hold them in; therefore, digital stimulation and irrigation is the better choice to manage constipation (Ray & McFall, 2010). If a colostomy is not functioning, the cause could include constipation from narcotics, dehydration, or blockage from tumor. An enema of 250–600 ml of tap water may be beneficial. A loop colostomy has a proximal and distal end; therefore, the proximal end would need to be used for an enema. A nonfunctioning ileostomy can be caused by food obstruction or tumor. A small lavage of 50–100 ml of normal saline can be administered to alleviate the obstruction (Ray & McFall, 2010).

Pouches are odorproof and waterproof, yet additional odor-absorbing products are on the market, such as pills to be taken by mouth and lubricating deodorant liquids to be put into the pouch; these have varying degrees of success. Dietary tips, such as which foods tend to produce greater odor and gas, and management strategies can help the patient to adjust to the ostomy. Examples include using pouches with gas filters to absorb the odor and laying the forearm over the stoma site if gas is felt to silence the noise (Snyder et al., 2010).

Clothing options for patients with colostomies are similar to those for individuals who do not have a colostomy. Dress shirt and tie, skirt, sweater, and jeans are all possible. Location of the ostomy may determine how shirts and pants are worn. Suspenders may be an option if the ostomy is occluded by a belt. Suggested swimming attire includes wearing a print as opposed to a solid; women can wear a skirted bathing suit, and men may opt to wear a shirt with swimtrunks.

Diet or Food Selection

Intake of food prior to the diversion is relatively unchanged following ostomy surgery. If the ostomy was for ruptured diverticula, avoiding seeds and nuts may be helpful, although little evidence supports this (Tarleton & DiBaise, 2011). New ileostomies are more likely to be obstructed by Chinese vegetables, apple peels, and orange pulp the first month after surgery. It is important to slowly add foods to the diet and eat in moderation. Dehydration can be a concern for ileostomy patients because of the large amounts of liquid stool that drain daily; therefore, signs of dehydration should be part of the patient education.

Medications

The need for medication adjustments depends on the amount of gastrointestinal anatomy that has been affected by the ostomy surgery (Sliesoraitis & Tawfik, 2011). If sufficient bowel remains for an oral medication to be absorbed, no adjustments will be necessary. However, in the patient with an ileostomy, medication adjustment may be necessary, particularly with long-acting or sustained-release medications, which may not be completely absorbed before excreted. Cardiac medications and analgesics may need to be given in liquid or transdermal form. A patient with an ileostomy will not need bowel preparation before a test, procedure, or surgery; therefore, having nothing by mouth or taking only liquids is usually sufficient (Kim et al., 2012).

Conclusions

Wound and ostomy care is common when working with the surgical oncology patient population, so developing these skills is an important part of nursing care. Wound and ostomy care nursing is a specialized field, and accessing these professionals when a complex wound or ostomy requires it can improve the patient's quality of life.

References

Benbow, M. (2011). Debridement: Wound bed preparation. *Journal of Community Nursing, 25,* 18–23.

Black, J.M., Edsberg, L.E., Baharestani, M.M., Langemo, D., Goldberg, M., McNichol, L., & National Pressure Ulcer Advisory Panel. (2011). Pressure ulcers: Avoidable or unavoidable? Results of the National Pressure Ulcer Advisory Panel Consensus Conference. *Ostomy/Wound Management, 57,* 24–37.

Cherry, C., & Moss, J. (2011). Best practices for preventing hospital-acquired pressure injuries in surgical patients. *ORNAC Journal, 29,* 6–8, 22–26.

Cook, L., & Ousey, K. (2011). Demystifying wound infection: Identification and management. Wound care series. Part 2: Infection. *Practice Nursing, 22,* 424–428.

Copeland-Fields, L.D., & Hoshiko, B.R. (1989). Clinical validation of Braden and Bergstrom's conceptual schema of pressure sore risk factors. *Rehabilitation Nursing, 14,* 257–260.

Degnim, A.C., Scow, J.S., Hoskin, T.L., Miller, J.P., Loprinzi, M., Boughey, J.C., ... Baddour, L.M. (2013). Randomized controlled trial to reduce bacterial colonization of surgical drains after breast and axillary operations. *Annals of Surgery, 258,* 240–247. doi:10.1097/SLA.0b013e31828c0b85

Dendaas, N. (2012). Toward evidence and theory-based skin care in radiation oncology. *Clinical Journal of Oncology Nursing, 16,* 520–525. doi:10.1188/12.CJON.520-525

Doughty, D.B., & Sparks-Defiese, B. (2012). Wound-healing physiology. In R.A. Bryant & D.P. Nix (Eds.), *Acute and chronic wounds: Current management concepts* (4th ed., pp. 63–82). St. Louis, MO: Elsevier Mosby.

Farren, M., & Martelly-Kebreau, Y. (2011). Wound assessment and management: Wound care fundamentals and OASIS-C. *Home Healthcare Nurse, 29,* 233–245.

Feight, D., Baney, T., Bruce, S., & McQuestion, M. (2011). Putting evidence into practice: Evidence-based interventions for radiation dermatitis. *Clinical Journal of Oncology Nursing, 15,* 481–492. doi:10.1188/11.CJON.481-492

Flores, A. (2008). Sterile versus non-sterile glove use and aseptic technique. *Nursing Standard, 23,* 35–39.

Kim, H.J., Kim, T.O., Shin, B.C., Woo, J.G., Seo, E.H., Joo, H.R., ... Lee, N.Y. (2012). Efficacy of prokinetics with a split-dose of polyethylene glycol in bowel preparation for morning colonoscopy: A randomized controlled trial. *Digestion, 86,* 194–200. doi:10.1159/000339780

Mangram, A.J, Horan, T.C., Pearson, M.L., Silver, L.C., Jarvis, W.R., & the Hospital Infection Control Practices Advisory Committee. (1999). Guideline for the prevention of surgical site infection. *Infection Control and Hospital Epidemiology, 20,* 247–280.

Myles, J. (2006). Wound dressing types and dressing selection. *Practice Nurse, 32*(9), 53–62.

Nix, D.P. (2012). Skin and wound inspection and assessment. In R.A. Bryant & D.P. Nix (Eds.), *Acute and chronic wounds: Current management concepts* (4th ed., pp. 108–121). St. Louis, MO: Elsevier Mosby.

Ousey, K., & Cook, L. (2011). Understanding the importance of holistic wound assessment. Wound care series. Part 1: Assessment. *Practice Nursing, 22,* 308–314.

Pieper, B. (2012). Pressure ulcers: Impact, etiology, and classification. In R.A. Bryant & D.P. Nix (Eds.), *Acute and chronic wounds: Current management concepts* (4th ed., pp. 123–136). St. Louis, MO: Elsevier Mosby.

Pittman, J. (2011). Characteristics of the patient with an ostomy. *Journal of Wound, Ostomy and Continence Nursing, 38,* 271–279. doi:10.1097/WON.0b013e3182152bbf

Ramundo, J.M. (2012). Wound debridement. In R.A. Bryant & D.P. Nix (Eds.), *Acute and chronic wounds: Current management concepts* (4th ed., pp. 279–288). St. Louis, MO: Elsevier Mosby.

Ray, K., & McFall, M. (2010). Large bowel enema through colostomy with a Foley catheter: A simple and effective technique. *Annals of the Royal College of Surgeons in England, 92,* 263. doi:10.1308/003588410X12664192075134h

Rolstad, B.S., Bryant, R.A., & Nix, D.P. (2012). Topical management. In R.A. Bryant & D.P. Nix (Eds.), *Acute and chronic wounds: Current management concepts* (4th ed., pp. 289–306). St. Louis, MO: Elsevier Mosby.

Ryan, M. (2008). The issues surrounding the continued use of saline soaked gauze dressings. *Wound Practice and Research, 16*(2), 16–21.

Sliesoraitis, S., & Tawfik, B. (2011). Bevacizumab-induced bowel perforation. *Journal of the American Osteopathic Association, 111,* 437–441.

Snyder, R., Richter, D., & Hill, M. (2010). A retrospective study of sequential therapy with advanced wound care products versus saline gauze dressings: Comparing healing and cost. *Ostomy/Wound Management, 56*(11A), 9–15.

Tarleton, S., & DiBaise, J.K. (2011). Low-residue diet in diverticular disease: Putting an end to the myth. *Nutrition in Clinical Practice, 2,* 137–142.

United Ostomy Associations of America. (n.d.). About us. Retrieved from http://www.ostomy.org

U.S. National Library of Medicine. (2013). 2012AB Braden Scale source information. Retrieved from http://www.nlm.nih.gov/research/umls/sourcereleasedocs/current/LNC_BRADEN

CHAPTER 24

Survivorship Issues in Surgical Oncology Nursing

Joanne L. Lester, PhD, CNP, AOCN®

Introduction

People with cancer are identified as "survivors" at the moment of diagnosis. Treatment interventions may have life-saving results for the survivors, but in turn they may cause short- and long-term side effects that negatively affect quality of life. At the time of diagnosis, most survivors are willing to accept whatever treatments are offered in an effort to cure their cancer and prevent or ameliorate metastatic disease. Short- and long-term side effects are reviewed in detail with verbal and written education; however, long-term memory of these interactions may be clouded. This disconnect and the reality of changes such as appearance, intimacy, emotions, and body functioning may cause distress for the survivor and his or her family. Nurses are in an opportune position to help survivors as they grapple with the short- and long-term realities of a cancer diagnosis and side effects of treatment. Although not inclusive of all potential survivorship concerns that may be experienced, this chapter will highlight common issues that occur secondary to surgical interventions for cancer.

Physical Issues

Fatigue

Fatigue is one of the most frustrating side effects that survivors encounter and is often coupled with sleep-wake disturbances. Fatigue can affect a host of other survivorship issues, such as functioning in daily life, at work, with children, and in relationships. Fatigue can negatively affect mood changes, emotional issues, social situations, and physical symptoms (Berger & Mitchell, 2011). Sleep habits can be altered by despair, worry, pain, positional changes, and many other issues that people normally take for granted.

Nearly all cancer surgical procedures involve the use of general anesthesia. Often, survivors will require more than one surgery, whether to obtain clear margins around a tumor, to rectify an infectious process or abscess, or to resect metastatic disease. Women with extensive breast reconstruction secondary to absence of the breasts from cancer may require several surgeries to complete the reconstructive process. General anesthesia can affect one's circadian clock, alter time perception, disrupt sleep, and cause fatigue. Alterations in a person's circadian rhythm can have negative effects on multiple physiologic and behavioral aspects of body functioning (Cheeseman et al., 2012). The additive effects of surgical procedures, multiple anesthesia administrations, worry, and the physiologic energy that is required to heal can significantly increase fatigue and sleep deprivation in the surgical patient.

Voice Quality

Removal of the larynx for laryngeal carcinoma can cause instantaneous issues for the survivor and family. Dysphonia interferes with communication and successful social interaction with even the closest loved ones. New ways of communication must be established as soon as the patient awakes from surgery. Early glottic cancers may result in laryngeal preservation, although voice quality may permanently be affected (Jotic et al., 2012). Speech therapy, vocal assessment, and emotional support are necessary during this difficult challenge for survivors and their families.

Surgical procedures for advanced head and neck cancers can affect swallowing, speech, and voice with symptoms of dry mucosa, muscle atrophy, and fibrosis. These significant anatomic changes can alter a survivor's quality of life, communication, risk of aspiration, and personal identity (van der Molen et al., 2012). Early rehabilitation with a multidisciplinary team is essential to preserve function and prevent additional morbidity in this population.

Nutrition

The cancer diagnosis and surgical interventions may influence nutrition based on multiple etiologic factors. Surgical interventions can alter the alimentary tract from the oropharynx to the rectum, as discussed previously in this book. These alterations may affect the physical intake of liquid or solid nutrition as well as the manipulation and elimination of liquids and solids. For example, survivors with an ileostomy or incontinent cutaneous pouch may not eat or drink during certain times if they want to avoid the drainage of liquid stool or urine. Some survivors who work outside the home may make a habit of this controlled fasting that can be harmful to nutritional and electrolyte balances, as well as their level of hydration.

Protein malnutrition is also a significant problem in patients with altered alimentary tracts (Isidro & Lima, 2012). A persistent state of protein malnutrition can affect tissue integrity, healing, and the immune system (Icard & Lincet, 2013). Survivors may know the *what* and the *how* of dietary management but may struggle with their new food identity and eating with family or in public or may suffer from fatigue or cognitive disorders that mitigate their comprehension of nutritional instructions. Survivors of head and neck, esophageal, and gastric cancers may rely on caretakers to administer enteral nutrition, or they may receive parenteral nutrition from caretaker or home health nurse. These significant alterations isolate the survivor who may rely on this type of nutrition for the remainder of his or her life.

Stoma Issues

Survivors of rectal cancer may undergo a low anterior resection or an abdominoperineal resection to surgically treat their cancer. These cancer-related surgical procedures may also include an ostomy for evacuation of formed stool when the lower rectum and perhaps the anus have been removed. Sexual dysfunction can occur secondary to the presence of a stoma because of body image changes, concern about odor, and defecation issues (Orsini et al., 2013). Survivors may never reinstate, renew, or reinvent partner intimacy because of the fear of bag dislocation, the presence of fecal matter, odor, and their overall body image.

Survivors who experience altered urinary functioning secondary to cancer surgery may undergo restorative surgery to enable drainage of urine. Urinary diversion procedures include incontinent cutaneous diversion that creates an abdominal stoma, continent cutaneous diversion with an internal pouch, bladder reconstruction, neobladder reconstruction, or ureterocutaneostomy (Lester, 2012). The everyday normal body function to remove urine is significantly altered. Survivors may require private facilities while in public to adequately drain their urine (or feces) and reattach their pouch. Patients who undergo a pelvic exenteration have two stomas: one for urine and one for stool. One can imagine the potential difficulties and learning curve these survivors may face as they attempt to reenter socialization in public places.

Psychosocial Issues

Sexuality

The psychosocial impact of a cancer diagnosis and side effects from treatment modalities cannot be underestimated. Prostate cancer survivors report multiple unmet psychosexual needs after surgical treatment and the gaps in physician-to-patient discussion, rapport with the healthcare team, concealment of problems, and age-related sexual function issues compound the problem (O'Brien et al., 2011). Psychosexual issues involve both the survivor and his or her partner. The partner is often struggling to stay strong and accept changes and cannot effectively communicate and move forward with new sexual and intimacy challenges.

Testicular cancer survivors must often deal with challenges such as fertility, body image, sexual desire, and sexual performance that are altered by surgical procedures. Oncology nurses may choose a passive communication approach and wait for patients to ask about sexuality or self-image concerns versus taking an active role and openly discussing some of the common issues (Moore, Higgins, & Sharek, 2013). In the event that a nurse expresses a knowledge gap, additional education should be provided to enhance this communication. To meet the common needs of testicular and prostate cancer survivors, nurses should subsume sexuality as a necessary component of routine care (Moore et al., 2013). For survivors who require more complex sexuality counseling, referral options should be in place.

Emotional Response

A cancer diagnosis and pending or completed surgical interventions can elicit emotional responses that are intense and interfere with daily life. Anxiety and anxiety-related emotions such as worry, fear of recurrence, and fear of dying can negatively affect daily life, relationships, and employment. High levels of anxiety have been observed in up to 30% of patients with cancer (Jarrett et al., 2013). Anxiety prior to a surgical procedure can increase biophysical stress changes that may impede initial healing and recovery. Anxiety does not typically resolve after surgery because the survivor and family must anxiously wait for the surgical pathology results and perhaps experience angst over these findings and future treatment.

Patients with breast cancer report feelings of vulnerability, loss of control, uncertainty, stress, and loss of energy (Schmid-Büchi, Halfens, Müller, Dassen, & van den Borne, 2013). Psychosocial support before and after surgery from family and friends may not be effective if these individuals are also experiencing emotional responses that impede their support mechanism for the survivor. Therefore, it is important for nurses to understand the experiences of survivors and screen for distress, assess identified sources of distress, and provide interventions and referrals to help patients move forward and gain control of their situation. These steps are important to help survivors cope with the challenges they face and adjust effectively with identification of their new normal (Schmid-Büchi et al., 2013).

Self-Image

Breast cancer survivors can suffer from multiple self-image issues related to body image and body dissatisfaction both before and after surgery. Appearance issues may include a defect in remaining breast tissue or a loss of one or both breasts secondary to surgical interventions. Other issues of self-image include tissue damage, decreased range of motion, lymphedema (Brunet, Sabiston, & Burke, 2013), and persistent seromas. Other bothersome matters include changes in muscle definition secondary to surgery, breast tenderness, and frustration that the body looks and functions differently than before surgery (Brunet et al., 2013).

Men with breast cancer have a difficult time in choosing and wearing clothes because even a soft golf shirt can illuminate the absence of the nipple after a total or modified radical mastectomy. Men struggle with their self-image secondary to surgical changes to internal and external male organs, specifically the prostate, testicles, and penis. Following a partial or total penectomy, significant changes occur with self-image, sexuality, appearance, masculinity, and function (Held-Warmkessel, 2012). As discussed, men with testicular and advanced prostate cancers suffer from body image changes secondary to a unilateral or bilateral orchiectomy. A testicular prosthesis can be placed in the scrotum; however, restorative surgery is not always discussed with prostate and testicular cancer survivors.

Survivors who have experienced disfigurement from extensive head and neck surgery have significant issues with body image that lead to social isolation from both family and friends. Their disfigurement is highly visible and difficult to disguise. Head and neck cancer survivors also face social isolation in both personal and work settings (Rhoten, Murphy, & Ridner, 2013). Surgical removal of tissue, bone, nerves, and vasculature can result in highly visible scars, change in facial shape, and alterations in facial communications secondary to muscular deficits.

Conclusions

Survivors who undergo surgical procedures as primary or secondary treatment for their cancer can experience physical and psychosocial changes from internal and external alterations of their bodies. Short- and long-term side effects of these life-saving yet life-altering surgeries can negatively affect survivors, social relationships, and overall quality of life. Family and friends also feel the impact of these changes. Minimally invasive surgical procedures may result in fewer visible changes but may not be successful in resolving functional issues that alter daily living and communication. This chapter merely touched on a few of the most common alterations caused by surgical intervention. Nurses should actively explore common issues with survivors, screen and assess patients' and families' level and source of distress, and provide interventions or referrals that rehabilitate, restore, and resolve issues.

References

Berger, A.M., & Mitchell, S.A. (2011). Cancer-related fatigue and sleep-wake disturbances. In J.L. Lester & P. Schmitt (Eds.), *Cancer rehabilitation and survivorship: Transdisciplinary approaches to personalized care* (pp. 101–112). Pittsburgh, PA: Oncology Nursing Society.

Brunet, J., Sabiston, C.M., & Burke, S. (2013). Surviving breast cancer: Women's experiences with their changed bodies. *Body Image, 10,* 344–351. doi:10.1016/j.bodyim.2013.02.002

Cheeseman, J.F., Winnebeck, E.C., Millar, C.D., Kirkland, L.S., Sleigh, L., Goodwin, M., ... Warman, G.R. (2012). General anesthesia alters time perception by phase shifting the circadian clock. *Proceedings of the National Academy of Sciences of the USA, 109,* 7061–7066. doi:10.1073/pnas.1201734109

Held-Warmkessel, J. (2012). Penile cancer. *Seminars in Oncology Nursing, 28,* 190–201. doi:10.1016/j.soncn.2012.05.008

Icard, P., & Lincet, H. (2013). The cancer tumor: A metabolic parasite? *Bulletin du Cancer, 100,* 427–433. doi:10.1684/bdc.2013.1742

Isidro, M.F., & Lima, D.S. (2012). Protein-calorie adequacy of enteral nutrition therapy in surgical patients. *Revista da Associação Médica Brasileira, 58,* 580–586. doi:10.1590/S0104-42302012000500016

Jarrett, N., Scott, I., Addington-Hall, J., Amir, Z., Brearley, S., Hodges, L., ... Foster, C. (2013). Informing future research priorities into the psychological and social problems faced by cancer survivors: A rapid review and synthesis of the literature. *European Journal of Oncology Nursing, 17,* 510–520. doi:10.1016/j.ejon.2013.03.003

Jotic, A., Stankovic, P., Jesic, S., Milovanovic, M., Stojanovic, M., & Djukic, V. (2012). Voice quality after treatment of early glottic carcinoma. *Journal of Voice, 26,* 381–389. doi:10.1016/j.voice.2011.04.004

Lester, J. (2012). Restoring and maintaining urinary function. *Seminars in Oncology Nursing, 28,* 163–169. doi:10.1016/j.soncn.2012.05.005

Moore, A., Higgins, A., & Sharek, D. (2013). Barriers and facilitators for oncology nurses discussing sexual issues with men diagnosed with testicular cancer. *European Journal of Oncology Nursing, 17,* 416–422. doi:10.1016/j.ejon.2012.11.008

O'Brien, R., Rose, P., Campbell, C., Weller, D., Neal, R.D., Wilkinson, C., ... Watson, E. (2011). "I wish I'd told them": A qualitative study examining the unmet psychosexual needs of prostate cancer patients during follow-up after treatment. *Patient Education and Counseling, 84,* 200–207. doi:10.1016/j.pec.2010.07.006

Orsini, R.G., Thong, M.S.Y., van de Poll-Franse, L.V., Slooter, G.D., Nieuwenhuijzen, G.A.P., Rutten, H.J.T., & de Hingh, I.H.J.T. (2013). Quality of life of older rectal cancer patients is not impaired by a permanent stoma. *European Journal of Surgical Oncology, 39,* 164–170. doi:10.1016/j.ejso.2012.10.005

Rhoten, B.A., Murphy, B., & Ridner, S.H. (2013). Body image in patients with head and neck cancer: A review of the literature. *Oral Oncology, 49,* 753–760. doi:10.1016/j.oraloncology.2013.04.005

Schmid-Büchi, S., Halfens, R.J., Müller, M., Dassen, T., & van den Borne, B. (2013). Factors associated with supportive care needs of patients under treatment for breast cancer. *European Journal of Oncology Nursing, 17,* 22–29. doi:10.1016/j.ejon.2012.02.003

van der Molen, L., van Rossum, M.A., Jacobi, I., van Son, R.J.J.H., Smeele, L.E., Rasch, C.R.N., & Hilgers, F.J.M. (2012). Pre- and posttreatment voice and speech outcomes in patients with advanced head and neck cancer treated with chemoradiotherapy: Expert listeners' and patient's perception. *Journal of Voice, 26,* 664.e25–664.e33. doi:10.1016/j.jvoice.2011.08.016

Index

The letter f after a page number indicates that relevant content appears in a figure; the letter t, in a table.

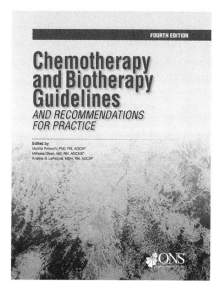
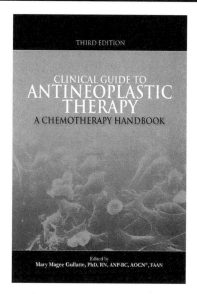
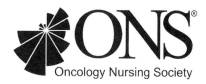

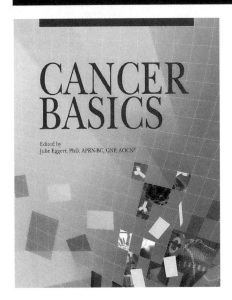
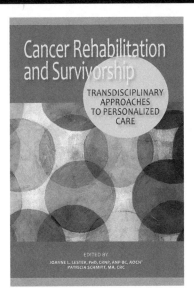
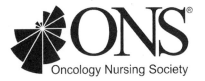